International Research on Poverty Reduction

Series Editors

Xiaolin Wang, Fudan University, Shanghai, China

Qianqian Liu, Finance Center for South-South Cooperation, Hong Kong, China

This book series covers poverty reduction practices and experience, knowledge mobilization, poverty reduction strategy analysis, and comparative research of different poverty reduction models. By analyzing China's poverty reduction approaches and experiences, and comparing them with those of other countries, this book series provides policy makers, researchers and practitioners in poverty reduction with theoretical and technical support, as well asproviding a new channel for sharing experiences as well as facilitating collaboration and communication in poverty reduction development fields between China and the rest of the world. Poverty remains a crucial development issue for the world, and China has become an important player in the global endeavor in poverty reduction and development. China has made a substantial contribution to the achievement of the Millennium Development Goals (MDGs) by reducing half of its poverty population.

Editorial Team of Case Studies of Targeted Poverty Reduction and Alleviation in 100 Villages
Editor

Case Studies of Targeted Poverty Reduction and Alleviation in 100 Villages

Selection of 18 Village Cases

SSAP

Springer

Editor
Editorial Team of Case Studies of Targeted Poverty Reduction and Alleviation in 100 Villages
Chinese Academy of Social Sciences
Beijing, China

Translated by
Fang Xie
Beijing, China

ISSN 2195-9781 ISSN 2195-979X (electronic)
International Research on Poverty Reduction
ISBN 978-981-95-0548-7 ISBN 978-981-95-0549-4 (eBook)
https://doi.org/10.1007/978-981-95-0549-4

Jointly published with Social Sciences Academic Press

The print edition is not for sale in China (Mainland). Customers from China (Mainland) please order the print book from: Social Sciences Academic Press.

This Springer imprint is published by the registered company Springer Nature Singapore Pte Ltd.
The registered company address is: 152 Beach Road, #21-01/04 Gateway East, Singapore 189721, Singapore

Foreword

Investigation and research is the fine tradition and work style of the Communist Party of China (CPC). Under the leadership of the CPC Central Committee, Chinese Academy of Social Sciences (CASS) has been consistently adhering to the style of study of "linking theory with practice" in a long tradition of conducting investigation and research of national conditions. In 1988, together with nationwide social sciences circles, CASS carried out social and economic surveys of one hundred cities and counties in China, which were successively listed as the National Key Projects of Philosophy and Social Sciences during the 7th and 8th five-year period, and published *China's National Conditions Book Series: Social and Economic Surveys of One Hundred Cities and Counties.* In 1998, the survey's horizon developing from meso-level to micro-level, CASS conducted social and economic surveys of one hundred villages under the sponsorship of the National Social Science Fund of China, which was the National Key Project of Philosophy and Social Sciences during the 9th five-year period, and published *China's National Conditions Book Series: Social and Economic Surveys of One Hundred Villages.* In 2006, CASS launched a series of comprehensive surveys of national conditions, and implemented national condition survey projects one after another in a total number of more than 1000, and established 12 academy-level as well as 59 institute-level bases for investigation and research of national conditions in cooperation with local authorities. The conduct of the investigation and research of national conditions has made important contributions to the full play of CASS as both think tank and brainpower by bringing the Marxist epistemology and style of study into practice, and it entails linking theory with practice and treating practice as the sole criterion for testing truth.

Since the 18th National Congress of the CPC, and under the guidance of the goal for building a moderately prosperous society in all respects, the CPC Central Committee has put forward the aim that by the end of 2020, all the rural poor population will be lifted out of poverty, and all the poverty-stricken counties will be eradicated to resolve overall regional poverty under the current standards. China has made remarkable achievements in poverty alleviation to complete such an unprecedented goal of grandeur rarely seen in the world. One of the three critical battles raised in the Report to the 19th National Congress of the CPC is to achieve comprehensive targeted poverty reduction by 2020, and it is a major social goal and political mission of great significance. During the process of poverty alleviation, the poverty-stricken areas across the country will experience even greater changes, and the changing process itself is not destined to be all plain sailing or smooth and easy. It is the due responsibility of social science workers to make a record of such a great process, to summarize the experience of resolving this world-class problem, and to provide suggestions and advice on how to win this battle.

In 2016, following the strategy of "to win the critical battle against poverty" deployed by the CPC Central Committee, CASS made its decision to set up this mega project for the investigation and research of national conditions titled "targeted poverty reduction and alleviation in 100 villages". Under the subject of targeted poverty alleviation, and by concentrating the superior resources of intelligence and materials, CASS conducted the investigation and research of 100 villages for two years. As a CASS mega project for the investigation and research of national conditions, with clear goals and unified work schedule of investigation and research, the project of "Investigation and Research of Targeted Poverty Reduction and Alleviation in 100 Villages" has both a unified standard of choosing sample villages and widespread sampling. Of all the 104 sample villages, those in western, central, and eastern region respectively account for 57%, 27%, and 16%, with particular considerations of different ethnic regions, borderline regions, special areas, and severely impoverished areas in hopes of presenting basic characteristics and representativeness of poverty-stricken villages, as well as a cross-sectional panorama of the status quo of poverty, poverty reduction, and development in rural areas of China.

Under the strong leadership of CPC central committee with Comrade Xi Jinping at the core, since the 18th National Congress of the Communist Party of China, the socialist practice with Chinese characteristics has ushered China into a new era of socialism with Chinese characteristics, and the economic and social landscape in China is experiencing profound changes: the poverty eradication campaign is successfully advancing, making more than 10 million people out of poverty each year, reducing the poverty-stricken population from 98.99 million in 2012 to 30.46 million, and achieved a huge improvement over the appearance of poverty-stricken villages in a relatively short period of time. The Chinese Academy of Social Sciences has organized 100 research teams, mobilized no less than 500 research staffs, committed no less than 3,000 working days into this, and recorded with footsteps, pen tips and lenses the great changes that have occurred in more than 100 poverty-stricken villages in recent years.

According to the plan, each poor village sub-subject group is not only supposed to provide data for the general subject group, but also write and publish the village's investigation and research report, all of which are presented to the readers as the "Investigation and Research of Targeted Poverty Reduction and Alleviation in 100 Villages Book Series". In order to reach the basic goal of understanding the national conditions, the general subject group formulated a research outline and questionnaire, which stipulates that the investigation and research of every village is supposed to implement the basic "prescribed actions" and carry out the "optional actions" that vary from village to village so as to understand and grasp the characteristics of each village, and write down the weal and woe on the road out of poverty! We organized an expert team to review of every report, and the author made some revisions according to the review comments until it met the publication requirements. We hope that the publication of this book series can add a lot of color to the great undertaking of poverty eradication.

The success of holding 19th National Congress of the Communist Party of China (CPC) lies in the establishment of Xi Jinping Thought on Socialism with Chinese Characteristics for a New Era as the guiding thought for all the work, the announcement that socialism with Chinese characteristics has entered a new era, as well as a major judgment the central government has made that the main contradiction facing Chinese society has evolved. From now until 2020, it is not only the decisive period to build a moderately prosperous society in all aspects, but also the period in which the timeframes of the Two Centenary Goals will converge. During this period, the country emphasizes that the three tough battles must be won, respectively referring to the battle of preventing and defusing financial risks, the battle of targeted poverty alleviation, and the battle of pollution control. On the eve of the Chinese New Year in 2018, General Secretary Xi Jinping visited the deeply impoverished Liangshan region of Sichuan Province and put forward eight requirements on fighting the battle of targeted poverty alleviation, and all of these requirements were implemented through a three-year action plan to eradicate poverty. In the meanwhile, in order to address imbalances and inadequacies in rural development, the country launched the rural revitalization strategy at the right time, requiring that important progress be made in rural revitalization by 2020 and the smooth transition between the implementation of the rural revitalization strategy and the battle of targeted poverty alleviation be ensured. We also found in our research that many places have already carried out the fight against poverty in combination with the construction of Beautiful Countryside and the integration of urban and rural development in actual work. It is foreseeable that winning the fight against poverty in poverty-stricken areas will not be limited to poverty alleviation of poor households, and we have full confidence to see the dawn and bright future of rural revitalization out of the development of poverty-stricken villages.

Thank you for your attention!

October 2018

Li Peilin
Vice-Chairperson of the Social Construction Committee, National People's Congress of the Republic China & Vice President and Academician, Chinese Academy of Social Sciences

"Investigation and Research of Targeted Poverty Reduction and Alleviation in 100 Villages Book Series"

Editorial Committee

Editor-in-Chief:
Li Peilin

Deputy Editor-in-Chief:
Ma Yuan, Wei Houkai, Chen Guangjin

Member:
Wang Zihao,Wang Yanzhong, Li Ping, Zhang Ping, Zhang Yi, Zhang Juwei, Jing Linbo, Xie Shouguang, Pan Jiahua
(in the order of stroke number of Chinese characters of those family names above)

CASS[1] Mega Project

"Investigation and Research of Targeted Poverty Reduction and Alleviation in 100 Villages"
Program Coordination Office

Director:
Wang Zihao

Member:
Tan Xuewen, Diao Pengfei, Yan Jun, Tian Tian, Qu Haiyan

[1] CASS is the abbreviation for"Chinese Academy of Social Sciences".--Trans.

Contents

Chapter 1
Opportunities and Challenges in the Birthplace of "Targeted Poverty Alleviation": Observations from Shibadong Village in Hunan Province

Yanhong Liu

Abstract Shibadong Village in Huayuan County, Hunan Province, is the birthplace to initiate the "Targeted Poverty Alleviation" in China, when Xi Jinping, General Secretary of the CPC Central Committee and President of the People's Republic of China, visited Shibadong Village on November 13, 2013, and made the important remarks on "Targeted Poverty Alleviation" for the first time. Henceforth it opened the new chapter of nationwide poverty alleviation and development. In order to implement the instruction spirit of General Secretary Xi Jinping's visit to Shibadong Village, CPC Party Committee as well as the people's government of Huayuan County took Shibadong Village as a pilot village to explore the replicable and promotable experience of targeted poverty alleviation in the county. And it also creatively explored and yielded positive results in resident work and industrial alleviation mechanism. In this paper, we discuss the three major development opportunities for Shibadong Village as the birthplace of "targeted poverty alleviation", and the risks and challenges encountered in the rapid transformation and development of industries, from the perspective of development opportunities and realistic challenges. We argue that the visit of the General Secretary Xi to Shibadong Village and the continuous and extensive coverage of Shibadong Village by the Central Media of the Central Government of the People's Republic of China in support of the national poverty elimination campaign have provided very critical and rare external opportunities for the development of Shibadong Village. In the process of rapid transformation from traditional farming and breeding industries to the modern manufacturing and tourism service industries, the more and more pressing problems such as the bottleneck problem of the collective economy of Shibadong Village, the lack of private capital, and the negative impact on traditional industries caused by policy changes are posing real challenges to the independent and sustainable development of the village, which cannot be ignored.

Y. Liu (✉)
University of Chinese Academy of Social Sciences, Beijing, China

Case Studies of Targeted Poverty Reduction and Alleviation in 100 Villages, International Research on Poverty Reduction, https://doi.org/10.1007/978-981-95-0549-4_1

Keywords Birthplace of "Targeted Poverty Alleviation" · Collective economy · Private capital · Policy risk · Shibadong Village

Situated on the triple boundaries point of Hunan Province, Guizhou Province, and Chongqing City, Shibadong is a village of the Miao people, located in Huayuan County, in the west of Hunan Province. It belongs to the contiguous areas of dire poverty in Wuling Mountains, and there are more mountains than land and it is economically backward. On November 3, 2013, Xi Jinping, General Secretary of the CPC Central Committee and President of the People's Republic of China, visited Shibadong Village, where he first made the important remarks of "targeted poverty alleviation", opening a new chapter in the national poverty alleviation and development work. Taking this opportunity, the local government took Shibadong Village as a pilot village for the county to explore the replicable and exemplary experience of targeted poverty alleviation, and made bold and leading explorations in such aspects as targeted identification, targeted assignment, targeted policy implementation and targeted industrial development, and achieved a series of positive results. After 3 years of efforts, the per capita net income of Shibadong Village increased from 1668 yuan in 2013 to 8313 yuan in 2016, and took the lead in shaking off the poverty of village in Hunan Province in 2017. In 2019, the per capita net income of Shibadong Village increased to 14,668 yuan, and the collective economic income reached 1,264,000 yuan, achieving the goal of a well-off society ahead of schedule.

In the process of implementing the instructions and requirements of the General Secretary and exploring and practicing the effective path of targeted poverty alleviation, Shibadong Village has firmly grasped the development opportunities brought about by the visit of General Secretary Xi Jinping to Shibadong Village and his advocacy of the strategy of targeted poverty alleviation, as well as the popularity effect brought about by the continuous news reporting on the practice of poverty alleviation in Shibadong Village where it has established the development of special farming and breeding industries in order to achieve the short goal of income growth; the mid- to long-term income as well as asset income will be insured through large-scale cultivation of kiwi fruit project; and the in-depth development of tourist resources and the countryside tourism will make it happen that the mid- to long-term industrial poverty alleviation and development plan will promote internally driven development and sustainable income, and it has achieved remarkable results in infrastructure and industrial system construction. Just over the past 6 years, Shibadong Village has turned a Miao cottage in dire poverty into a red tourist attraction receiving more than 500,000 visitors annually. However, in the process of rapid development, the collective economy of the village has encountered bottlenecks in development, it is difficult to seek external capital to invest, and the risks brought by policy changes to industrial development have gradually become highlighted, posing challenges to the transformation of the village from targeted poverty elimination to rural revitalization and from "outside-leveraged" development to the self- and sustainable development.

1.1 Three Opportunities for Shibadong Village

1.1.1 General Secretary's Visit

From the opening of 18th CPC National Congress to the 5th Plenary Session of the 18th CPC Central Committee which explicitly specified the targeted poverty alleviation as the basic strategy in fighting the battle of poverty elimination, the Party's thoughts on targeted poverty alleviation have undergone a gradual deepening and systematization process. During the evolution of targeted poverty alleviation from discourses to thoughts and then to the strategy to be implemented, Shibadong Village is undoubtedly of great significance. On the afternoon of November 3, 2013, General Secretary Xi Jinping and his entourage came to Lizi stockade of Shibadong Village in Huayuan County, and after visiting the homes of two villagers, Shi Bazhuan and Shi Chengfu, he chaired an on-site colloquium on a piece of flat ground in front of Shi Chengfu's house. It was in this colloquium that the General Secretary first put forward the important thesis of "targeted poverty alleviation". He stressed in front of the cadres and people on the spot, "Poverty alleviation must be practical and tailored to local conditions. To implement targeted poverty alleviation strategy, not to chant slogans, nor set overly ambitious goals".

The visit of the General Secretary has brought unprecedented development opportunities to this ancient Miao stockade village, which has long suffered from poverty. In order to implement the important instructions of "seeking truth from facts, acting according to local conditions, giving targeted guidance to different categories, and targeted poverty alleviation" and the requirement of "no special but different treatment", CPC Party Committee and Government of Huayuan County made a decision to take Shibadong Village as a pilot project for exploring a new path of poverty elimination and getting rich in dire poverty of ethnic regions. Shibadong Village has become a "pilot village" of poverty alleviation and a "sample village" for exploring replicable and exemplary experience in practicing targeted poverty alleviation in the county. According to this decision, the Party Committee of Huayuan County drafted in five cadres (all section-level cadres) from five departments, namely the Publicity Department, the United Front Work Department, the Forestry Bureau, the Civil Affairs Bureau, and the Natural Resources Bureau, to form the first Targeted Poverty Alleviation Task Force in the Huayuan County, which was officially assigned to Shibadong Village on January 23, 2014. Without precedent to learn, the CPC Party Committee and government of Huayuan County, the deployed village task force and the two committees of the village[1] worked together to focus on the implementation of "target" and to make pioneering efforts to identify poor households, implement measures of poverty alleviation, develop industries, and have achieved remarkable results. The Shibadong Village was the first to explore and finally establish the poverty identification standards and methods in the "targeted" way, which is the first template,

[1] Namely, the CPC Party branch of village as well as the villager's committee. -Trans.

namely the "nine ineligibilities" + "seven procedures" for identifying poor households, which has been promoted throughout the county and further the province. In terms of industrial development, in view of the basic fact of Shibadong Village that there is lack of land resources and management talents, the local community also established the characteristic plantation development idea of "driven by leading enterprises" + "to develop outside the village". Located on a 1000 mu[2] of transferred land in Dao'er town, 30 miles away from the Shibadong Village, a kiwifruit planting base was established to explore a new way of special industry poverty alleviation that can be copied and promoted.

When inspected Shibadong Village, the General Secretary praised it as a "small Zhangjiajie[3]", which aroused local cadres and people to develop the rural tourism. But how to establish their own characteristics on the basis of the natural landscape of the peaks and mountains and the tourist elements such as the Miao villages? With the gradual establishment and implementation of the CPC Central Committee's strategic concept of winning the battle against poverty with the strategy of targeted poverty alleviation, they realized that the remarks of "targeted poverty alleviation" first made by the General Secretary in Shibadong Village was a unique milestone in the strategic deployment of winning the battle against poverty, so the concept of "the first place to advocate targeted poverty alleviation" was refined and then became the unique label of Shibadong Village. In order to highlight the characteristic of the birthplace of "Targeted Poverty Alleviation", the Shibadong Village not only protected and restored the scene where the General Secretary held the colloquium at that time, but also built a "targeted level ground" square for tourists to visit, and appointed the two old men, Shi Bazhuan and Long Decheng, who were visited by the General Secretary, as the "tourism ambassadors" of the village. By introducing to the tourists all the details and their memory clips of the General Secretary's visit to their families, Shi Bazhuan, who was affectionately called "Big Sister" by the General Secretary, appeared on various advertisements for kiwifruit and spring water in Shibadong Village, has become a veritable "spokesperson" for the village.

The General Secretary's visit not only brought the special mission of "a pilot field for targeted poverty alleviation" to the Shibadong Village, but also awoke the people in this stockaded village like a spring thunder. Some young people in the village who were working outside the village watched the General Secretary's visit to the village via TV channel and keenly caught the opportunity to change their own fate and that of their hometown. Shi Jinlan was one of the first to take action. In his recollection, he and his wife were still working in an enterprise in Wenling, Zhejiang, at that time. He was a workshop director in charge of CNC[4] lathe in the factory. Because his work was relatively technical, he could earn 7000–8000 yuan a month. When he learned from the TV news that the General Secretary had inspected the Shibadong Village, he made the decision to return to his hometown that night. The next day, despite his wife's opposition and his boss's try to retain him, he resolutely embarked on his return

[2] Mu, a unit of area (=0.0667 hectares). - Trans.

[3] Zhang Jiajie, a famous tourist attraction in China. - Trans.

[4] CNC: Computerized Numerical Control. - Trans.

journey. In the spring of the next year, he was successfully elected as the head of the villager's committee of Shibadong Village in the general election of the villager's committee by virtue of his talents accumulated through years of working outside and his campaign slogan of "three years of hard work, with or without money", and became the leader of income-increasing undertakings in the village. Three years later, he saw a more suitable development opportunity in the development of tourism industry in the village, so he resigned from the post of the head of villager's committee to become a deputy general manager of Shibadong Tourism Company, responsible for the reception and tour guide work of the whole village tourism team. Following Shi Jinlan's footsteps, some young and middle-aged people who have also worked outside and seen the world, and even some "post-80 s" and "post-90 s" who have received secondary and higher education have also returned to the village, setting up farmhouses and homestays, and taking advantage of the trend of online sales by doing live-streaming promotion of homestay rentals and local product sales...

1.1.2 A Series of Reports by China Central Television (CCTV)

In November 2015, the Conference of the CPC Central Committee on Poverty Alleviation and Development was held in Beijing, officially blowing the charge to win the battle against poverty. General Secretary Xi Jinping systematically elaborated the basic strategy of winning the battle against poverty with targeted poverty alleviation and poverty elimination at the conference. In support of the central government's comprehensive deployment of targeted poverty alleviation and poverty elimination actions, major news media began to search every corner of the country to collect and report the experience and practices of targeted poverty alleviation practices and poverty elimination at the grassroots level. In this context, the Shibadong Village, where the General Secretary once visited and made the first important remarks on "targeted poverty alleviation", attracted the attention of major central media once again. At the end of 2015, People's Daily, Xinhua News Agency, China National Radio, Guangming Daily, Economic Daily, and other mainstream media reported on the changes in the village over the past 2 years, making the village's popularity out of the Western Hunan and further the Hunan Province again, and becoming a hotspot for national public opinion. Nonetheless, the Shibadong Village has become a model village for targeted poverty alleviation and a household name thanks to CCTV's focused coverage during the Spring Festival in 2016.

According to the recollection of Long Zhiyin, a member of the first task force stationed in the village, at the end of 2015, the CCTV news team came to the village to do the on-the-spot reporting, when Long Xiulin, the leader of task force, was still on the business trip outside and came back to the village as soon as possible, and made a detailed introduction about the practical explorations in poverty alleviation and changes had made over the past 2 years for the reporters from CCTV. In the introduction, a "matchmaking" plan being made in the village immediately attracted the reporters' attention. It turns out that since the task force was stationed in the village, it was found that in the village of less than 1000 people, there were as many as 38 "bachelor men" who had never got married. In order to solve the problem of these older young men in starting new families to improve the life quality of poor villagers, the task force came up with the original idea of using the collective matchmaking approach to attract young men and women from the surrounding villages and even further from the counties to find a match in the village. According to Long Zhiyin, the "matchmaking for poverty alleviation", an innovation unprecedented in the history of poverty alleviation work in China, immediately caught the eye of reporters. The CCTV news team decided to replace the original interview plan of only one episode by taking "Matchmaking" as the entry point, and reported a series of poverty alleviation stories in the Shibadong Village in terms of ideological construction, infrastructure construction, industrial development, and helping older youths with getting married in five consecutive episodes. From January 16 to 20, 2016, CCTV Channel One and News Channel aired five episodes of the special report "New Answer Sheet at the Grassroots Level: Chronicles of Poverty Alleviation in Shibadong" for five consecutive days in the columns of "Morning News", "Newsroom Live", "News 30 min", and "Common Concern", which caused strong responses at home and abroad. From February 13 to 17, 2016, "CCTV News" aired "Shibadong Village's poverty alleviation story" series in the column of "New Practices in State Governance", further expanding the influence of the Shibadong Village. Through CCTV's huge communication network, the "nine invalid conditions" and "seven procedures" implemented by the village in the targeted identification of poor households, the practice of using star-rating to enhance villagers' mutual help and collective consciousness, and the "enclave" model of developing the kiwi industry of the Shibadong Village among other practical explorations have quickly spread throughout the country and even overseas furthermore. The "Shibadong Experience" of targeted poverty alleviation has not only provided the nation with a "Hunan sample" of the practice of targeted poverty alleviation at the grassroots level, but also made Shibadong Village a banner of targeted poverty alleviation in China.

1.1.3 A National Flag for Targeted Poverty Alleviation

The concentrated and continuous coverage by CCTV in 2016 has made the image of Shibadong Village as the first place to initiate targeted poverty alleviation and a model of innovation in targeted poverty alleviation in China deeply popular. Shibadong Village has become a national banner for targeted poverty alleviation, and while earning honors in all aspects, it has also brought unprecedented opportunities for its own development. These development opportunities are focused on the following three aspects.

First of all, Shibadong Village has become an object of national study and red tourism scenic spot. With the establishment of the Shibadong Village as the first place to initiate targeted poverty alleviation and the image of advanced model in the country, it has rapidly become the object for study and research of targeted poverty alleviation and the grassroots Party building for the Party and government departments at all levels and even enterprises and public institutions across the country, and the number of people coming to the Shibadong Village for study, visit, and tourism has been rising year by year. According to Xiang Jingwen, the former general manager of the Shibadong Travel Company, who told the media, the number of visitors to the Shibadong reached 100,000 in 2015, 160,000 in 2016, and 250,000 in 2017. Another media report said that in 2018, the number of visitors to the Shibadong Village exceeded 300,000. According to Peng Yong, head of the tourism working group of Huayuan County stationed in Shibadong Village, after Shibadong Tourism Company officially opened for business in May 2019, the number of tourists counted through the tourism company's ticket system alone reached 30,000–32,000 each month, and the number of tourists received for the whole year could reach 450,000. This figure does not include the official inspection teams that are received by local Party and government departments without the tourism company system. According to Peng Yong's estimation, the latter category of visitors can account for about 1/3 of the total number of visitors to Shibadong Village.

Secondly, the Shibadong Village has become the focus of social support. Under the powerful call of the central government to mobilize the whole society and make joint efforts to promote poverty elimination, Shibadong Village has become a priority target for many enterprises and public institutions to fulfill their social support responsibilities. Thanks to the massive investment of all social forces in infrastructure construction, industrial development, market matching, and technical support, the infrastructure and production and living conditions of Shibadong Village have been significantly improved, completely changing the old look of the former poor and dilapidated village. According to Long Zhiyin, after the CCTV broadcast of the 5 serial episodes in 2016, the popularity of Shibadong Village was further enhanced, which brought a lot of benefits to the village's infrastructure construction. One of the best examples is that Shibadong Village needed to ask for help in internet access before then, but after 2016, it successfully realized internet access to the village, a full year ahead of the surrounding villages. In 2018, China Construction Fifth Bureau and China Shipping Group supported the construction of a new village headquarters and parking lot in Shibadong Village, which integrates comprehensive service functions such as villagers' service center, exhibition hall, video room, library and medical room, etc. The whole construction project took less than 4 months, with an investment of nearly 20 million RMB.

Finally, Shibadong Village has become a hot spot for private capital investment. The potential business opportunities that come with the increasing influence and popularity of Shibadong Village have also attracted the attention of many private capitals inside and outside the province, creating huge opportunities for Shibadong Village to develop industries with external forces. It is understood that in 2016–2017, private enterprises such as Consumer Treasure (Beijing) Asset Management Company, Hunan retail chain company BBK Group, and Hunan Earth Warehouse Technology Co. Ltd., were jointly signed cooperation agreement with Shibadong Village, respectively. At the end of 2016, the Consumer Treasure (Beijing) Asset Management Company and the Miaojiang Tourism Development Co. Ltd of Huayuan county (a wholly-owned subsidiary of the State-owned Assets Supervision and Administration Commission of Huayuan county) co-funded a Shibadong Tourism Development Co. Ltd, in which Consumer Treasure takes 51% of the shares and Miaojiang Tourism takes 49% of the shares, to cooperate in the development of the big caves of Shibadong tourism scenic spot in the Shibadong Village and the surrounding villages, including Yelang Shibadong karst cave. According to the tourism development cooperation agreement reached between the two sides, the total investment of Consumer Treasure is not less than 600 million yuan; in terms of the distribution of investment income, the Shibadong Village (collective) can enjoy 10% of the equity dividend entitlement for 30 consecutive years. On April 27, 2017, Wang Zhen, the chairman of the Hunan retail chain company BBK Group, inspected the industrial projects of poverty alleviation in Shibadong Village, and immediately made the decision to build a mountain spring water plant in Shibadong Village after knowing the spring water quality was very good for drink through test. It only takes 161 days to complete the whole process from the location of water source, project setup, program planning, purchase, plant building, and the operation of the plant on October 8 of that year. Ten days after the plant was put into operation, the bottled mountain spring water with the Shibadong logo was brought to the venue of the Hunan delegation to the19th National Congress of the Communist Party of China. At the end of that year, the spring water plant honored its commitment to Shibadong Village by fulfilling the "500,000 + 1" dividend commitment, that is, the water plant is supposed to give Shibadong Village collectives 500,000 yuan as the guaranteed income each year, where 1 cent of dividend comes from each bottle of water to be produced.

1.2 The Three Challenges of Shibadong Village

1.2.1 The Way Out of Collective Economy

With the implementation of industrial projects and the revenues being produced, the collective income began to make zero breakthrough. In 2016, the village collective received its first rental income of 70,000 yuan by renting out its collective house, and in 2017, with the dividends distributed from mountain spring water plant invested by Hunan BBK Group and the kiwifruit project with Miao Hanzi company, the village collective income exceeded 500,000 yuan, and further increased to 700,000 yuan in 2018. In 2018, it further increased to 700,000 yuan. In 2019, after the Shibadong Tourism Development Company officially came into operation, it also began to fulfill its guaranteed dividend promise of 300,000 yuan. According to Long Shuwu, the former secretary of village Party branch, in 2019, the collective income of the village exceeded the million yuan threshold, reaching 1.264 million yuan. With the gradual increase in collective income, how to achieve asset preservation and appreciation through the development of collective industries began to be put on the agenda of Shibadong Village.

In the second half of 2018, Shibadong Village established a rural tourism farmer cooperative, which transferred 80% of the village's land and tried to embark on the large-scale planting and operation of crops such as peppers and rice. But after only 1 year, it broke and ended in a loss. The land transferred from each family was also returned to the villagers. Some villagers therefore complained that their own paddy fields were abandoned after being transferred, and it was difficult to grow crops again, and they asked for compensation from the cooperative but failed. According to Long Shuwu, there are three causes leading to the failure of the planting project of the rural tourism cooperative. First, the market for agricultural products is not stable, and it is not easy to grasp market opportunities. Second, there is the problem of "presenteeism and not work", and there is a lack of collective responsibility for the collective planting and management of the project. Third, there is adventurous in the scale of land transfer, and some land is not effectively used after the transfer, but increases the operating costs of the collective project. After this failed attempt, Long Shuwu realized that "it is better to return the planting to the people to do self-operated business".

In 2019, in response to the call of the Organization Department of the county Party committee, Shibadong Village set up an economic association, with the veteran secretary of village Party branch, Long Shuwu as the chairman of the board, in the hope that he could oversee the development of specialized cooperatives and collective economy in the village. On August 1 of that year, Siyuan Restaurant, which was invested by the village collective with nearly 700,000 yuan, was officially opened to the public. The location of the restaurant is right next to the new village headquarter, close to the shuttle bus stop for tourists. Plus, it is the village's collective enterprise, so it has the distance advantage in the tourist reception. According to Long Shuwu, the restaurant has opened for 6 months and achieved a profit of 120,000 yuan. He believes that in this year (2020), the annual profit of restaurant is expected to reach 400,000–500,000 yuan, plus the dividends from water plant, kiwifruit, and tourism company; this year's collective income will exceed 2 million yuan, which is not a problem.

As the chairman of the village economic association and the leader of the village collective economy, Long Shuwu realized that only relying on the dividends from several existing industrial projects in the village is not a long-term solution to sustainable development and hoped to further develop and expand the village's own industries. He mentioned several ideas for the next development of collective industries: first, to focus on tourism derivative products and services, and develop some tourism entertainment projects and cultural and creative products in the village. Second, by using the brand name of Shibadong and mountain spring water resources, they can open their own bacon processing factory and winery. The third is to use the consumer poverty alleviation channel in Shibadong Village to cooperate with the neighboring Jiwei Town in the marketing of Chinese Snake Gourd seeds. When asked how to make these projects on the ground, he thinks the lack of relevant business talents is a bottleneck, and how to break through this bottleneck is one of the issues he has to focus on at the moment.

1.2.2 The Landing of Private Capital

The year 2017 was an important turning point in the development process of targeted poverty alleviation and targeted poverty elimination in Shibadong Village. In that year, Shibadong Village not only officially lifted out of poverty, but also the kiwifruit project cooperated with Miao Hanzi Company 3 years ago was officially mature and realized the first dividend. Also in that year, three major industrial projects invested or operated by foreign capital were signed or landed in Shibadong Village, which are respectively the tourism development project of big Shibadong in cooperation between the Consumer Treasure (Beijing) Asset Management Company and the Miaojiang Tourism Development Co. Ltd of Huayuan county and Huayuan County Miaojiang Tourism Development Co. Ltd., the spring water plant wholly invested by the Hunan BBK Group, and the construction of the Earth Warehouse Hotel project constructed by Hunan Earth Warehouse Technology Co. Ltd. According to the cooperation agreement at that time, Consumer Treasure, as the controlling shareholder, will invest no less than 600 million yuan in the Shibadong and strive to complete the construction of a national 4A-level scenic spot within 3 years, and commit to building a 5A-level scenic spot. And Shibadong Village will receive 10% of the dividend income during the 30-year operation period of the tourism project.

After 3 years, when I came to Shibadong Village again to see the progress made by these three industrial projects, I found some intriguing changes. First of all, the controlling shareholder, Consumer Treasure, and the Xiangxi Tourism Company, which later succeeded Consumer Treasure, have withdrawn from the Shibadong Tourism Company. The later became the sole proprietorship of Miaojiang Tourism Development Company under Huayuan County State-owned Assets Supervision and Administration Commission. When asked about the reasons for the withdrawal of these two companies, Peng Yong, head of the tourism working group of Huayuan County in the Shibadong Village, gave two explanations: the first one is that the Shibadong Village cannot charge entrance fees to tourists since it became the eight red scenic spots in Hunan Province in 2018, which affects the return expectations of investors; the second is that private funds tend to be more cautious when the development of scenic spots is still in the market cultivation stage. Compared to the withdrawal of the consumption treasure and Xiangxi Tourism Company, the Shibadong development undertaker Huayuan Shuanglong tourism development company, which is another private enterprise (invested by two Fujian businessmen), although not withdrawn, but was also in the face of difficulties in promoting the project. The person in charge of Shuanglong told me that since 2017, the company had completed the first phase of investment of 47 million yuan for the construction of internal cave footpath and lighting, as well as compensation for land acquisition of 70 acres of land around the cave. The second phase of the project will also invest 120 million yuan for the construction of the wind and rain bridge connecting the village road and the cave, as well as the construction of integrated tourism facilities such as B&B and catering. According to the person in charge of the project, the Shibadong tourism company is responsible for the cave development project approval and other related procedures.

Because the project development involved prime farmland, the relevant land transfer work was not completed until 2019, resulting in the supporting facilities construction of wind and rain bridge among others in the second phase unable to carry out, and the opening of the cave to the public also delayed. At present, although the approval procedures for the second phase of the project have been completed, no agreement has been reached between Shuanglong Company and the Shibadong Tourism Company on the mode of cooperation and benefit sharing. Secondly, since the first phase of seven barn-style rooms of the Shibadong Earth Warehouse Ecological Hotel, which was constructed and operated by Hunan Earth Warehouse Technology Company, was completed and operated to the public at the end of 2018, it has also not achieved satisfactory business performance. According to Peng Yong, the occupancy rate of the Earth Warehouse is only thirty to forty percent even in the current peak travel season. Due to the low occupancy rate of the hotel, the Earth Warehouse has also adopted the operation mode of cooperation with travel agencies in order to reduce the company's employment costs. Finally, compared to the difficulties encountered in tourism development and eco-hotels, the investment and operation of the mountain spring water plant is in a much better position. 2017 saw the construction and production trial of the water plant by BBG in just under 6 months. Although the plant has only one production line and two packaging sizes, the average daily output can also reach 80,000 bottles. I noted during the workshop visit that nearly 50 central and local enterprises have joined the Shibadong Spring Water Plant's "Love Brand Alliance", and these enterprises have underwritten a significant proportion of the Shibadong Spring Water in the form of poverty alleviation through consumption (PAC).

1.2.3 Risk from Policy Changes

The low literacy level of villagers and the lack of entrepreneurial individuals are not only major causes of poverty in the village for a long time, but also an important bottleneck that restricts the internally driven development momentum of the village to achieve independent and sustainable development. In the absence of knowledge and talent, only a few entrepreneurial individuals in the village are particularly valued. In 2017, when we paid our first visit to the village for research, we heard that there was a pig raiser Long Yingzu in the village with large-scale production. In the interview, Long Yingzu told us that she learned pig-breeding technology while working in Changsha, and in 2003, she returned to her hometown with 8000 yuan to start a pig farm. In 2014, Long Yingqi responded to the village's call and set up a professional cooperative for raising Xiangxi pigs, leading 21 poor households in the village to raise pigs together, with Long Yingzu providing piglets and feed as well as technical guidance at first, and then collecting the capital after the pigs matured and sold. In 2016, she was elected as a deputy to the county people's congress.

However, surprisingly, after more than a year, the fate of this pig raiser has changed dramatically. In 2017, Huayuan County started the work of closing down the farms in the livestock breeding ban area. In 2018, the new village plan (2018 ~ 2035) of Shibadong Village included large-scale breeding as the negative list of industrial access in Shibadong Village, and the pig farm run by Long Yingzu located in the scope of the ban area. Early in 2019, Huayuan County Livestock Breeding Regulation Office reached an agreement with Long Yingzu who closed her pig farm and received 797,000 yuan in compensation after being promised by the local authorities that she could switch to local production. According to the proposal of the relevant departments during the consultation process, Long Yingzu, who "can only raise pigs", was prepared to invest 2 million yuan to open an ecological farm providing accommodation, catering, and agricultural experience after closing the pig farm, and completed the company registration and project filing in April 2019. However, just when the two sisters, Long Yingzu and Long Yinglan, invested nearly one million yuan and were close to completing the construction of the main building of the farm as well as the supporting concrete wall facilities, a paper seal from the Natural Resources Bureau called a halt to the project. At this time, the two sisters learned that their pig farm belongs to the category of basic arable land, so the farm development and construction is contrary to the land use. Seeing that the huge investment in the early stage was about to go down the drain, the two sisters had to ask for help from the village, town, and the relevant departments in the county. They believed that the original proposal to switch to production was given by the relevant government departments, and now the project is halted, and the government should hold the responsibility to help them out. According to Long Yinglan, the relevant departments told her that they could apply for the land planning adjustment for the farm, but the application must be done through the tourism company in the village, so a more realistic solution is that the tourism company needs to acquire the farm's assets at first. The two sisters said that they were still waiting for news from the relevant departments, and whether they could reach an acquisition agreement with the tourism company was still a question.

1.3 Summaries

As the birthplace to initiate the "Targeted Poverty Alleviation" and a banner of its practice in China, the development of Shibadong Village has always attracted much attention. In the course of exploring effective ways to targeted alleviate poverty, the local government, the task force stationed in the village, the two committees of Shibadong Village, and all villagers have exerted great initiative and creativity; and make bold exploration as well as prominent achievements in the targeted identification of poor households, building villagers' ideology and morality, building grassroots organizations, poverty alleviation through marriage, developing the kiwifruit industry and rural tourism, and so on. These invaluable grassroots explorations are the main cause for casting the banner of targeted poverty alleviation in Shibadong Village. At the same time, we should also see that the popularity and influence brought by the General Secretary's visit to Shibadong Village and the extensive media coverage, which provided rare external opportunities for the development of the village, especially the infrastructure construction and related industrial development of the village. To a certain extent, these external opportunities have contributed to the success of the "leveraged" development model of Shibadong Village. In the rapid development of the village, we cannot ignore the constraints that may affect the transition from targeted poverty elimination to rural revitalization and from "leveraged" development to independent and sustainable development. How to better cultivate the internal development momentum of Shibadong Village and find a suitable collective industrial development model based on its own advantages; how to let foreign private capital land better and play its advantageous role in the development of tourism-related industries in Shibadong; how to improve the policy implementation level of government departments and villagers' awareness and ability of risk avoidance, and protect the entrepreneurial talent and enthusiasm of entrepreneurial individuals, may be the problem that needs to be faced and paid attention to for Shibadong Village.

References

Chen, Z. (2017). The Shibadong village visited by the General Secretary has a mountain spring water plant!. Huaxia Times, October 21, 2017.

Luo, M. (2014). Exploring targeted poverty alleviation with Shibadong villages as a pilot. *Xinxiang Review, No., 23*, 2014.

Pan, S. (2015). Central media focus on Shibadong village, report on all-round experience of targeted poverty alleviation. Unity Daily, March 2, 2015.

Shibadong. (2018). Introducing the "Earth Warehouse" to revolutionize the travel and residence model in the first place of precise poverty alleviation. Huasheng Online, September 30, 2018.

A series of reports on the poverty alleviation stories of the Shibadong villages. CCTV.com, February 13, 2016.

Yanhong Liu is an associate professor at the University of Chinese Academy of Social Sciences, whose main research interests are political economy, public policy, and sustainable development.

Chapter 2
Dual Poverty Reduction of Good-Neighbor Sharing: Physical and Spiritual Poverty Reduction: Social Benefits of a Farmer's Self-Employment in Jiangjia Village, Zhejiang

Wei Jiang

Abstract From poverty to moderate prosperity, the progress is not only the increase of material wealth, but also the increase of happiness index, and a joyful and harmonious rural community is an important source of happiness. Based on a field survey in Jiangjia Village, this paper takes the bamboo processing production chain of the village as a clue to play back the experience of a poor household who started his own business in 1991. While getting rid of poverty himself, he drove his neighbors to get rich together, reflecting the unity of economic and social benefits, and the unity of material and spiritual poverty reduction in the targeted poverty reduction.

Keywords Good-neighbor sharing · Bamboo processing · Spiritual poverty reduction · Jiangjia Village

In September 2015, the United Nations officially announced the Sustainable Development Goals (SDGs), which consist of 17 subgoals that are closely interlinked and aim to make a shift to a sustainable development path in an integrated way, emphasizing the harmonious development among economy, environment, and society. The progress from poverty to moderate prosperity is not only the increase of material wealth, but also the increase of happiness index, suggesting that a joyful and harmonious rural community is one of the important sources of happiness. Based on field survey and household interviews, this paper takes the bamboo processing production chain as a clue to truly replay the experience of a poor household in Jiangjia Village, Longyou County, Zhejiang Province, who started his own business since 1993 and got rid of poverty himself, while driving his surrounding neighbors to get rich together, reflecting the unity of economic and social benefits, material wealth and spiritual poverty reduction in the targeted poverty reduction.

W. Jiang (✉)
Institute of Ethnology and Anthropology, Chinese Academy of Social Sciences, Beijing, China

Case Studies of Targeted Poverty Reduction and Alleviation in 100 Villages, International Research on Poverty Reduction, https://doi.org/10.1007/978-981-95-0549-4_2

Located in the mountainous area of Longnan, the Jiangjia village is a beautiful village in the farthest southwest of Luojia Town, Longyou County, Quzhou City, Zhejiang Province. The whole village takes the shape of a long snake, about 4.5 km long, with a mountainous forest area of 8,933 mu,[1] including more than 3,900 mu of bamboo forest, 827 mu of arable land, and more than 600 mu of tea plantation. Jiangjia Village was named Jiyu[2] Village in 1982, the name is derived from the early stage of reform and opening up in hope of collective economic prosperity and thus adopt the name. Jiangjia Village is well known for its famous mountain, Shengtang[3] Mountain, also known as Shengdeng[4] Mountain. In the mountains, there are Tianchi,[5] Shizhang,[6] and Shengdeng, which are serene and elegant. There are also "passageway of bird hovering, the name of 18 tortuous paths, climbing to the peak and the scenery at far is secured". And the top of the mountain is also called "Wanglong[7] Mountain Tip" (Wanlu[8] Mountain Tip) where you could see the hills and streams, as well as the villages and fields by looking around. Jiangjia Creek runs through the village from south to north and merges into the Qiantang River, along which are scattered paddy fields and bamboo seas, dotted at intervals with tea plantations, nursery-grown plants, and orchards. Bamboo seas, rice plants, tea plantations, flowering woods, and fruit-bearing forests are the village's green resources. And to turn lucid waters and lush mountains into invaluable assets has always been the desire of the villagers by the mountains and water. The interviewee of this paper, a villager called Lao Xia is carrying this desire to lead the neighbors and friends to the path of green development, and successfully lead his villagers to achieve the dual goals of both material and spiritual poverty alleviation.

2.1 Good-Neighbor Sharing Model for Dual Poverty Reduction: From a Lively Network of Neighborhood Friends and Relatives to a Green Industry Chain

At the beginning of the 2017, when the project of investigation and research of 100 villages launched, our team moved into villager Youzhen and Qiusheng's house and lived with them in Jiangjia Village, and we lived very close to the Lao Xia's house. Their houses along with five or six peasant households' buildings are arrayed close together on either side of the Jiangjia Village Cultural Hall, located in the center of the long strip of land in Jiangjia Village. We visited each other's homes all the

[1] 1 mu equals 1/15 hectare. –Trans.

[2] Jiyu means the collective economic prosperity in Chinese. – Trans.

[3] Literally it means sanctuary.–Trans.

[4] Literally it means sanctuary lamp.–Trans.

[5] Literally it means Heaven Lake.–Trans.

[6] Literally it means stone dhanari column.–Trans.

[7] Literally it means watching the dragon.–Trans.

[8] Sounding similar but means tens of thousands of censers.–Trans.

time, had meals and chats together, and had reunions with relatives and friends from the city on holidays. On every weekend there is full of friends and laughter. Among those villagers, Lao Xia and Qiusheng are the type of people who are the most warm-hearted and hospitable ones. They have always been in a sharing state like good neighbors and kith and kin, from sitting around the poor enough meal in the difficult time to tasting delicious food after getting rich.

When we arrived at Jiangjia Village, Youzhen treated us in a warm and welcoming way as always. It was at noon on Saturday, Youzhen and Qiusheng prepared sumptuous meal once again with their own home-raised chicken, wild bamboo shoots from their own land at the mountain, and fruits and vegetables from their own vegetable plantations on their private plots. And they warmly called their neighbors and friends to join us. As we were about to have the meal, a cheerful laughter was coming from the door.

> *"Hahahaha ...... oops, did all of you see my car? I remembered it was parked in front of the door of Jianhong's house, but no car was there......". It turned out to be Lao Xia striding over to us again.*
>
> *"And where did you just go? Did you stop at the door of the plant where the bamboo branches got sun exposure?" A neighbor reminded Lao Xia.*
>
> *"No!"*
>
> *"Then let's have meal first, just leave it alone for now, you can't lose it anyway......"*

The village security has been well guarded, so it is not necessary to lock the car's door. The laughing Lao Xia joined everyone at meals, and began to chat lively with them. All of them said, he is a true happy man everyday for he never holds disturbing things in his heart overnight, and he chooses to solve problems in an optimistic way. If a problem cannot be solved, he would simply forget it, so everyday he is happy.

> *"Will you still have the day off tomorrow? I have a large flock of flying birds (a local type of cage-free native chicken raised in the hills), and I will kill a few tomorrow. At noon of tomorrow, all of you are welcome to my house for meals!" Lao Xia made another arrangement with his neighbors for Sunday.*

In short, "it is a happy thing to share together" is the philosophy of life of the people like Lao Xia. They used to yearn for and be curious about city life, but once they left the house, they could not see the lush mountains and lucid water, and did not have their own vegetable gardens and private plots, so they felt that they did not belong to the city; especially, they were not accustomed to and did not appreciate the lifestyle that neighbors did not know each other nor did not interact with each other, and the rule of their interaction is that people tended to "seek profit and avoid loss". In the Lao Xia's dictionary, the city life, short of lucid water, lush mountains, and the milk of human kindness, is a kind of "spiritual poverty"; they believed that neighbors, relatives, and friends should visit each other, and get along with each other. It is common to have conflicts, but only if make a compromise to each other, any conflict can be resolved. Therefore, they are satisfied with their cozy community. The seamless interaction and mutual help have always been the community mainstream of Jiangjia Village, which is also their cherished "spiritual wealth".

It is under the influence of this philosophy of life that the lively network of neighbors and friends gradually extends to the network of Lao Xia's production chain in green industry. Jiangjia Village, which is located near the mountains and water, has a strong resource endowment for green industry, in which moso bamboo has always been an important part of the villagers' income. During every spring, after spring thunderstorms and the spring rains, at the foot of the mountain, there is full of yellow and green colors of tea plantations, and on the mountain, there are spring bamboo shoots racing to emerge from the soil. Both add radiance and beauty to each other. Especially in the big year of the mountain bamboo shoots, the spring shoots will grow in density, and the idiom "spring shoots after the rain" is derived from this scene. Villagers dig up the bamboo shoots to prevent the overdensity, and then blanch and dry them in the sun to make dried bamboo shoots, which are rare mountain delicacies. Moso bamboo is also the raw material for bamboo ware processing and building industry. Consequently, the villagers have a good plan for the bamboo hills and will cut the moso bamboo in batches for sale. The waste branches from the bamboo processing are the raw material for brooms. Since 1991, Lao Xia has been collecting the discarded bamboo branches from the mountain, inviting neighbors and friends to make brooms together, and then seeking markets to sell them. With the expansion of production, and more neighbors and friends joined this cause, the lively network of neighbors and friends gradually developed into a network of production chain in green industry, creating more than 30 jobs (in addition to those of collecting bamboo branches in the hills). If we count the non-fixed collectors, all the farming households in this village are basically the network nodes of this production chain.

2.2 The Trajectory of Dual Poverty Reduction: From the Network of Production Chain in Green Industry to the Social Sharing of Economic Benefits

Lao Xia is born in 1960s and a big crowded peasant family. His father and all of those people of his father's generation have lively and helpful personal character. When neighbors are in trouble, they would not hesitate to lend a hand, while his mother and aunts are all hardworking with household chores, raising poultry and managing vegetable gardens. They will help each other to plow the land, plant seedlings and reap the harvest during the busy farming season, and gather together to share joy and talk about the daily trifles as well as hardships in the old days during the slack season. Lao Xia grew up in the atmosphere of this big family. There were five children in his family, and the poverty would not allow all of them to accept higher education, so the family had to take care of his brother, who had a leg injury, and his youngest sister, and merely supported these two children to go to high school. The other three siblings, including Lao Xia, had to work on the land at home after they graduated from primary school. They had to make a living by selling moso bamboo occasionally and two pigs every year, and struggled to survive on low incomes, i.e., they were typical low-income people.

In the 1990s, the real estate industry began to boom rapidly and the construction industry flourished. As a result, the moso bamboo, which is the raw material for the scaffolding to be heavily demanded by the industry, and had been always in short supply. Consequently, the villagers would sell moso bamboo more frequently, leaving bamboo branches in huge quantities in the hills. Most of the brooms that people used to make at home were made of these discarded branches, and those people who were skillful in making brooms would often make a few more not only for themselves but for their neighbors, as was the case with Lao Xia. At first, he made a few brooms for himself and his neighbors, but later he noticed that the discarded bamboo branches in the hills were not only wasteful, but also when branches were piled up, it often blocked the way to the mountain and made it inconvenient to dig bamboo shoots, which seriously affected the management of their private hills; also, he thought that brooms were a necessary daily commodity, so he came up with the idea of making brooms for sale. Keeping that in mind, Lao Xia started to organize neighbors by dividing the labor and they made the discarded bamboo branches into brooms for sale.

The whole process of making and selling brooms, from collecting bamboo branches in the hills to selling the brooms, can be roughly divided into the following five steps, which forms a production and marketing network, as shown in Fig. 1a; meanwhile, the neighbors and friends who invested their labor in the process also received corresponding income, as shown in Fig. 1b.

We asked Lao Xia about the cost of each step, and knew that in all the steps or processes workers are paid on a piecework basis. The first step is to collect bamboo branches and divide them into small bundles, making the cost of each bundle as 0.5 RMB; the second step is to turn and bake the bundles collected in the first step to remove the bamboo leaves, adding the cost of each bundle 0.1 RMB, and one

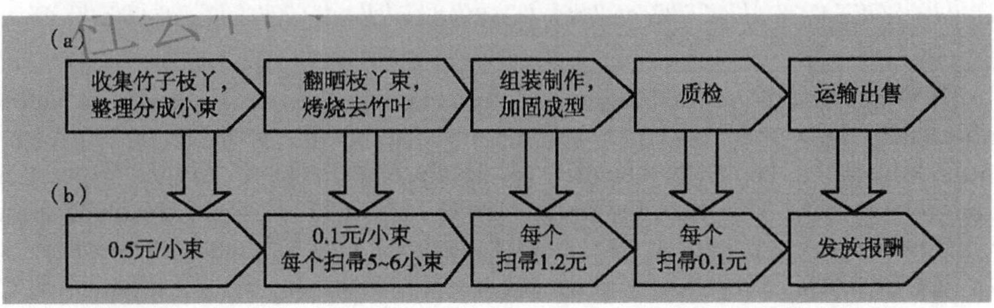

Fig. 2.1 Schematic diagram of broom production and marketing process. 收集竹子枝丫，整理分成小束:collect bamboo branches and divide them into small bundles, 翻晒枝丫束,烤烧去竹叶:turn and bake the dundles to remove the bamboo leaves, 组装制作,加固成型:assemble and manufacture, fasten and complete, 质检:quality inspection, 运输出售:transport and sale, 0.5元/小束:0.5 RMB/ small bundle, 0.1元/小束,每个扫帚5-6束:0.5 RMB/ small bundle,a broom is made of 5–6 bundles, 每个扫帚1.2元:1.2 RMB/ broom, 每个扫帚0.1元:0.1 RMB/ broom, 发放报酬:pay the wages

broom needs 5 ~ 6 bundles; the third step is to assemble the brooms with standard bundles, the purchased straps, and broom sticks, making each broom cost 1.2 RMB. The fourth step is to inspect the brooms, if there are too many leaves, remove them, if the length difference of the branches is too obvious, trim them slightly and organize them into a regular and good-looking broom, and increase the cost of each broom 0.1 RMB because the time and effort required for this step are very little as everyone takes the work very seriously in each step before, so basically there are only a few brooms that people need to remove the leaves and cut the branches. The last step is the transportation and sale, along with the wage payment for each person. In addition to the mentioned payment, Lao Xia also needs to invest in other assembly materials, such as broom sticks and straps, which cost about 1.00 RMB per broom; electricity fees, depreciation cost of equipment, and freight costs are all shared on average, costing about 1.30 RMB per broom. The selling price of a broom is 7.00 ~ 7.50 RMB, so the profit of each broom is only 0.70 ~ 1.20 RMB.

In spare time, Lao Xia also planted a total of about 50 mu[9] of kiwifruits and raspberries. We remembered that in the first year, after the trees bore fruits, they reaped the harvest. Afterward, he felt too busy to manage and take care of the harvest, so left the fruits to those villagers whoever like to pick for free. Later, a non-native businessman passed by there and wanted to buy kiwifruits, and Lao Xia let him to pick on his own for free. And after picked 2,000 jin,[10] that man felt it inappropriate and paid him at the price of 2 RMB per jin, Lao Xia also felt sorry because he thought he overcharged that man. He seems to be a person who does not know how to calculate the profits as the market price of the kiwifruit is 30 RMB per jin (his first year's harvest is sold at the price of 30 RMB). If he does business well, the income of kiwifruit will far exceed that of broom.

> *That season happens to be very busy for all of us, I know the first harvest has got me a lot, so the next thing is to let people pick fruits themselves to taste. This is too difficult for me to run this business, hahaha, so I leave it here ...... hmmmm, yes, this can pay me more than doing brooms, but we are used to doing brooms, and every day we have things to do together, and it feels quite good. Making broom makes me earn less, but it is enough for me, hahaha, we are all happy for doing business together.*

He thinks that the profitability of kiwifruits and raspberries is unstable, which is affected by the weather, and there is sometimes bad harvest, and sometimes even no fruits to bear, thus he just let it be there carelessly. Now the kiwifruits and raspberries are growing wild. This year, the raspberries bore fruits a lot, so he organized those villagers to pick a batch for sale, and let everyone pick and eat the rest of fruits. In fact, he knows very clearly about the profit calculation, but his approach is of Buddha-like. What the most important thing is that his philosophy calls for him to do things together with everyone and to make money together because everyone thinks this is a happy way to go on living. Only in this way, what they do will not only economically lift them out of poverty, but also spiritually make them rich.

---

[9] 1 mu equals 0.067 hectares.–Trans.

[10] 1 jin equals 500 g.–Trans.

2.2.1 The First Session of Interviews

In the afternoon, we walked along the Jiangjia Creek on the way to Lao Xia's simple factory, and came across Zhang Youshu and his wife, who happened to be driving a small tractor back from collecting bamboo branches in the hills. The old couple were both in their 70 s, but looked much younger than their actual age. The young lady told us about the day's harvest.

Usually we, the old couple, are at home. Our son and daughter have got married and formed new family. They work outside the village, and will come home to spend time with us on holidays. There is not much to do in daily work, such as to water the vegetable garden; to feed the chickens and ducks; and occasionally weeding the tea plantation and so on. Now there is nothing to do anyway, so we prefer doing more work than being idle when we are still fit as a fiddle. If left in the hills ,these bamboo branches will block the normal passage in the hills. Before Lao Xia led us to make brooms with him, we took the branches back home to burn as firewood, and it was a total waste. Since Lao Xia started to make brooms, the bamboo branches could be fully utilized. We do not work outside every day, and as it happens, today we have to cut down some bamboos (because new bamboo grows a lot every year, so it is necessary to cut down some mature bamboos in case that the bamboos will grow in density and thus affect the growth of bamboo shoots), or Lao Xia contacts us about where bamboo branches are, and then we will collect those branches and make them bundled up, and each bunch is worth 50 cents, 5~6 bunches is almost made into one broom. This is good. Look, we have enough raw materials for making 50 brooms in one cart, 2.5 RMB each, so that's 125 RMB in one cart. We can fill one cart in the morning and another in the afternoon, which is about 200 RMB. Such a workload is still a bit tiring, but we can have a rest when we feel tired, which is unlike working outside, where we can't have a rest when we get tired. Nowadays, we are old and we are almost illiterate, so it is not easy for us to find a job outside. We think this is good for us by helping Lao Xia collect bamboo branches, and we can also take care of our work at home as well as our grandchildren when they are back home, so we are satisfied with our lives now.

2.2.2 Second Session of Interview

Before we walked into the simple factory of Lao Xia, a fresh smell of bamboo leaves refreshed us, making it feel like we were embraced by nature. It was very hot then, and Aiting and Rumei, who were baking the bamboo leaves, greeted us warmly with electric fans. Along with several other women, such as Youzhen and Juxiang, they are respectively the wives of Lao Xia's cousins and have been the permanent employees of Lao Xia's broom production network for more than 20 years.

Interview with Youzhen

It was a Sunday, and the couple Youzhen and her husband happened to invite their neighborhood friends and family relatives to her house, and she made the day off that day. She has adapted to the pace of work in Lao Xia's broom production and is happy to work in her small community and enjoy the country life.

Now, it's hot in summer, and the hottest period of time is between 11:00 a.m and the whole afternoon, so it makes you very hot to bake bamboo leaves. We usually get up at 1:00 a.m., stop working until 11:00 a.m., and after having lunch, we take the whole afternoon off to avoid the hottest time. It is very tiring to do it day after day, so we often take some time off after working for a few consecutive days. Having done this for 20 years, we are all skilled and work very fast. We can complete the process of baking bamboo branches and removing leaves, and it is about 600-800 brooms' workload a day (from 1:00 am to 11:00 am), so that we can basically get 300-400 RMB. Because it is very tiring to work every day in a row, we take a few days off every month, but even so, we get 6,000-7,000 RMB a month. Although it is tiring to work, but it is certainly better than working outside, because you can have more freedom to arrange working hours. Of course, sometimes we work overtime when Lao Xia is in a hurry to deliver brooms, but it's still convenient to be at home. We help Lao Xia make brooms, and it usually does not affect the farming work, such as planting vegetables and picking tea leaves when it is needed. Moreover, it is also convenient to live at home, we pick fresh vegetables and fruits in our own plantation. And we do not need to worry about whatever chemical fertilizers and pesticides on them. Here we can also take care of outselves, and feel secure and safe. If work outside without any skills, I could at best serve in the hotel as a waiter and doing washing dishes or take other jobs like that, with a maximum salary of 3,000 RMB a month. And the first is low wages, and then the second is all the farming work at home will have to be delayed, and furthermore, there are no friends and neighbors with me to work, chat, and eat together. All day long it keeps me in suspense, and it is not secure . So I think this is good now.

Every time came Jiangjia Village for research, we lived in Youzhen's house, and found that she usually expressed her optimism and contentment with the state of life when she chatted subconsciously. The woman in is Youzhen.

Her family built a finely decorated three-story house 6 years ago. The house is clean and tidy, and in front of the door is 10 mu of camellias, and across the road is a factory for baking bamboo leaves. In every spring when the camellia flowers blossom, there will be many people coming to the village to enjoy taking pictures of flowers.

Interview with Juxiang

Juxiang also did not go to work that day, because her daughter took her nephew and niece home to play at home. Because the youngest one was just born, she helped look after the baby. Juxiang once went to Yiwu to work, but she is a homesick person, so after a few days later, she came back home. Thereafter, she started her work life in the small community of Jiangjia Village. Later, her life is gradually getting better, and her family also built a three-story building, which is decorated beautifully.

When Bobo (Juxiang's son) was still very young, then he was not yet 5, I was introduced by the village's employment agency to work in Yiwu. At that time, I went to work as a nanny, to take care of children, because I am a person who loves children by nature, so it was a good job for me, and the treatment was also good, and the employer was very good to me as well. But when I hugged someone else's child, I couldn't help but think of my own child, and I didn't know how he was at home, then my tears fell down naturally (I heard Juxiang more than once about this experience, and saw Juxiang's eyes wet and watery every time when she talked about it). I was also very patient with child, and a nice and neat person, so the employer was particularly satisfied with my work, and then once they saw me falling tears, but I did not dare to explain because I just came to work for not long, and how embarrassing it is to explain. Again, at that time I was bound by a contract, which means my breach of contract is to lose my money, so I did not say anything. Afterwards, they repeatedly asked me to explain the tears. After they knew the reason, the employer showed sympathy and understanding for me, and let me go back home. They not only did not report my breach of contract nor cut my salary, to whom I am very grateful. Not long after I came back home from Yiwu, the business of the Lao Xia's brooms thrived, so I went with Rumei and some old ladies to give help, and gradually we could do more and more work, and our salaries also increased. The most important thing is that I can be with my children every day, so I won't have to worry about them like what I did outside, and I feel more secure.

2.2.3 Third Session of Interview

The third step is to assemble and manufacture, fasten and complete the brooms. Lao Xia renovated the old school building into a factory. The school was very dilapidated but it has a large, open, and well-ventilated field, which meets the environmental requirements for broom production. When we walked into the old school, we found that there were still many chickens in the playground running around to chase flying insects or compete for eating bugs on the ground. Tugen told us that to assemble and fasten the brooms is a laborious task, so there are usually arranged 5–6 male workers.

My wife Xuemei and I spent a lot of money in curing us of diseases a few years ago and accordingly owed a lot of debt, when the children were small, so the whole family was short of labor, and became a poverty-stricken family, which I felt quite humiliated. When it got better, we began to wok-dry Longjing tea. In Jiangjia Village, raw materials of planted tea has very good quality, and the tea is particularly fragrant. In addition to making tea, we would help Lao Xia with his broom business in the spare time, as I could do the assembling and making the broom, while she would do the baking branches to remove the bamboo leaves. Gradually, the economic situation of my family went better; afterwards, we felt that the tea business involved all kinds of things, including picking tea leaves in our tea plantations, the purchase of other villagers' tea leaves, the repair and update of equipment, the contact of dealers, as well as the ups and downs of the price that bothered us among other things. There were too much work to do, making us fatigued. So we thought it would be better if we just worked in Lao Xia' broom factory, which is the most simple and reliable job for us.

Xuemei's health is not very good, so she occasionally helps Lao Xia to bake branches to remove the leaves, and she can earn about 200 RMB a day. If she works more than ten days per month, then she can earn more than 3,000 RMB, which is quite a lot, because she can not only take care of household chores as usual, but also do some like a piece of cake (i.e., a little amount of) tea work, raise chickens, take care of the bamboo shoots on the mountain, and so on. She can do all these works without any delay. While in the Lao Xia's factory, when the work is urgent, I will work overtime without some intermittent breaks, but if the work is not urgent, I will take turns with several other workers to rest several days, because to work in assembly production for a month in a row will be quite fatiguesome, we need to shift a few days to rest. My job is to assemble and make the brooms, that is, to assemble brooms by fastening the bunches of bamboo branches without leaves to the broom handle to make a complete broom. Usually it takes 5 bunches of branches to make a normal size broom, if you want to make a larger broom, then you need 6 bunches of branches. These broom handles are made either from wooden or bamboo sticks, and they are more costly to buy, about 0.5 ~ 0.7 RMB a stick, or even 1 RMB when the price is at the highest. Also, buying some reinforcement materials such as straps will cost almost 1 RMB. My income is like this, the reward of each broom is 1.2 RMB, we can usually make more than 250 brooms a day, and to make more than 300 brooms is too exhausting, so it is good enough to make more than 200, and not too much more. Have a rest when you get tired. Of course, when Lao Xia is in a hurry to deliver the goods, we will work overtime and not rest so early to help him deliver the goods on time. Lao Xia doesn't earn much money per broom, but he must always take care of these things, and we can't help him, so when he has to hurry up the delivery, we will work more overtime to make sure that he can deliver in time. In the past, I also went out to work for the construction team, that kind of tiredness is that you are not only unable to arrange your own time, but also not respected, and sometimes you will not get paid, so I think now in our own Jiangjia village my job is quite good, and Lao Xia's factory is like our own home, so I am quite satisfied.

2.2.4 Fourth Session of Interview

The fourth step is quality inspection, and relatively speaking, it is the easiest to do, because they usually do it very carefully, so basically there is no problem in quality. Just directly put the brooms neatly on the line. It occasionally happens that there are single branches particularly longer, it simply needs a trim, so this process is also the fastest, and the pay is also low, that is, a broom rewards 10 cents. Qingsheng is the staff for the third step. He will use his day off to help do the quality inspection.

This step is not tiresome, but it has little rewards anyway, so Lao Xia will do it himself. Sometimes when we have time, and he is busy, we will do this for him. I used to go to the city to work, and I went to pedal the yellow cart (ricksha). Because I was pulling a human-powered yellow cart, not an electric driven one, so it was a labor-intensive job. I was very tired at the end of the day, but the day pay was not more than 80 RMB. At the end of month, after paying the rent and spending some for food, there was not much left. And in the city, this work is not respected. We often met scoundrels sitting in the cart, who did not pay after reaching the destination. Although this situation is very rare, but after all, almost everyone pulling the yellow cart more or less encountered them. In short, it was not much money, and we were discriminated against there, as well as not able to take care of the family, so one or two years later, I returned to the Jiangjia Village. Usually I help Lao Xia with broom, which I feel very satisfied because I can find job in my own village, and it does not affect my farming work, as well as I could take care of my family, so how can I find such a job elsewhere? Of course, when we are in a hurry to deliver, we work overtime that is exhausting, but if you do not deliver on time, you will not have orders anymore, then our factory will have no future! So, when it comes to urgent delivery, Lao Xia does not need to say anything, and we will voluntarily work overtime to work around the clock. We cannot help anything else, so we work overtime, and as long as we can do, we will try to help him as much as possible.

2.3 Conclusion: Radiation Effect of Social Benefits and Dual Poverty Reduction of Good-Neighbor Sharing

Judging from the net income of brooms, Lao Xia, as a local business owner, does not gain much economic benefits, but he thinks it is very satisfying himself because the neighbors and friends are very satisfied, so the greatest harvest in this way is not the economic benefits, but the social benefits.

From the interview, we all know that Lao Xia does not make much profit in broom business, but he needs to take care of everything, so we are willing to do our best to reduce Lao Xia's workload. And Lao Xia is trying his best to create opportunities for everyone and provide convenience. In Lao Xia's production network, the actual working hours also change according to the changes in broom orders and temporary changes in the employees' farming work at home. When there are a small number of orders, everyone will have more time to rest; when the orders are in large numbers, everyone will voluntarily work overtime so that Lao Xia can deliver on time. When the farming season is busy, Xia will take fewer orders or cancel some so that the staff can free up some time to complete the farming work in the fields. At the maximum of the broom demand, there were more than 30 employees and nearly 20 at the minimum of the demand. As a result, almost more than a dozen households of the Jiangjia village's production squad (community) are included in his network of production chain. If we count in those temporary workers who collect bamboo branches in the hills, it includes more than 80% of the people in Jiangjia village, because almost everyone has a moso bamboo hill and sells their unused and discarded moso bamboo branches to Lao Xia who will make raw materials for brooms. With the expansion of Lao Xia's broom industry, neighbors and friends also became busy with their jobs and saw their income increased, and the elderly people would occasionally help to work together who often chat together while working.

As this form of labor is relatively flexible and it allows people to take care of the farming work at home without leaving the elderly and children, and the income is not lower than that of working outside, and more importantly, one does not have to leave the familiar and cordial community life with neighbors and friends, so people say they feel more comfortable to work here than to work outside, and especially people will enjoy the leisure time and family network together here. The broom production chain of Lao Xia has developed into a green industrial network encircling broom production, in which everyone, including women and the elderly, can get paid for their work and find their own existence in their work, and through this production network, people have become more cooperative and the community more harmonious.

Therefore, to a certain extent, it can be argued that Lao Xia's broom production chain has created a good-neighbor sharing model of dual poverty eradication in the community, i.e., a lively network of neighborhood friends and relatives has turned into a green industrial chain. Its advantages are at least reflected in the following aspects.

(1) People are locally employed, which reduces the number of elderly people and children left behind and makes it possible to take care of the family, the most important unit of society.
(2) Increasing income while maintaining the lucid water and lush mountains. The whole process of broom making is almost pollution-free, and bamboo branches are the use of waste; broom handles and straps are also recyclable.

The bamboo leaves removed in the second step are also used as fertilizer or domestic fuel which makes no waste. Therefore, Lao Xia's broom production is a process of utilizing and maintaining the green ecology of the resources from the lucid water and lush mountains.

(3) While taking a common path to get out of poverty and become rich, it reinforces the traditional living pattern of neighbors and friends in the local countryside,

and it keeps people in a state of "spiritual wealth". Here, everyone is happy and optimistic, which avoids the "crowded and lonely" state of "spiritual poverty" in modern life, where people are crowded in a flat but neighbors are indifferent and strangers to each other. And this is a way to achieve "spiritual poverty reduction" in modern society.

2.4 Policy Recommendations

The UN SDGs goals emphasize harmonious development of economy, environment, and society. The process from poverty to prosperity is not only the increase of material wealth, but also the rise of happiness index, and a happy and harmonious rural community is one of the important sources of happiness. In a modern society where the number of people suffering from mental illnesses is increasing day by day, "mental poverty reduction" is as important as "material poverty reduction", or even more important, as I insist. As a poverty-stricken household member, Lao Xia, through his self-employed business, has been able to lift himself out of poverty, and at the same time, he has been able to lead his neighbors around him to work and increase their income. This model of unifying economic and social benefits, material enrichment and spiritual poverty eradication should be supported for further promotion and publication. To this end, shall we create more conditions to promote the emergence and development of entrepreneurs like Lao Xia? For example, giving certain subsidies to the development of industries alike to update equipment, build plants, and provide a safer and more comfortable production environment; reducing the corresponding taxes with certain policies to increase their profit margins; as well as giving certain incentives for providing local jobs; providing more order channels; and so on. In short, the corresponding policies will surely inspire more people like Lao Xia to lead their neighbors toward the economic growth by good-neighbor sharing and to achieve both material and spiritual poverty reduction.

Let us wait and see……

References

Elvey, A., & Gormley-O'Brien, D. P. (2013). *Climate Change—Cultural Change: Religious Responses and Responsibilities*. Mosaic Press.

Fu, C. (2006). China's Rural Cooperative Economy: Organizational Forms and Institutional Changes. *China Economic Press, 2006*, 136.

Pan, J., & Liu, W. (Eds.). (2012). *Economic Law* (4th ed.). People's University of China Press.

UNDP. (2019). China Human Development Report Special Edition, China Publishing Group, China Translation Press.

Wang, X. (2017). Actively promoting the combination of precise poverty alleviation and green development. China Social Science Journal, December 15, 2017.

Zhou, Y. (2007). Xi Jinping's research in Quzhou Lishui emphasizes the in-depth promotion of "underdeveloped townships to run a well-off project" to accelerate the process of building a well-off society in Zhejiang. Zhejiang Daily, January 24, 2007.

Wei Jiang is an associate researcher at the Institute of Ethnology and Anthropology of Chinese Academy of Social Sciences, whose main research interests are climate change and sustainable development. Appreciation to Salahan Sun, a student, for designing the questionnaire about the production chain of bamboo processing industry, as well as the contribution to the home interviews and to writing the first draft.

Chapter 3
Poverty Reduction Model of "Industry + Welfare + Collective Transfer Payment": Poverty Alleviation Experience of Asset Income Project in Wangma Village, Jiangsu

Haijun Xu, Zongshuai Zhang, and Yanmei Dong

Abstract As a poverty-stricken village in an economically developed area, Wangma Village seems to be more like a relative poverty village from an overall perspective, and the definition standard of poverty line is higher than the national level, so the model of poverty reduction also has certain characteristics. Based on the analysis of the features and causes of poverty in Wangma Village, this paper analyzes the poverty reduction model of Wangma Village. Through investigation and analysis, the poverty reduction model of Wangma Village can be concisely summarized into the model of "industry + welfare + collective transfer payment", which provides income opportunities for poverty-stricken households through employment driven by industrial development. At the same time, industrial development promotes the growth of collective income and enhances the ability to use collective income to make transfer payments to poverty-stricken households, which becomes one of the important ways for those households to get out of poverty. The welfare model, on the other hand, consists of the policy guarantee and transfer payments provided by the government at all levels and society, which is also an important support for most poverty-stricken households to get out of poverty. Based on this model, the specific policies implemented in Wangma Village are introduced, and the effects of these policies are illustrated with corresponding case studies. At the end of this study, the future development of the "industry + welfare + collective transfer payment" model of poverty reduction in Wangma Village is presented.

Keywords Poverty reduction model · Industrial development · Poverty alleviation experience · Wangma Village

---

H. Xu · Y. Dong (✉)
Business School of Jiangnan University, Wuxi, China

Z. Zhang
University of Chinese Academy of Social Sciences, Beijing, China

Case Studies of Targeted Poverty Reduction and Alleviation in 100 Villages, International Research on Poverty Reduction, https://doi.org/10.1007/978-981-95-0549-4_3

3.1 The Basic Situation of Wangma Village and the Causes of Poverty

Located in the eastern part of Jianghuai Plain, Wangma Village is under the jurisdiction of Xisongji Town, Huaiyin District, Huai'an City, Jiangsu Province. It is always called the "a place where its crow reached three counties".[1] It is a relatively small administrative village in the plain area, with an administrative area of only 4 square kilometers and there are 7 groups of villagers distributed in 16 natural villages and stockaded villages. Wangma Village is 1.5 km away from the nearest station and about 40 km away from Huaiyin urban area. It is connected to the outside world by National Highway 205 and Provincial Highway 328, while there is also a new long railroad passing through, so the traffic condition is relatively convenient. As of 2017, Wangma Village has 617 households with a total population of 2452, all of whom are Han Chinese, with a resident population of about 1000 and about 70 households with 300 people entirely working and living outside. The number of labor force in the village registered population is about 350, of which about 280 are working outside the village, and only about 70 are working at home for a long time or taking care of their families. The outgoing workers are mainly concentrated in labor-intensive factories and construction sites, mainly engaged in the service industry. New laborers are not highly educated. The number of new laborers who graduated from middle school and did not receive higher education is about 30, and the number of new laborers who graduated from high school and did not receive higher education is about 80. There are about 300 villagers who are illiterate or semi-literate, and 55 are disabled and most of them became disabled as a result of diseases. In 2016, there were 137 poor households in the village according to the provincial poverty standards, 289 people officially registered as poverty-stricken population, and the actual poverty incidence rate was 11.79%. Among the poverty-stricken households, there are 34 households enjoying minimum living guarantee, involving 49 people; 20 households enjoying the five guarantees,[2] involving 20 people.

Wangma Village is a typical agricultural village in the plain area of northern Jiangsu Province, with a weak overall economic situation. The village's economic activities are basically focused on the production of bulk agricultural products, and there is neither industry nor specialty cash crops. The income of the villagers mainly comes from agricultural activities, outworking, and doing business. In 2016, according to the estimated data of the villager's committee, the per capita net income of Wangma Villagers is about 12,000 RMB per year, 1.3 mu[3] of arable land per capita, and the average net income per mu is about 600 RMB per year. The net income mainly comes from working or doing business outside, and if the family lacks laborers who go out to work, they are bound to fall into poverty. Judging from the provincial poverty line standard of 6000 RMB per capita, and the average per

[1] It means it locates at the intersection of three counties.–Trans.

[2] "Five guarantees" summarizing the State guarantee on proper food, clothing, medical care, housing, and funeral expenses for residents. –Trans.

[3] 1 mu equals 1/15 hectare. –Trans.

capita arable land in Wangma Village is 1.3 mu, and the average net income from agriculture is less than 1000 RMB, we can conclude that the main cause of poverty is lack of labor force working or doing business outside. There are more relative poverty cases than absolute poverty ones in this village. In terms of per capita net income level, the provincial standard for identifying poverty-stricken households in Jiangsu is less than 6000 RMB, which is much higher than the national level, and there was no poverty-stricken household without basic living guarantee found during the research. The absolute income of poverty-stricken households in Wangma Village is not low, and their basic lives can be guaranteed, but the regional economic level is relatively low, and their living standard decreases due to the necessary expenses such as medical care and education.

The main cause of poverty is the lack of labor force, followed by disease and education. In the sample of 31 households surveyed, 27 households responded, among which 10 households directly attributed the poverty to lack of labor force, 9 to disease, and 2 to disability. In fact, the ultimate result of poverty due to disease and disability is still the lack of labor force. Going out to work is the main way to get income, but poverty-stricken households generally lack labor force and the percentage of going out to work is not big. Due to the lack of family labor force, poverty-stricken households have fewer opportunities to go out to work and accordingly earn less income, which is the most important cause for the emergence of rural poverty. Among the poverty-stricken households interviewed, 2 people worked in the township, 1 person worked outside the township but still in the county, 1 person worked outside the county yet remained in the province, 2 people worked outside the province. The remaining 25 households have no one going out to work. There are 2 people who have been out to work for less than 3 months and 4 people who have been out to work for 6–12 months, which means that poverty-stricken households who work nearby can only work this way due to the lack of labor force at home and have to take care of their families and agricultural production. In summary, Wangma Village, as a provincial economically weak village in the eastern region, has certain differences in poverty features from the poverty symptoms in the central and western regions. Poverty in Wangma Village is more reflected in relative poverty, and the percentage of absolute poverty is relatively low; the main poverty cause is lack of labor force, and then successively the family structure, disease, disability, and education, which prevents people from going out to work for income.

3.2 Four Poverty Reduction Cases of Typical Poverty-Stricken Households

Case 1

Dai Jiayong, male, is 64 years old. Dai and his wife have a son and a daughter, who are now in their 30 s. His wife died of asthma when her daughter was 3 years old.

Dai Jiayong worked in Shenzhen when he was young, and the money he earned from his job was used up for his wife's medical treatment. After the death of his wife, the two children were brought up by their mother in their hometown, and due to poverty, both children did not attend middle school. Now that his daughter is married, there are four people with registered permanent residence: Dai Jiayong, his son, and two granddaughters. The son is also in poor health, inherited his mother's asthma, and has difficulty breathing when it rains. Dai Jiayong's daughter-in-law is a non-local, who met Dai Jiayong's son when he was working outside. The daughter-in-law gave birth to two children and shortly afterward, she came back to her hometown and left this family. And Dai Jiayong's son always does odd jobs, so he takes care of the two granddaughters usually, one of whom is now 9 years old and a student of the second grade at the elementary school, and the other is 10 years old and of the fourth grade at elementary school. The two granddaughters spend a lot of money on books and learning materials for school, which becomes a considerable economic burden for Dai Jiayong. Moreover, because he needs to put more energy into taking care of the children, picking them up and dropping them off at school and cooking for them, Dai Jiayong is unable to spare much time to work to earn money. Due to the lack of manpower at home to take care of the family, and plus the agricultural production, he can only choose to work nearby, and the working hours are limited. Before enjoying the poverty alleviation policy, the main economic source of the family depended on the son's working outside and the family's 3 mu of crops.

Through the industrial poverty alleviation, Wangma Village has vigorously developed the planting industry of Chinese Snake Gourd (Trichosanthes kirilowii), enabling Dai Jiayong to work odd hours at the Chinese Snake Gourd production base at his doorstep. By weeding and spraying insecticide, he can earn more than 50 RMB a day and several thousand RMB a year. Dai Jiayong's two granddaughters also enjoy the education poverty alleviation policy, and each of them receives 500 RMB from education subsidies every quarter. This poverty alleviation measure has helped Dai the most. In addition, the "City Celebrity" hotel in Huaiyin District gives him an annual dividend of 500 RMB. After being removed from the poverty tag, Dai Jiayong said, "Let's just get out of poverty" because he was "unsure" about the policies and specific poverty alleviation practices he would enjoy after being removed from poverty tag. Then, Dai Jiayong was worried that he would not be able to enjoy these poverty alleviation policies after he got out of poverty, but at the same time, he also expressed that he was satisfied, saying, "We are grateful to the Communist Party, the Party can take care of us as much as possible, which is already the biggest help to us, and we can't always rely on reliefs". Dai Jiayong's desire to make a fortune is not strong, he said his own conditions were already here, and it is good enough to raise two young granddaughters, "when the two children grow up, I will be 70 years old, and will not be able to take care of themselves, and what wealth I will make".

Dai Jiayong's two children left at home did not complete their compulsory education due to the poverty that his wife's disease induced, and their grandchildren's generation repeated the same fate as their father's. However, education poverty alleviation policies ease Dai Jiayong's family burden and make it possible for his two grandchildren to receive a complete education. Education is the main way to accumulate human capital. In Wangma Village, the overall education level of the interviewed poverty-stricken households over 35 years old is low, and the education level of the interviewed poverty-stricken household objects over 60 years old in Wangma Village is below elementary school, and the education situation of the 50–60 age group is not optimistic, as 6 out of 14 people belong to the illiterate category, 4 with elementary school education, and 4 with middle school level. This is the most fundamental cause of poverty. Poverty leads to early school dropout and low-skilled labor for subsistence, which in turn leads to low income levels, and lower income levels lead to low education levels for children, thus trapping them in a vicious cycle of intergenerational poverty transmission. Dai Jiayong's granddaughters are obviously able to change their fate and break this cycle through education, and the effect of the education poverty alleviation policy on Dai Jiayong's family is remarkable. Even in poor families, people attach great value to the education of the next generation, which is the most powerful weapon we have to break the intergenerational transmission of the poverty cycle in the future. Because he is over 60 years old, and his son is in poor health, and plus a lack of labor in the family, Dai Jiayong's motivation and aspiration to get out of poverty and become rich is not strong, and the effect of the poverty alleviation measure "helping the poor's spirit first and then reducing the poverty itself" is not significant in Dai Jiayong's case. It is because of his own lack of endogenous motivation to get out of poverty, and the publication and promotion of "to get out of poverty, but will not be removed of the support policy" are not put in place, Dai Jiayong worried that the current policy would not continue in his life after the poverty reduction.

Case 2

Chen Aiju, female, is 47 years old, with a family of four including two children: the daughter is 20 years old and studying in junior college, and the younger son is 12 years old and studying in the fifth grade of elementary school. Although Chen Aiju's husband has legs paralyzed, he still works outside all year round and works as a tailor in a garment factory, earning more than 2000 RMB a month, while Chen Aiju is left at home taking care of their children. The biggest expense of the family is the education of the children, she has to give the college daughter 1000 RMB a month for the living cost. After becoming a officially registered poverty-stricken household, Chen Aiju's family enjoys the poverty alleviation policy of ensuring minimum living guarantee: her husband, daughter, and son enjoy a monthly subsidy of more than 400 RMB. The two children enjoy the education poverty alleviation policy at school: her daughter receives an education poverty alleviation subsidy of more than 1000 RMB a quarter, and her son receives an education poverty alleviation subsidy of 500 RMB a quarter. Chen Aiju herself enjoys a poverty alleviation policy of public welfare job, and is responsible for cleaning the village arterial roads in the village, earning more than 400 RMB a month. At the end of each year, Chen Aiju's family can also get the dividends from the poverty alleviation of the Chinese Snake Gourd industry, with each person getting more than 400 RMB of dividends each year. For Chen Aiju's family, due to the lack of labor force, the children's education expenses have become the biggest burden on the family economy. These combined measures of minimum living guarantee, education poverty alleviation, public welfare jobs, and industrial dividends have solved the economic problem of children's education, eased the family's economic burden, and guaranteed the children's rights to education, with remarkable results in poverty alleviation and poverty reduction, and the family's living conditions are greatly improved. According to the education poverty alleviation policy of Huaiyin District, in 2019, poverty-stricken households in Wangma Village received a total of 11,125 RMB in government education subsidies, with an average household education subsidy of about 200 RMB, which effectively eased the pressure of poverty-stricken households' education expenses and enabled the children of those households to obtain regular education resources and allowed them not to drop out of school too early, improving the endogenous capacity for their own future development. It is worth noting that, due to her illiteracy and being a non-native, Chen Aiju did not understand the poverty alleviation policies, and thus answered "I don't know" and "I don't understand" when asked about many of the poverty alleviation measures she enjoyed. Therefore, more work needs to be done to the promotion and publication of the poverty alleviation policies.

Case 3

Shi Conghe, male, 61 years old. Shi Conghe has a physical disability that prevents him from doing heavy physical labor, and his wife has a mental disability, and the family has two daughters, one 15 years old who is now in the first grade at middle school and the other 13 years old who is in the sixth grade at elementary school. Because his wife got ill very often, Shi has to stay by his wife's side and cannot go out to work, but he can only do some odd jobs. Before enjoying the poverty alleviation policies, Shi felt a lot of pressure. The children's daily expenses were too much, and they had to pay more than 1600 RMB a semester for food, as well as other expenses for covering the school bus transportation fee and weekly allowance for the children. Each time his wife got mentally ill, it will cost more than 10,000 RMB to make treatment. All these expenses usually depend on relatives to cover. After becoming officially registered poverty-stricken households, all four members of the family enjoy the minimum living guarantee policy, with a total of more than 1200 RMB a month for the four members of the family, and this has become the main source of income for Shi Conghe's family. Each of the two children in school receives education subsidies of 500 RMB per quarter for poverty alleviation. In addition, Shi and his family can get a dividend of about 1200 RMB from the Chinese Snake Gourd industry poverty alleviation project at the end of each year.[4] On New Year's Day and other festivals, the person in charge of Shi Conghe's poverty alleviation will also bring some gifts to Shi's family. Shi Conghe is satisfied with this series of poverty alleviation policies, which have greatly reduced his economic burden and guaranteed

[4] The data here should be about 2,000 RMB, and the amount of Chinese Snake Gourd industry dividends paid to the bank account is 495 RMB per capita, and 4 people should be 1,980 RMB in total. The data were not changed accordingly due to the lack of deep memory and to respect the authenticity of the interviewer's records.

the education of his two children. Shi Conghe's greatest wish is to raise two children to adulthood. About the children's education, he said he would do his best to support his daughters in their studies in high school till college if they want and can do.

Case 4

Bi Weiping, female, 60 years old, whose husband died of disease in earlier years. Bi Weiping independently raise her son to adulthood, and then the son married and had his own daughter. In 2015, the son died from car accident, and the daughter-in-law left the family because she did not think there was a future in life, and the granddaughter was left at home. Thereafter, Bi Weiping lost her source of livelihood, had to take care of the granddaughter, could not work outside, and thus got into trouble. The villager's committee verified the situation and identified her family as a poverty-stricken household. In 2016, after the villager's committee verified the situation and in accordance with the procedures for identifying poverty-stricken households, Bi Weiping's family was recognized as a poverty-stricken household, and her family was included in the scope of minimum living guarantees. From the 2016 onward, Bi Weiping could receive about 500 RMB per month, which eased the pressure of life. Moreover, thanks to the implementation of education poverty alleviation measures, Bi Weiping can also receive an education poverty alleviation subsidies of 625 RMB per year; in addition, there are 500 RMB from social assistance grants every year. However, the per capita income of Bi Weiping's family of two people is only about 3550 RMB, which is far from 6000 RMB/year, the per capita net income of local standard poverty line, and her life is still very difficult.

In 2017, after the Chinese Snake Gourd industry project was officially launched and brought benefits, the village "two committees"[5] decided to hire Bi Weiping to work in the Chinese Snake Gourd farmland. The work in the Chinese Snake Gourd farmland is mostly manual work, which is not very labor-intensive, and the work is done during the day when the children are at school, so the work time does not affect the care of children. The work in the Chinese Snake Gourd farmland is about 10 months a year, and the daily labor pay is 60 RMB, which amounts to an annual labor income of 18,000 RMB. In addition, the collective income of the Chinese Snake Gourd project gives the poverty-stricken households a transfer payment of 495 RMB per capita per year, so the two members of Bi Weiping's family get a total income of 990 RMB. During the period of working in the Chinese Snake Gourd farmland, Bi Weiping transferred 2.8 mu of her own arable land to the village collective, and received nearly 2000 RMB of land transfer income each year. In 2018, the income of Bi Weiping's family included 18,000 RMB of labor income from the Chinese Snake Gourd farmland, 990 RMB of village collective transfer payment from the Chinese Snake Gourd project, 625 RMB of education poverty alleviation subsidies, 500 RMB of social assistance grants, and about 6000 RMB of minimum living guarantee, as well as the income from arable land transfer is 2000 RMB, so to sum it up, the annual income of the family is as high as 28,115 RMB, and the per capita income of the family is 14,057.5 RMB, successfully realizing the poverty reduction. Within

[5] Aka villagers' committee and the village's Party committee.–Trans.

3 years, according to the policy of "to get out of poverty, but will not be removed of the support policy", this family will keep the income level. And they will not only improve their lives, but also have some savings to provide guarantees for their future. After 3 years, even if the relevant welfare transfer payments for poverty-stricken households will be withdrawn, given the current age and health condition of Bi Weiping, she will continue to work in Chinese Snake Gourd farmland or other village collective industries to maintain this level of income for 5 years, and after 5 years her granddaughter will grow up and the family will enter a virtuous cycle to achieve long-term poverty reduction. During the interview, Bi Weiping, this old woman with eyes full of tears, excitedly told us, "Thanks to the Communist Party and the secretary, I never thought I could have such a good life today". In fact, there are many cases of getting out of poverty in the similar ways in Wangma Village.

In Wangma Village, poverty-stricken households are mainly the elderly people living alone who have lost their working ability and families who are poor due to diseases and disability. It is difficult to achieve lasting poverty reduction through existing welfare transfer payments, and in the long run, industrial development bringing about endogenous growth mechanism is the long-term mechanism for poverty alleviation. It is the industrial development that brings employment opportunities and enhances the transfer capacity of the collective economy of the village to poverty-stricken households, while poverty-stricken households can activate their land assets and bring lasting income. With the gradual removal of poverty-stricken households with working ability, the number of poverty-stricken households that the village collective needs to support will gradually decrease, and the per capita village collective transfer payments received by poverty-stricken households will rise, and their living conditions will further improve, truly realizing that the first grew rich will lead the others to wealth together and sharing the fruits of the village collective economic development.

3.3 Problems Encountered in the Process of Poverty Alleviation in Wangma Village[6]

In the more economically developed eastern regions like Jiangsu Province, there is no worry about various related subsidies from the higher levels in winning the fight against poverty; in addition to the financial subsidies from the central government, the local government can also provide a lot of financial subsidies. In the rural areas of northern Jiangsu Province, represented by Wangma Village, from 2016 to now, after five years of poverty alleviation, the low-income peasant households among the officially registered poverty-stricken households have gained real benefits: as the last safety net, the rural minimum living guarantee has been expanded to cover all eligible low-income peasant families, so that they can be insured as much as possible.

[6] Obtained through an interview with Lu Kexiang, deputy town mayor in charge of poverty alleviation in Xuliu town.

For adults with severe disabilities who lead difficult lives, depend on family support, and still cannot establish a separate household, they can be included in the scope of minimum living guarantee as a single-person household upon individual application. The number of households participating in pension insurance in Wangma Village in 2016 was about 200, involving about 300 people, with a low participation rate; 49 households enjoyed the minimum living guarantee policy, and 20 people were provided for by the five guarantees. In addition, both the elderly aged 60 and above and those aged 70 and above, in 2016, will receive the unified pension subsidies from the government. In 2016, the village received a total of 256,000 RMB of state aid funds, which were distributed by the town as the minimum living guarantee for the low-income households enjoying minimum living guarantee, and the living allowance and support for the households enjoying the five guarantees; all of the officially registered poverty-stricken households were included in the new rural cooperative medical care system. In 2017, the due part that should be paid by the poverty-stricken households of Wangma Village was paid by the town. Under the unified planning, the participation rate of pension insurance began to rise, and in 2019, it made the basic realization of "new rural cooperative medical care, new rural insurance, and full coverage". Since 2017, Huaiyin District has set up a "first get treatment and then make payment" policy for the low-income population in the whole district; since 2018, the supposed individual contribution to the new rural cooperative medical care is actually paid by the Huaiyin District government through financial expenditure. In terms of poverty alleviation in education, Huaiyin District subsidizes at respective levels the schooling of children from officially registered poverty-stricken households in the district, from kindergarten kids to university students: 500 RMB for every student per semester at kindergarten and elementary school, 625 RMB at middle school, 500–1000 RMB at high school (differentiated by low-income levels), and 1000 RMB for vocational high school. And one-time subsidies for enrollment in public universities or colleges are given as follows: 2000 RMB for college students and 4000 RMB for undergraduates. Plus, children from the low-income households are given subsidies of 750 RMB and 1000 RMB at the elementary and middle school levels to cut off the intergenerational transmission of poverty in education.

The fight against poverty has increased the income of the low-income population, expanded social demand, and alleviated social conflicts caused by the excessive gap between the rich and the poor. One of the relatively prominent problems in the process of poverty alleviation in Wangma Village is, without bogus case of poverty reduction, there is a risk of poverty reduction by making up numbers, because the poverty reduction line is set at an annual per capita income of more than 6000 RMB. Governments at various levels attempt to increase peasants' income and help them to get out of poverty, but there is still a lack in poverty alleviation measures such as "reducing the poverty itself by helping the poor's spirit and giving intellectual support", which are mainly reflected in the following three aspects.

3.3.1 Low Acceptance Percentage of Poverty Reduction

A large number of the low-income population have been included as officially registered poverty-stricken households with the national preferential policies, but their acceptance of the policies is not as high as we think, and the percentage of acceptance of poverty reduction realities from those who have already have been lifted out of poverty is 60% to 70%. This is because those peasants consider themselves to have enjoyed less social security than they should do, and they would rather show that they are still living in difficulty in the hope that these poverty alleviation policies will continue and they will receive greater social security. For example, a district leader had just visited a poor household and expressed sympathy to them at the Mid-Autumn Festival, and when the town leader paid a revisit to ask them if anyone had come to visit them, the household would answer: no one came, no one ever came, and the new quilt presented by the district leader was put on the bed. Although there is a policy "to get out of poverty, but will not be removed of the support policy", that is, the poor households will continue to enjoy the policy of poverty alleviation after "removing the poverty tag", due to the distrust between cadres and the masses accumulated over the years, some poor households do not believe in the continuity of the policy and do not accept the work of poverty alleviation.

3.3.2 Inadequate Understanding of Poverty Alleviation Policies

The reason why many low-income households become the bottom of society is largely due to their obvious physical or mental disadvantages, e.g., they have difficulties in understanding the policies, even though they enjoy many poverty alleviation policies, but they "don't know" and "can't say too much" about the policies they enjoy. They attach more importance to intuitive help, such as the gifts brought by the poverty support cadres at the Mid-Autumn Festival, to which they pay more attention and forget the alleviation measures in education and health care which bring more benefits to them in reality. And the money sent to their bank account is more like abstract numbers to them, which is not as intuitive as giving cash directly, but the current financial system is not permitted to subsidize them in cash directly. Therefore, to solve this problem, we need to make more efforts in publication and explanation of the poverty alleviation policies clearly to them, so that they can accept the policies and work of poverty alleviation and thus resolve the distrust between cadres of village and township and the peasants.

3.3.3 Poverty-Stricken Households Are not Motivated to Get Out of Poverty

After the poverty alleviation industrial project is implemented, according to the requirements of the poverty alleviation office of Jiangsu Province, more than 50% of the project income will be allocated as dividends to the officially registered poverty-stricken households, and each household can get more than 2000 RMB on average. But this time the villager's committee is worried that some poor households will not go to work for the poverty alleviation project after getting the dividends, and will not come back to continue working until they spend all the money. In terms of poverty alleviation through employment, when employment training is provided to the officially registered poverty-stricken households, the focus of work review is on the number of poor households to be trained, but the employment rate after the training is rarely included in the poverty alleviation work review. At the government level, it spends a lot on employment training, and the officially registered poverty-stricken households who get trained will receive a daily subsidy of 50 RMB during the employment training, and the result of training is not satisfactory. It is not only the lack of vocational relevance of the training content, but also to a large extent, the poor households are not highly motivated to get out of poverty. Therefore, it is necessary to establish a long-term mechanism for poverty alleviation in which we need to find ways to change the mindset of poor households, which is the most difficult problem encountered in the process of poverty alleviation, and is also the most worthy of brainwork.

3.4 The Successful Experience of Poverty Alleviation Process in Wangma Village

In order to solve the above-mentioned problems in the fight against poverty, Wangma Village and the Government of Xuliu Town have explored a series of relatively successful experiences and practices.

3.4.1 Poverty Alleviation Projects as Pillars to Enhance the Sense of Gain of Poor Households

Through agricultural projects, industrial projects, and fixed asset investment projects, poor households can get a relatively sustainable and stable income and receive real benefits. Since 2017, Wangma Village has focused on developing the Chinese Snake Gourd project, which is an industrial prosperity project invested by the Municipal Bureau of Agriculture and Rural Development. The reason for choosing to plant

Chinese Snake Gourd is that when the secretary of the village's CPC[7] Party branch from the neighboring village of Wangma Village was visiting the Chinese herbal medicine market in Bozhou, Anhui Province, he heard about this Chinese Snake Gourd project and came back to plant it on a trial basis, and it turned out to be very good benefits. As an economically weak village, Wangma Village got the investment of the industrial prosperity project from the Municipal Bureau of Agriculture and Rural Development, and in 2016, when the Chinese Snake Gourd project was officially launched, the first phase of the Chinese Snake Gourd project was implemented with the help of the Municipal Party Committee's Department of Agriculture and Industry, which transferred 140 mu of village land. Based on the successful experience of the first phase of the Chinese Snake Gourd project, it enjoyed a good harvest in 2017, and brought about the income increase of 150,000 RMB for the village collective. The second phase was developed with the strong support of the government of Huaiyin District and Xuliu Town. The project received a financial investment of 1.2 million RMB, and established the base of Chinese Snake Gourd, which covered 254 mu. The Chinese Snake Gourd project is entrusted by the village collective to carry out daily operation and management, and after deducting the operating costs, all the proceeds belong to the village collective and allocated by the village collective. 50% of the proceeds will go into the collective economic account as collective development funds, and the other 50% are distributed directly by Wangma Village according to the poverty-stricken population as poverty alleviation funds. In 2018, the second phase of this project yielded 110,000 RMB additional income, among which 55,000 RMB was collective account funds, and the other 55,000 RMB was equally distributed by the poverty-stricken households members either in cash or to their bank accounts, and the remaining funds were carried forward to the next distribution. The Chinese Snake Gourd project not only strengthens the collective economy and directly increases the village collective's drive to pull the poverty-stricken households out of poverty, but also provides low-income households with more opportunities to reduce poverty by providing work opportunities and rental income from land transfer. In 2018, the project drove 9 low-income households to realize rental income from land transfer amounting to 34,239 RMB, and provided employment opportunities for 17 low-income households to realize labor income of 10,730 RMB. In 2019, the Chinese Snake Gourd project further expanded its scale and enhanced the employment drive for Wangma Village, adding 60–70 people employed in this village, including 14 people from poverty-stricken households, and bringing an average of 10,000 RMB/year of labor income to participating poor households based on a calculation of daily income of 60 RMB.

In combination of the development of poverty alleviation projects with the development of the village collective economy, it strives to increase the collective income of the village, and spends 60% of the new financial resources of the village collective economic income on people's livelihood. Take the neighboring village, Hongbei Village, as an example, by using the dividends of the imported enterprises, it increases

[7] Aka Communist Party of China – Trans.

the village collective income, and by using the collective income to cover the self-payment cost of participating the villagers' cooperative medical care services, it will eliminate the risks of poverty caused by getting diseases. The villagers have a strong sense of gain in comparison with the surrounding villages and get motivated in developing the village collective economy.

3.4.2 Industrial Projects and Fixed Asset Investment to Supplement Agriculture Projects

Since only the Chinese Snake Gourd project was developed in the early years, the collective economic income source of Wangma Village is still relatively limited. Moreover, the upstream and downstream of the Chinese Snake Gourd industry are controlled by other places, and both ends are out of reach of Wangma Village. The seedlings of Chinese Snake Gourd are monopolized by large households in Anhui seedling market, which control the pricing right of Chinese Snake Gourd seedlings. After the harvest, it is those people who sell the seedlings that purchase the Gourds. Wangma Village is just in charge of the plantation, which leads to the limited profitability. In order to obtain higher income from the Chinese Snake Gourd project, it is necessary to carry out deep processing, but the members of the "two committees" of Wangma Village are relatively old aged, with five members of the Party committee over 60 years old, one member between 50 and 60 years old, three members between 40 and 50 years old, and one member between 30 and 40 years old, which is an old-age structure. Excluding the overlapping candidates of cross-appointment, there are 3 members of the villager's committee over 60 years old, 1 person who is 50–60 years old, 2 people who are 40–50 years old, and 1 person who is 30–40 years old. Plus, the cultural quality of the members of the two villager's committees is relatively low. In terms of the education background, most of them just received high school and even lower education. In terms of the social status, only one is a physician, and the rest are peasants, lacking professional personnel. In addition to the limited talents in the village, limited technology, limited ideas, young people are not willing to contribute intelligence and energy to the development of the village, and the age structure brings rigidity of thinking and the slow acceptance of new things, which cannot keep up with the requirements of the development of the times, and it is difficult to develop the deep processing of Chinese Snake Gourd. In the supplementary investigation and research conducted in April 2019, it found that, after 2 years, the list of the "two committees" of Wangma Village did not change, and the average age accordingly increased by 2 years. In the conversation with the secretary of the village's Communist Party branch, Secretary Ni also expressed his concern. As the income of village cadres is very low, young people do not want to be a village cadre. Although the older ones have the will to work, they lack the ability to work and the attitude of acceptance of new things, resulting in his shouldering the whole village's working pressure alone, and his own health also had problems caused by the pressure in the past few years. This shows that the village cadres of Wangma Village are and will be still facing this problem in the foreseeable future. In view of this, the Xuliu town is actively selecting reserve cadres for poverty-stricken villages, and selecting young people as reserve candidates for village cadres who have certain cultural quality and are willing to be rooted in the countryside to provide services for peasants. But the training of reserve cadres is not done overnight. For the Wangma Village, the development of agricultural projects in the absence of talents involves certain risks, such as the development of vegetable greenhouse project through land transfer failed, because the contractor of the vegetable greenhouse is an amateur, and spoiled the greenhouse facilities and soil, and it turned out to be a business failure and the contractor became a deadbeat. Therefore, in order to reduce the risk from business operation of agricultural projects, the Wangma Village and the Xuliu town changed the way of thinking and tried to help fight poverty through industrial projects and investment in fixed assets. Industrial land is used in the town to build small industrial projects, and the proceeds from these industrial projects will be used as a stable source of income for poverty-stricken households, which has in fact achieved relatively good results. Xuliu town built three photovoltaic projects on the roofs of factory buildings of industrial enterprises in 2019, and those enterprises equipped with photovoltaic panels have priority to use the electricity generated by photovoltaic systems. For enterprises, photovoltaic projects reduce the original electricity cost of 1.13 RMB/unit to 0.70 RMB; for the village, there is income of 0.20 ~ 0.30 RMB/unit which is sustainable as the life of power generation of photovoltaic panels is 20 years, so that the village can yield about 100,000 RMB of electricity revenue in a stable way from industrial enterprises every year.

In addition to industrial projects, Xuliu town also invested in fixed assets, and use the asset income to drive the poverty alleviation. Led by the Poverty Alleviation Office, in coordination with the Bureau of Finance, the Department of Agriculture and Industry, the Bureau of Agricultural Machinery, Supply and Marketing Cooperatives among other departments, a comprehensive cleanup and mapping work of all the assets owned by the town collectives is conducted, and all the factory buildings, storefronts, etc., constructed or purchased by special financial funds are for lease. At least 50% of the rental income generated are used for low-income households in distribution; the assets in form of investment in facilities for agriculture, breeding industries, photovoltaic industry, agricultural machinery, rural tourism among other projects can be quantified as shares and the dividends of these shares will be given to economically weak villages and low-income peasants, especially those who lost their working capacity, so as to establish and improve the income distribution mechanism to ensure that the income from assets is returned to the low-income peasants who hold shares in a timely manner; support peasants' cooperatives and other business entities to drive low-income peasants to increase their income and get rid of poverty through land trusteeship by converting peasants' land management rights into shares; etc. Take Huaiyin District's City Celebrity Hotel project as an example, through the purchase of the hotel rooms (more than 500,000 RMB per room), the annual dividends of one room are paid more than 30,000 RMB, the village that bought the most rooms has purchased five hotel rooms, so in a year it can earn more than 100,000 RMB. The six villages of Xuliu town bought enterprise plants in Huaiyin's high-tech zone, and those plants also generate a lot of annual rental income. Xuliu town also invested in two pilot projects, including the Hujiang pastoral business, whose investments are in shares, and it does not participate in the operation, but only buy pig sheds which are leased to large households, and the annual income is 210,000 RMB; in Zhihe's duck factory, they bought three duck houses for 1.05 million RMB, left alone the facilities and equipment in duck houses, and only bought assets fixed on the land, and the annual rental income is 120,000 RMB. Compared with agricultural planting projects, the income of such fixed assets projects is more stable.

References

[India] Amartya, S. (2002). Looking at Development with Freedom, translated by Ren Ze and Yu Zhen. People's University of China Press (2002)

Tan, X., Luan, J., Shi, H., et al. (2019). Targeted Poverty Reduction and Alleviation in 100 Villages - Yongshun Village Volume. Social Sciences Academic Press (China)

Tang, X., Liu, C., et al. (2013). How Xiaokeng is Made—A Survey of Xiaokeng Village in Anhui Province. Social Sciences Academic Press (China) (2013)

Luo, X. (2019). Improving the System of Resident Cadres to Help Promote Rural Revitalization. *Journal of China Agricultural University (Social Science Edition)*, No. 3.

Hu, L., & Sun, Y. S. (2011). A Review of Research on the Formation Mechanism of Poverty. *Ecological Economics*, No. 11.

Wang, G., Zhang, N., & Yang, Y. (2017). Poverty Vulnerability Deconstruction and Precise Poverty Eradication System Reconstruction—Based on Western Rural Areas. Social Science Research, No. 5.

Haijun Xu, an associate professor at the business school of Jiangnan University, whose main research interests are agricultural economic management and multinational corporation.

Zongshuai Zhang, a PhD candidate at the University of Chinese Academy of Social Sciences, whose main research interest is rural society and regional culture.

Yanmei Dong, a 2017 enrolled finance student at the business school of Jiangnan University, whose research interest is rural finance.

Chapter 4
Understanding the Village by Tea Leaves: Community Governance is also Productivity—Case Study of Poverty Alleviation in Organic Tea Industry in Jinlongping Village, Hubei Province

Fang Lv

Abstract Based on field observations and in-depth interviews, this paper attempts to tell a story about the "co-change" of agricultural industry development and poverty-stricken rural communities. Unlike the knowledge landscape of existing studies on the social basis of rural industrial development, industrial development in rural area, and the polarization of community, the case of Jinlongping Village organic tea industry poverty alleviation project reveals that the community, as the main body of action, can effectively use national policy support and market resources to realize the industrial development in the community. At the same time, the changes in the village "for development" and the results of "development" have a complex impact in shaping community organization, community governance, and community culture.

Keywords Community governance · Countryside industry · Targeted poverty alleviation · Jinlongping Village

Hubei tea is, well known to the people, such as Enshi Yulu, Wufeng Maojian, Lichuan black tea and Wujiatai Gong Cha. Among them, Wujiatai Gong Chais named after the village, and has become a business card for the development of Xuan'en County industry. When I first arrived in Xuan'en, the local cadres gave me some introduction to this county.The agricultural industry development in Xuan'en County takes the decisive and well-considered steps, and they don't do much ado about nothing.Although the cadres at the county and town levels have been changed several times, the original aspiration to develop organic tea industry has never changed, which has been deeply pushing forward the product quality and industrial upgrading for decades. Especially within the years of targeted poverty alleviation, the county's tea industry developed rapidly, with planting area of 242,000 mu, tea production of

F. Lv (✉)
School of Social Sciences, Central China Normal University, Shanghai, China

Case Studies of Targeted Poverty Reduction and Alleviation in 100 Villages, International Research on Poverty Reduction, https://doi.org/10.1007/978-981-95-0549-4_4

1.71 tons, and the comprehensive output value reaching 1.76 billion yuan.Tea has become a pillar industry to drive the poor households out of poverty and increase their income. Among those tea industries, the tea industry in Wanzhai Town is the most successful, as Wujiatai Village belongs to Wanzhai Town. Through the brand building of Gong Cha, the town has gradually become the famous "Gong Cha town" in Hubei Province. At present, the total scale of tea plantations in the town exceeds 56,000 mu[1]with the per capita tea garden area of 1.8 mu, and there are more than 20 tea speciality villageswith 74 tea processing enterprises, including 8 enterprises above designated size and 2 enterprises with self-support export rights.[2] Undoubtedly, these industrial development fruits are not only certainly inseparable from the national policy support, but also benefit from the urban consumption revolution and industrial and commercial capital flowing to the countryside in recent years. However, if we look at the course, some questions will be asked like how do the specific villages "seize" the policy and market development opportunities? How can we promote the rapid rise of rural industries? What kind of changes did this course bring about to the villages? Based on the case of targeted poverty alleviation in the organic tea industry of Jinlongping Village in Xuan'en County, this paper will try to understand the "village" by the "leaves" and provide a possible answer to these questions.

4.1 Prelude: The Change of Industry in Jinlongping

Jinlongping Village, which belongs to Wanzhai Township, Xuan'en County, Enshi Prefecture, Hubei Province, is located in the hinterland of the Wuling Mountains and is a typical poverty-stricken village deep in mountains. Before the targeted poverty alleviation, Jinlongping was one of the poorest villages, and the agricultural production was dominated by traditional grain crops, but there were seldom large-scale industries. To work outside is the livelihood choice for the majority of families.If the family labor has some professional skills to do carpenter and renovation work, the family will lead a well-off life, so most of the young and healthy villagers choose to leave their hometowns to work in Fujian province and Zhejiang Province. As most villages in Wanzhai Township made rich through the development of organic tea, why Jinlongping Villagecould not catch the "express train" of the development of organic tea just as other villages did in the township? And it is quite surprising that Jinlongping Village is the earliest local village to develop organic tea.In other words, the local organic tea industry with a great success was originated in Jinlongping.

In contrast, targeted poverty alleviation has brought the noteworthy changes toJinlongping Village over the past few years. Not only have the established goals of "Two

[1] 1 mu equals 1/15 hectare. –Trans.

[2] Based on the interview materials collected in Wanzhai Township, Xuan'en County, April 26, 2017.

Assurances and Three Guarantees"[3] for poverty alleviation been fully realized, but also the infrastructure of the village has been significantly improved, and the tea industry has gradually scaled up, with nearly 2,000 mu[4] of tea gardens in the village as of the end of 2019, realizing nearly 2 mu per capita. And all of those tea gardens have passed the stringent organic tea garden certification, becoming a demonstration area of organic tea gardens in Wanzhai Township. Only in 2019, the enterprises of the village processed and produced more than 400,000 jin[5] of dried tea, achieving an output value worth more than 6 million yuan, with the village income of more than 12 million yuan from the fresh leaves. Under the order-based production cooperation with "Yusheng"Company, the tea merchants from all over the world come to visit the tea base of Jinlongping all the time, and the tea of Jinlongping is sold to all over the world, makingsuch a situation where the supply falls short of the demand. In 2019, the "Green Needle"tea produced by Jinlongping Tea Cooperative won the bronze medal as an International Organic and Fair Trade Food, and more than 90% of the "Green Needle" tea was exported to Europe. In particular, just in 2020, the Jinlongping Village also successfully introduced an ecological agricultural investment company that settled in the village and invested in the project of "Golden Dragon Valley Ecological Health Care". Now both sides have signed an investment contract, and it is expected to invest 200 million yuan.

Such a huge change in Jinlongping Village before and after the targeted poverty alleviation provides an excellent case for us to answer the questions raised above. On the one hand, we need to explain why before the targeted poverty alleviation, the development of Jinlongping Village was relatively lagging behind, unable to secure policy resources, unable to seize the opportunity to develop organic tea in the "first wave" of development. On the other hand, we will understand from the case of Jinlongping Village how the state intervention and the subject action of village reshaped the implementation path of policy and industry in the countryside during the period of targeted poverty alleviation, what changes prompted Jinlongping Village to enter the "fast lane" of development, and what knowledge logic this change reveals.

---

[3] The Two Assurances and Three Guarantees refer to assurances of adequate food and clothing, and guarantees of access to compulsory education, basic medical services and safe housing for impoverished rural residents. –Trans.

[4] 1 mu equals 1/15 hectare. –Trans.

[5] 1 jin equals about one and a half pounds. –Trans.

4.2 "Get up Early Morning to Catch up with a Late Show"

At the house of Gong Jiagang, the former CPC[6] branch secretary of Jinlongping Village, the research team met the boss of Yusheng Company, Mr. Bian, who came to the village to investigate the tea garden. And the Yusheng Company is the China-based institution of World Fair Trade Organization.[7] The organic tea industry in Xuan'en County originated from several organic tea projects carried out by Yusheng in 2003. Having been observing and investigating the tea industry in Xuan'en for a long time, I heard a lot about Mr. Bian. I began to chat with him about the hearth of the secretary Gong's home. Mr. Bian and the secretary Gong are long-time friends, so Mr. Bian went to secretary Gong's home to show his cooking skills, and after a brief introduction I sat in front of the hearth to add firewood while chatting with him. Mr. Bian told me that as early as in 2003, Yusheng Company came to Wanzhai Town and took the lead in cooperating with Gong Jiagang, who was then the secretary of the village's CPC Party branch, and mobilized villagers to plant organic tea. At the same time,there were also projects carried out in Wujiatai, Ma'anshan, and several other villages, but compared with Wujiatai and Ma'anshan, Jinlongping's development has been lagging behind, only in recent years Jinlongping Village organic tea industry has been gradually growing stronger. The earliest to start, but the last to develop, could be considered to be "get up early morning to catch up with a late show". As Secretary Gong introduced, having seen the Wujiatai organic tea making a fortune, the villagers were eager to develop this industry, but it has not been successful. I then asked the reason, Secretary Gong just said that the infrastructure conditions in the village were poor at that time, etc., but he did not want to say more about it. So to find the real answer to this question became an important question that we are aware of in our research activities.

During the research, the county, township, village cadres, and villagers mostly expressed concern about the limitation brought about by transportation problems, and some cadres and villagers even believed that as long as the road is built, the foundation of village development will be good enough to make rich which comes naturally. Of course, this understanding carries with quite limitations, but it does reflect the biggest dilemma of the poverty-stricken villages in the deep mountains. Especially the words of the township cadres brought a deep touch to the research group.

---

[6] Aka Communist Party of China – Trans.

[7] The so-called fair trade is an important form of social and economic movement that started in the 1940s and has been developing into a dominant project model since the 1960s in the participation of international organizations in economic justice initiatives. The "Fair Trade" movement emphasizes the need to reshape the existing global agricultural trade system, especially the dismantling of the complex supply chain, so that the end sellers and consumers can establish more direct links with smallholder peasants who engaged in agricultural production, thus expanding the benefits of smallholder peasants' production and business activities to support community economic development on the one hand, and it provides consumers with more safe and high-quality agricultural products on the other hand. Over the past few decades, fair trade products have covered a wide range of categories such as coffee, bananas, cocoa, and tea among other things.

Road, for our mountainous villages, is the most important thing. It was probably in 1998, during the national poverty alleviation program (the seven-year program to help 80 million people out of poverty), Jinlongping Village only built a township road to the village, yet this road has not been completely concreted, so when it is a sunny day, you will get a lot of dust; when it is a rainy day, get two feet of mud, which belongs to the typical "three choice road"[8] *. In the past, whenever we went to the village, village cadres and villagers would raise the issue of road repair. But we can't make a commitment*[9] *, we can only say that we will definitely reflect it to the county for support. (Why is it important to build roads? --Interviewer asks)*

Let's say, in the past, the village farmers raised pigs. When it is time to sell, due to inconvenient roads, it is often needed to ask for a few helpers to carry the pigs to the township fair, and the selling proceeds are not even enough to hire people. Of course, we are also helping each other, but if you think about it, the road is broke that naturally limits the production. The development of tea is located deeply inside the village, and the road for machinery vehicles is paved many years ago, where agricultural vehicles cannot enter, so the production costs are much higher, because all rely on the labors' shoulder to carry. Even if the bosses from outside like this place (natural base for the development of tea industry is good - from author's note), but they are not willing to come to invest. In addition, the available money given by the county is also very limited, so it is natural to weigh the cost-effectiveness of development, so the project construction with low-cost and quick result in some villages will be prioritized. Deep mountain villages like Jinlongping, the construction costs are too high, and the small scale of financial funds finds it very limited to solve the problems in Jinlongping.

–Source: 20171205WZXZYL Interview.

It can be said that due to its remote location, Jinlongping Village has high production costs and many living inconveniences there. Due to its geographical location, Jinlongping Village is also in a marginal position in the development map of the whole township and county. Before the targeted poverty alleviation, although the state continued to increase the investment in the field of agricultural and rural work, the total amount of resources was still very limited compared to the huge demand. How to allocate the limited resources has become one of the core issues of the county development system. What is certain is that it is difficult for such poverty-stricken villages in deep mountains like Jinlongping to enjoy policy dividends. The reason is that local governments tend to invest limited resources in those villages with "better foundation" and "low construction costs and quick results", which not only can highlight political achievements, but also, in the words of local cadres, can also "serve as a model for other villages".[10] The complexity is that, also due to the "geographical

[8] It refers to the pick of weather, vehicle, and driver. Specifically, "pick the weather" means the need for sunny days to traffic, "pick a car" demands not a large car, nor a small car, but the car's chassis height must be high enough, "pick a driver" means the driver must be familiar with the road conditions.

[9] After the tax reform, the financial strength at the township level has declined significantly, especially in the central and western regions where township finances are often in a state of running empty and basically unable to arrange for public construction, and the administrative power of rural road construction has been incorporated into the county-level unified planning and overall arrangements accordingly.

[10] Lv Fang: "Analysis of Governance Context: Local Government Behavior under Risk Constraints: A Case Study of "Complaint" in Wuling City Poverty Alleviation Office, Sociological Studies, No. 2, 2013.

marginality", coupled with the difficulty of enjoying the sun and rain from policy support, villages such as Jinlongping, even with resource endowment, but in the eyes of capitalists there is still a lack of "potential", and thusit is difficult to attract bosses to invest.

More meaningfully, our research on Jinlongping Village revealed that the marginality of the location has an impact on community governance itself. In the past, Jinlongping Village was considered a "problem village" in the local area, and the relationship between the cadres and the people was occasionally tense, the prestige and cohesion of the "two committees" of the village were not good enough, and there were often petitions from the villagers. In our inquiry, we found that the so-called conflict is not how the village cadres are preferential to friends and relatives, nor to make unfair treatment, but originated from "misunderstanding", and this misunderstanding is also somewhat related to "a remote location".

> *In fact, you say that such things like infringements of the interests of farmers or what cadres do bad things, are not existed. To be precise, it is inconvenient for the people to do things, then they will think that the village cadres make things difficult. For example, the county education bureau wants to deliver education subsidies for children of poverty-stricken families in need, and thus there is a need to fill out some forms. After the village and the township review those forms and then report to the county. Previously, the transportation was difficult, and it took a whole day to shuttle between the township and the village. If a villager want to declare subsidies, he will have to cancel other things. If you could not complete the materials or forget something after getting to the township, it will be a wasted trip. Over and over again, in order to apply for two or three hundred yuan of subsidies, going to and from township many trips, the villagers would rather believe that the village cadres intentionally made it difficult, while village cadres also felt very wronged. In recent years, the village service construction has changed a lot, and this situation is very rare to see.*
>
> –Source: 20171205WZXZYL Interview.

Most of the things around the people seem to be very trivial and not a big deal, but it is these matters that affect people's views on national policies, and even more the views on village cadres and "two committees" in the village. In "remote villages", the village-level service positions lag behind in construction, which causes the villagers more inconveniences, and furthermore, adverse effects. It is often the villagers who cannot understand the specific reasons, and thus gradually turned into the distrust of village cadres and the village "two committees". In particular, this distrust is somewhat of a "Tacitus trap", which can sharpen the problematic orientation when it comes to conflicts and cause further weakening of community unity. Jinlongping was once known as a local "problem village" because several villagers had problems with the former village cadres and kept petitioning. The petitions were largely the result of an escalating sense of distrust and misunderstanding. The complexity is that when Jinlongping is considered a "problem village", its "marginality" is exacerbated. Both for the county and township governments and for enterprises that wish to go to the countryside, they tend not to deal with "problem villages". Director Chang, who was previously the branch secretary in the village of Jinlongping and later passed through the civil service examination to work in the township, sentimentally said, "infrastructure construction projects, as long as the people support, then it is not a problem for a village to spend 4 million yuan, 5 million yuan. However, if you could not make a mass work to support, such as road project, and the work cannot be done, and thus not a penny".[11]

It is not difficult to find that the reason why the industrial development of Jinlongping Village is "to get up early but to catch up with a late show". To a large extent, it is constrained by the remote location and weak infrastructure, from the generative "process perspective", Jinlongping Village "missed" development opportunities because of "marginalities multiplier effect". In other words, the remoteness of the village in terms of geographic location brings marginality in the development system of county and township, and determines the lack of attractiveness of the village to external capital. Also, the problems multiplied with organization construction and community unity further increase the marginalities. If we agree with the above explanation, it is not difficult to find out that the dramatic changes brought by targeted poverty alleviation to Jinlongping Village cannot be understood as the only answer from the single dimension of increased policy input from the state. In the following, we will take the case of Jinlongping Village to illustrate that targeted poverty alleviation can be called a "community governance revolution", and that the standardization of community power exercise, closer relations between the Party, cadres and ordinary people, and a positive community culture are not only the results of targeted poverty alleviation, but also the changes that have helped Jinlongping Village seize a new round of development opportunities and drive the development of the village. It is also these changes that helped Jinlongping Village to seize a new round of development opportunities and drive the policies and capital in rural areas.

4.3 To Make the Organic Tea Industry Work

After seeing other villages of the same township successively make rich themselves in the development of organic tea, the villagers' desire to develop organic tea industry is even stronger in Jinlongping Village. During the targeted poverty alleviation, the Party committee and government at county and township level, the resident work team and the village "two committees" determined that the tea industry in Jinlongping must be developed. However, there were at least two levels of problems to be solved in developing the organic tea industry. One is to solve the infrastructure bottlenecks of industrial development, in order to form a relatively complete industrial chain; the second is the need for all the villagers to follow the organic standards of agricultural production.

In terms of the required economic infrastructure and technical conditions, the development of the industry mainly includes the renovation of industrial roads and power grid, the tea factory construction, genetic improvement, technical training and several other aspects. Relatively speaking, power grid renovation, genetic improvement, technical training and several other worksare easier to carry out, while the renovation of industrial roads is necessarily involved in striving for government resources

[11] Based on interview data from Jinlongping Village.

and negotiation with the relevant villagers to occupy part of their land. During the poverty alleviation period, the state concentrated on ensuring poverty alleviation inputs, the money problem is relatively easy to solve, but the involving coordination with the people needs more efforts. Also, organic tea planting is different from other industries, which is the need for a concentrated and contiguous development, that is, all peasants in the village cannot use chemical fertilizers and pesticides in agricultural production, but have to use the organic fertilizers and ecological pesticide and weed control methods in replacement. As you can imagine, these tasks require the understanding and cooperation of the villagers, therefore, the primary challenge in front of the poverty alleviation cadres is to improve the villagers' attitude toward the village cadres, village "two committees", and then to mobilize villagers to participate and support the relevant work.

In fact, in the first one or two years after the start of targeted poverty alleviation, the situation inside the village still did not change significantly. The main reason was that the poverty alleviation cadres did not understand enough about the work of "build a profile and create a card" at that time, and thought that it was just a simple work in the previous way, just reporting a form and filling in the data. In addition, due to the policy design itself, the accuracy of the first round of targeted "profile and card" work in 2014 was not high, and there were even some "mistaken poverty identity households". Villagers were also quite disapproving of this.On the one hand, it took several times to fill in the information, which bothered villagers; on the other hand, the identification results were not objective and accurate to villagers. After several rounds of "retrospective re-examination" upon targeted poverty alleviation, there were still some problems. After the 2015 Central Conference on Poverty Alleviation and Development, the top-level design of the country's targeted poverty alleviation campaign became gradually clearer, Party committees and governments at all levels took the poverty alleviation as the first people's livelihood project to promote the fight against poverty. Among all the work, it becomes the primary work to do a good job of data verification and improve the quality of data of the "profile and card". With big data comparison, household visits and "negative list" system among other measures, Jinlongping Village invalidated the previous "mistaken poverty identity households", and the village "two committees" and the resident work team adhered to the work standards and procedures to achieve fairness and openness in the "retrospective re-examination" and "dynamic adjustment" work. In addition to self-correction and self-inspection of "wrong assessment" and "missing assessment", the village "two committees" and the resident work team also took the investigation of poverty causes and development aspirations as an important task. The process of completing this work, in the words from someone in the work teamof the village, is to visit people very often, so as to make the people trust you, in a way of talking to them and helping them solve their problems. Originally, the standard was not clear, and the work was done carelessly, coupled with repeated form filling, villagers have some misunderstanding and resistance. But it proved later that as long as we carry out the practical and careful work, pay attention to the difficulties and needs of the people, and sincerely help to solve the problem, the people will welcome us.In a substantive work, Cadres will psychologically have a sense of gain too. Doing a good job for "officially registered poverty-stricken households".For Jinlongping, is not only the completion of the "routine practices" of targeted poverty alleviation.More importantly, the villagers gradually enhance the sense of trust and affection for the village cadres and the resident work team. It can be said that this process has completed the first step of the "community governance revolution" in Jinlongping Village, and its direct results are reflected in better communication and it is more convenient to handle affairs in the village.

With the strong support of the county and township Party committees and governments, the village "two committees" and the resident work team actively mobilize resources in all aspects to carry out the village-level targeted poverty alleviation plan step by step. In terms of infrastructure, Jinlongping has secured more than 8 million yuan of funds from the electric power department and has been equipped with 7 transformers, which has significantly improved the power supply situation in the village and provided the basic conditions for local processing of tea leaves. Many farmers purchased tea dryers, kneading machines, and other equipment to earn part of the income from tea processing. With the processing capacity, there is no need to rush to sell fresh tea leaves in a short period of time, but it can wait for a higher price to sell after rough processing. All the roads of the 12 villagers' groups in the village are paved with concrete, which has greatly enhanced the convenience of production. In the meantime, a tea-specialized cooperative was established in the village to produce organic tea in cooperation with Yusheng Company and most of the products can be sold to the international market. Technical training, variety improvement, and quality control of organic tea garden management have also gained the support and recognition of villagers. These are a few of the small things that the resident work team remembers.

> *When it comes to the village's industrial road (loop road to villager groups- the author's note), at first the village cadres and the resident work team felt it difficult to implement. It is not easy to do the work when it comes to occupying people's arable land because the income from growing grain is not high. But the work time requirements are there, so we have to figure out a solution. Therefore, as we agreed through discussion, to promote the household joint consultation, that is, we build the road to somewhere, and then the farmers involved will decide the implementation in their own negotiation. As long as a consensus is reached, we will start to build the road. In this way, the villagers will also have pressure, as they will feel that the road is built elsewhere, and the road is not built here due to my situation. The village poverty alleviation cadres were surprised that the road project progressed very smoothly. The village did not have compensation funds, and the villagers did not have any objections, and even some villagers also took the lead in proposing that the project could occupy their land as much as it needed. This really makes us very moved.*
>
> *--Source: 20181107JLPMSJ Interview*

Perhaps the saying of the cadres in the village was an understatement. But in our visits to farmers, the "hearts" of cadres and people are indeed closer than before during the period of targeted poverty alleviation. To make the agricultural industry work, such as infrastructure investment, fine seed promotion, and technical services, all cannot be separated from government support, but to make these resources successfully go to the "countryside", it obviously needs the cooperation of the village and villagers. In this regard, if it was said that the local government tended to choose those villages with "good foundation" in the process of allocating limited resources before targeted poverty alleviation, then in the stage of targeted poverty alleviation, in order to make each poor village get out of poverty, a "community governance revolution" is inevitably required. As a matter of fact, this "revolution" of community governance has brought great changes to Jinlongping Village. Organic tea production requires the establishment of a strict quality control system.In particular, all agricultural production in the village is required to be organized in accordance with organic standards. In order to realize the goal of "transforming paddy to dry land", the cadres of the village"two committees" and the resident work team worked patiently and meticulously. There is a family in the village whose children have been working outside for a long time, and their income is quite good.Only the elderlyare left at home, who were more accustomed to planting rice, corn, and potatoes. In view of this, the village cadres repeatedly visited the elderly, telling them that food rations were guaranteed, and that if they were not willing to farm and manage, they can hand over the land to the cooperative, which will hire someone to manage it. And, in addition to the rent for the land shares (transfer), part of the proceeds from the planting and management will also go to the elderly. Village cadres often chattedwith the elderly, and brought with them some small gifts. They patiently explained why the village must "transform paddy to dry land", which gradually won the support of the elderly. There are also some families, who were hesitant to develop organic tea, then the supporting cadres found ways together with them to develop some other industries, such as the establishment of a specialized beekeeping cooperative,which drove some of the farmers who were not very enthusiastic about growing tea. It can be said that these "embroidery" efforts are not only the inherent requirements of the basic strategy of targeted poverty alleviation and targeted poverty alleviation, but also the emotional connection process in which the supporting cadres visit the farmers' homes, care for the things around farmers, and seek the poverty alleviation and development with farmers.

4.4 Community Governance is also Productive

In the process of targeted poverty alleviation, a lot of mass work is involved, and the people's recognition and satisfaction of the targeted poverty alleviation policy depend to a large extent on the cohesiveness and combat power of the village "two committees" and on the heart and soul of the poverty alleviation cadres. In this process, a "revolution" in community governance is realized at the village level, which helps them better seize development opportunities. Moreover, in the process of poverty alleviation, the "revolution" of community governance is still ongoing, with the prominent features emphasizing the need to regulate the operation of village-level power and to strengthen the cohesion and fighting power of grassroots Party organizations. In particular, the construction of village-level Party branch work and village-level rules of procedure, and the overall reshaping of the grassroots political ecology and the laws governing the operation of rural public affairs. These initiatives are a powerful guarantee to ensure the achievement of the goals of the targeted poverty alleviation campaign, and also lay a solid foundation to promote the modernization of the rural governance system and the enhancement of governance capacity. Through a series of intensive actions, the cohesion and combat power of the Party grassroots organizations have been significantly enhanced, forming a "militant bastion" leading the poverty reduction and development in rural communities, promoting community unity, reducing the transaction costs of external resources entering the countryside, and improving the performance of policy operation.

In accordance with the deployment of the province and the prefecture, Xuan'en County launched a series of actions to comprehensively strengthen the construction of grassroots Party organizations and regulate the operation of village-level power, with a set of "combination fists", including strengthening the village leadership by selecting and cultivating team members; implementation of the pioneering index of Party members with appraisal system; the consistent promotion of institutionalized, normalized, and programmed Party branch activities at grassroots level; and the implementation of work institutions of "Four Discussions and Two Openness"[12] and since the promulgation and implementation of the *CPC Work Rules on Rural Primary-level Organizations* in December 2018, the operation of village-level organizations has become more standardized and efficient. In the words of the cadres of the resident work team, the targeted poverty alleviation work has put forward higher requirements for village cadres' work:

> *We need to understand the difficulties and needs of poor households on a regular basis, and then bring these needs and problems to the meetings of the village "two committees", and if necessary, convene a meeting of Party representatives or a general meeting of Party members to discuss and decide some matters. In this way, if the usual work is not in place, the people's demands will not be responded to in a timely manner. Of course, when it comes to urgent matters, we also work on the principle that the interests of the people come first. For example, there was a house in the village caught on fire due to the aging electrical circuit. As you can see, our houses here are mainly wooden structures. When we went to the house, it was still burning with great cost. We immediately contacted the provincial salt company to coordinate funds to help this family to tide over the difficulties.*
>
> *– 20,171,202 Jin Long Ping Village Resident Team YYGSYB Interview*

To sum up, in the stage of targeted poverty alleviation, with regard to the implementation of the basic strategy of targeted poverty alleviation and targeted poverty eradication, the technical logic and protocol requirements of targeted poverty alleviation have brought fundamental changes to poverty alleviation work at the village level. The whole process of "file management" is significantly different from the previous "simple governance", and the degree of standardization and institutionalization of the behaviors of poverty alleviation cadres and village-level organizations is significantly enhanced. On the practical level, this "community governance revolution" is still ongoing and has shown its great significance. It is precisely in the

[12] The "four discussions" refer to the proposal of the village party branch, the discussion of the village "two committees", the deliberation of the party member congress, and the resolution of the villagers' representative meeting or the villagers' meeting; the "two openness" refer to the content of resolution and the results of the implementation must be open to all villagers.– Trans.

process of targeted poverty alleviation that the village organization, cadre-mass relationship, and community unity in Jinlongping Village have undergone great changes, enabling it to seize the policy and market opportunities to achieve poverty alleviation and sustainable development. Through the organic management of tea plantations, combined with livestock breeding, the "pig - swamp - tea" organic cycle ecological chain is formed, and the masses' income reaches to a new high through organic tea planting. Targeted poverty alleviation has brought great changes to the appearance of Jinlongping Village. Relying on the traditional Tujia architectural clusters and ancient trees, Jinlongping was successfully declared as a traditional Chinese village. In particular, this year has seen an ecological agricultural investment company successfully introduced to Jinlongping,and the development of the "Jinlong Valley Ecological Recreation" project. At present, an investment contract has been signed with an estimated investment of 200 million yuan. With the change of the village's development, many young people have returned to Jinlongping one after another, and the number of young people and children in the village has gradually increased. After Jinlongping got out of poverty, the work team did not leave, and continued to serve Jinlongping Village to consolidate the achievements of poverty alleviation and seize a new round of development opportunities. The tremendous changes have stayed in the heart of every villager in Jinlongping. At the annual Jinlongping "village spring festival gala", each family tells their story of poverty alleviation with great joy. The village holds brilliance selection activities (to vote for brilliance families, brilliance individuals, etc.), and selects and honors model people who have made great contributions to the development of the village and have gotten rich after poverty eradication, so that the people's sense of gain, satisfaction, and happiness in life is constantly increasing.

4.5 Conclusion

The case of Jinlongping Village is a microcosm of China's poverty eradication efforts. In the background of the era when large-scale policies going to the countryside and urban industrial and commercial capital going to the countryside provide a favorable environment for rural reform and development, how the village can seize the opportunity has become a question worth serious consideration. The intellectual value of the case of Jinlongping Village lies precisely in its reflection of the inner logic of the rural development system in the new era. In other words, if we admit that the policies and factors such as policies going to the countryside, capital going to the countryside, and finance going to the countryside have constituted a supportive system to promote the development of rural communities since the tax reform, then we can also see that a good state of "village governance" is the key to ensure that a village can seize the development opportunities and turn a good development environment into development achievements. For poor communities, improvement at the level of "village governance" can even be called a "first move" for development, and is one of the core elements of the community's endogenous dynamics.

References

Chen, Y. (2019). The Social Dilemma of Capital in the Countryside and Strategies to Solve it - Mobilization of Social Resources in Villages by Capital. *China Rural Economy, 8.*

Huang, Z. (2008). Centralized Parsimonious Governance—Semi-Formal Grassroots Administration with Para-Officials and Dispute Resolution in China. Open Times, No. 2, 2008.

Jiao, C., & Zhou, F. (2016). Capital to the Countryside" and the Re-engineering of Villages. *Chinese Social Science*, No. 1.

Lv, F. (2013). Analysis of Governance Context: Local Government Behavior under Risk Constraints: A Case Study of "Grievances" in Wuling City Poverty Alleviation Office. *Sociological Research*, No. 2.

Mei, L., & Lv, F. (2015). The New Social Economy Movement": NGOs and "Private Standards"—A Discussion Based on the Case of Fair Trade Labeling Organization (FLO). *Fujian Forum (Humanities and Social Sciences Edition)*, No. 10.

Wang, C. (2014). A Study on the Relationship between Poverty Alleviation and Village Solidarity. *Zhejiang Social Science*, No. 3.

Wang X. (2017). Social Governance and targeted poverty alleviation. *Journal of Guizhou University for Nationalities (Philosophy and Social Science Edition)*, No. 1.

Xu, Y. (2008). Policy to the Countryside" and Policy Integration of Rural Society. *Contemporary World and Socialism*, No. 1.

Xun, L. (2017). From "Resource Transfer" to "Local Governance"-targeted poverty Alleviation and Rural Reconstruction. *Culture Vertical*, No. 6.

Zhe, X., & Chen, Y. (2011). The Hierarchical Operation Mechanism and Governance Logic of the Project System: A Sociological Analysis of the Case of "Project in the Village". *Chinese Social Sciences*, No. 4.

Fang Lv is a professor at the School of Social Sciences, Central China Normal University, with research interests in poverty reduction and development.

Chapter 5
How Can Alpine Resources Be Turned into Capital for Poverty Alleviation? The Practice of Tea Industry Poverty Alleviation in Puling Village, Hubei

Yafang Ning

Abstract Puling Village is located in the northeast of the contiguous poor area of Wuling Mountains. It is 110 km away from the county, and a remote mountain village; as it is located in the deep mountains, with poor development conditions, it is one of the county's important "battlefields" of targeted poverty alleviation. Yet, this remote mountain village in the targeted poverty alleviation is precisely fortunate. In 2015, it became the county's targeted poverty alleviation identification pilot village, and in 2018, the Dapunong Company put into operation the construction of tea processing plant. Under the dual drive of the government and the market, the high mountain organic tea of Puling Village finally achieved the two major changes, i.e., the change from products to commodities, and the change from the scale planting to the integration of production and marketing. The development of tea industry not only helps poor households to get rid of absolute poverty, but more importantly, unites the vision and confidence of all villagers to build a better hometown. It is also due to the gradual development of the tea industry, the village, the villagers' endogenous development aspirations and capabilities continue to grow, and the effectiveness of strengthening the village and enriching the people has gradually emerged.

Keywords Tea · Industrial poverty alleviation · Industrial modernization · Puling Village

5.1 Big Mountain Barrier: Why It is Difficult for Puling to Get Rid of Poverty

In 2002, after the "abolition of townships and towns, and merging villages and villager groups", the former Puling Village, Neixi Village, and Xiaoping Village were merged into the current Puling Village. Puling Village is a remote agricultural village located

Y. Ning (✉)
Institute of Ethnology and Anthropology, Chinese Academy of Social Sciences, Beijing, China

Case Studies of Targeted Poverty Reduction and Alleviation in 100 Villages, International Research on Poverty Reduction, https://doi.org/10.1007/978-981-95-0549-4_5

in the southwest of Duzhenwan Town, Changyang Tujia Autonomous County, Hubei Province, with a village area of 32.7 square kilometers, 110 km from the county. As it is located deep in the Wuling Mountains, the natural environment is a very obvious constraint to the development of the village. In the words of local cadres and people themselves, "the mountains are large with sparse population, and the mountains are like roofs, in the middle are three streams (Inner Creek, Liujia Creek, Daxigou), three pings (East Ping, West Ping, Top Ping), and a dustpan", the village's eight villager groups are distributed in the mountains with altitude difference of 300 ~ 1800 m. For a long time, it took 4 h to drive from the village to the county town, and the distance from the villagers to the nearest Machi town was more than 10 km.The poor transportation made the Puling Village trudge on the way to reform and opening up and the building of a moderately prosperous society. As early as 2013, the village was listed as a whole village to promote poverty alleviation, and formed poverty alleviation industries based on walnuts and konjac planting. However, due to the failure to achieve large-scale production and the inconsequential effect on income generation, the village has been stagnant in the development of agricultural industry. According to the villagers, before the targeted poverty alleviation, the village has no agricultural industry with real economic benefits, including the old tea plantations built in the 1980s which no one cares for a long time, and agricultural products are basically self-produced and self-consumed, and people have to buy part of the staple food from the market town down the mountain such as rice due to its low yield. As a result, the majority of the village's young and middle-aged labor force has gone out to work or even moved away, leaving a quiet mountain village with occasional smoke from kitchen chimneys.

5.1.1 Constraints of the Great Mountain Barrier

The constraints of traffic are most obvious due to the large mountain barrier. Because of the mountain barrier and the location in the border area of the township, there is only one road that goes into the village and only one road out of the village, so the whole village has been inconveniently connected with the outside world, and the level of economic and social development of the village has been low for a long period of time. As of 2015, the village then had 50 km of main roads and 80 km of roads connecting households, but only 8 km of road paved with concrete (only 6% of the village roads). There were 53 households without access to roads. When the research team went deep into the villager groups in 2017, there were still many farmers in group 1, 2, and 3 whose household roads were mud roads and far away from the village roads, making it extremely inconvenient and unsafe for people and vehicles to pass. In addition, once encountered with heavy rain, gale, and other bad weather, road access will be blocked.

The constraints of mountain barriers on trade and commerce are also very serious. For a long time, because of the high mountains and remote location, vegetable vendors outside the Puling Village rarely come there to buy vegetables grown by farmers, so farmers often have to use agricultural vehicles or three-wheeled Mamu sack truck[1] and other means of transport for several times, to deliver the products to the Machi town for centralized load and transport. This costly mode of transportation leads to extremely high transportation costs for agricultural products.And the loss of freshness and completeness of agricultural products caused by transportation will reduce their selling prices. In the farming industry, the remote location and poor transportation cause farmers to be unaware of market information and often sell pigs and goats to vendors at a much lower price. It is estimated that the price of a pig or a goat sold by a farmer in Puling Village is about 300 yuan lower than the purchase price in the township where Puling Village is located.[2] As a result, villagers have long been seriously affected in market trading activities and hauling construction materials to build houses. Wang Chaodong, the village director, said: "In the past, 'big cars could not go inside, and in raining days, small cars will stop', nothing cannot sell a good price. Villagers planted vegetables, raised pigs and goats, and have to go through multiple transfers to sell, with high transport costs, long transit time, so the villagers were not motivated".[3] There was a lack of location advantage for commercial logistics and materials exchange, and industrial structure is relatively single.Farmers generally plant corn, potatoes, and other food crops with the average annual income of about 300 yuan / mu.[4] Villagers also do not have the habit of going to the market on a fixed date. In the interviews with elderly villagers, we learned that only when they ran out of production and living materials, would they go down to Machi (the location of the old Machi Township government, now it is incorporated into the Duzhenwan Town) to buy things.

The whole village's production service facilities are also restricted by the large mountain barrier. In terms of electricity, the village has 11 power transformers, but most of the poles are wooden poles, so the problem of low and unstable voltage is very serious, and villagers often need to alternatively use off-peak power when use grinding machine during the busy farming season, and production activities are severely restricted.[5] In 2013, the village has a bookstore, without any recreational facilities. There were still many villagers from group 1, 2, and 3 living in thatched houses.

---

[1] The common name of three-wheeled motorcycle in E'xi (i.e. West Hubei – Trans.) region, which belongs to local language. In China, except for the Exi region, there are regions where Tujia people live also have such a name.

[2] See "Puling Village Survey".

[3] Wen Kai: "Pu Yu Grows Gold - A Record of Poverty Alleviation in Puling Village, Changyang Tujia Autonomous County, Hubei Province," Jingchu Poverty Alleviation Website, http://hbfp.cnhubei.com/2019/0723/409897.shtml.

[4] 1 mu equals 1/15 hectare. – Trans.

[5] According to the investigation of targeted poverty alleviation in the town of Dojinwan, the problem of incomplete transformation of low voltage exists in Puling Village, the common voltage is around 160 V, barely lighting, washing machine, wet and dry mill, and other common rural appliances cannot be used normally, often "cannot turn", wooden poles, loose strands of wire still exist in large numbers.

At the beginning of reform and opening up, some villagers went out to work as tailors following the Zhejiang bosses who were building roads in the village at that time, which became a major highlight of the labor economy in Changyang Tujia Autonomous County. However, due to the influence of geographical location, residents in the village are restricted in the development of arable land, food crops plantation, and their access to medical care, education, communications, electricity, and other aspects for a long time.Coupled with the causes that the village is difficult to effectively develop processing industries, and the breeding industry affected by the poor infrastructure could not form a scale production, all these factors contributed to the development of the entire village lack economic vitality and social dynamics. Long lived in the mountains, the Puling villagers lack the information from the outer world. Although there is a relatively high degree of self-sufficiency, the villagers had a weak awareness of the market economy. As a result, the village has not been able to fully develop and improve itself in the process of socialist modernization since the reform and opening up. These combined factors have led to the overall poverty of Puling Village. Generally speaking, the mountain barrier not only restricts the material production and life of villagers, but also affects their spiritual world and development concept.

5.1.2 The "Appearance" of Poverty in Puling Village

In general, the remote location, poor infrastructure, more conservative thinking, lack of public service supply, and accelerated exodus of young laborers are the causes of poverty in Puling Village, and also important manifestations of the village's poverty problem. Specifically, they are mainly manifested in the following seven aspects.

Firstly, the infrastructure is poor and the villagers are not strong in market participation. Poor roads with poor safety is the primary constraint for the poverty of the whole village. The terrain surrounded by mountains on all sides leads to the low level of accessible roads in the village, with narrow and mostly sandy roads. In addition, the distance from the town and the county is very far, so the villagers' production and life are extremely inconvenient.

Secondly, the industrial structure is single, and it is difficult for farmers to rely on local agriculture to increase their income. For a long time, on the available arable land, more than half of the farmers grow corn on a large area (the yield is 300–500 kg per mu); there are also small areas of rice, potatoes, soybeans, etc., and the yields are not high. The poultry and livestock are raised for self-consumption, with only a small part will be sold on market. In 2015, only 4 households in the village slaughtered more than 100 pigs, with a low annual output and low income. In addition, tea, walnuts, medicinal herbs, and other cash crops have not become large-scale planting. Take tea as an example, in 2014, a villager in group 5 planted 8 mu of tea, but the annual income from tea is only 3000 yuan, and less than 400 yuan per mu.[6] In terms of

[6] See "Puling Village Survey".

walnut planting, supported by the whole village promotion project since 2013, the village planted 700 mu of walnuts, but due to the lack of professional cultivation and management techniques, many fruit trees could not bear fruits. In general, the industrial structure is single for a long time, resulting in the under-development of agricultural processing industry in the village. There is only one workshop tea factory in the village for primary processing of tea, and the tea processing capacity is very limited.

Thirdly, the supply of basic public services is insufficient and the development capacity of the village is weak. Due to the dual impact of being located in the deep mountains and the abolition of the township, public institutions such as the original Xiaoping Primary School and the Machi Township Office stationed in Puling were abolished one after another in the early twenty-first century. This had a negative impact on the villagers' access to education, medical care, and public services. There is only one health clinic left in Puling Village, and it is still renting a dilapidated building that was previously used as a supply and marketing cooperative, lacking the most basic hardware facilities for medical treatment.[7] There is only one retired doctor in the village health clinic, and the health clinic is only equipped with a blood pressure meter and other electronic equipment for daily monitoring. Medical resources are extremely scarce. Most of the time, villagers can only go down the mountain to the Machi Health Center for initial consultation, while it is a long way to the county hospital and very inconvenient to rent a car.[8] The lack of educational resources in the village has also led to a prevailing trend of escorting children to attend school in the township, which is more than 10 km away from their homes, starting from preschool education. This kind of escorting from kindergarten to high school is a way to "reduce income and increase expenses" for families in Puling Village. As a result, the cost of raising a student in Puling Village is significantly higher than that in other areas. In addition, the village has long lacked basic public recreational facilities due to the inadequate allocation of basic public services such as electricity and internet, and there was no village broadcaster, library or basic

[7] According to the division of the scope of consultation in the *Implementation Plan for Graded Medical Institutions in Changyang Tujia Autonomous County*, the scope of consultation in village health clinics is the outpatient treatment of common diseases and frequently-occurring diseases. The township health centers are mainly responsible for the prevention and treatment of common diseases, frequently-occurring diseases and chronic diseases, providing public health services, assisting the hospitals at higher level to provide intermediate or post-hospital services, and reasonably triaging patients. It mainly receives general outpatient and inpatient cases with simple diseases and stable conditions, as well as cases that are compatible with the technical level and facilities and equipment conditions, including: patients with common diseases and multiple diseases; patients with clear diagnosis who do not need special treatment; patients with stable conditions after acute treatment who need continued rehabilitation; chronic patients who need long-term treatment and management; elderly care patients; patients with various malignant tumors at the late stage needless to make non-surgical treatment and in need for hospice care; primary surgical treatment with conditions; patients in the rehabilitation period transferred from higher level hospitals.

[8] At present, there is a shuttle bus to the county town in the village in the morning and afternoon, and if there is a sudden illness, they can only rent a van or motorcycle to go down the mountain for medical treatment, which is very costly in terms of transportation and time.

cultural activity room before the targeted poverty alleviation. Except for the occasional game of Changyanghuapai.[9]There are almost no public recreational activities among villagers. In fact, since villagers have to leave early to work and return late to home in the mountains or on the slopes, they rarely have time to watch TV throughout the year, and they cannot access the internet on their smartphones due to the unstable signal. Therefore, villagers who have been working in the village for a long time have little knowledge of the world and information outside the village.

Fourthly, the problem with poverty due to illness is serious.The villagers are under pressure of catastrophic expenses. Puling Village is located in high mountains, so villagers suffer from rheumatism, lumbar spine injury, and other common chronic diseases in rural areas with a high proportion. And these chronic diseases have a greater impact on farmers engaged in agricultural farming, and physical labor can be seriously affected by the above-mentioned joint diseases, and it is more common for families to lose their main labor force due to illness. In addition to the serious shortage of medical resources at the primary level, many villagers in Puling Village also adopt the strategy of "carrying with small diseases and delaying the big ones" when they fall ill. In addition, since it is difficult for villagers' families to generate a significant and stable income, in the case of long-term chronic illness or sudden major illness, these vulnerable rural families not only face catastrophic medical expenses, but also it means their loss of labor income. The Puling Village Survey found that in 2015, there were 150 poor households suffering from major illnesses (treatment costs above 20,000 yuan) in the village, accounting for 20.20% of the total number of household registrations. As of the first half of 2015, the proportion of healthy population in the village was 64.25%, the proportion of poor people suffering from long-term chronic diseases was 26.81%, the proportion of poor people suffering from major diseases was 7.66%, and the proportion of poor people with disabilities was 1.28%. The health condition of the poor is worrisome, and the high rate of illness, disease, and disability has become the biggest obstacle for the poor to get out of poverty.[10] Many families in the village were initially "suffering from minor illnesses", and then had to face catastrophic medical expenses when it became difficult to treat major illnesses, which crushed many families in the village.

Fifthly, the villagers' human capital accumulation is weak due to their low education level. Since the 1980s, many young and middle-aged laborers in Puling Village have gone out to Beijing and other places to engage in the tailoring "profession", and these villagers also participated in the modern market industrial production activities earlier and completed a certain amount of family capital accumulation. However, in general, the education level of most villagers in Puling Village has been low for a long time, the human capital accumulation of villagers is weak, and the human resources of young and middle-aged laborers have not been well developed. The

[9] Changyanghuapai, a popular card game played in Yichang, Jingzhou, Tianmen, Hunan, and Sichuan. Huapai, aka "Shangdaren", is a kind of traditional Chinese long card game with long strips, about one span long and half inch wide, made of hard paper with varnish. Each deck has 110 cards, and in the 1980s, it was jokingly referred to as "learning to play the 110 articles".

[10] See "Puling Village Survey".

Puling Village Survey on the educational level of poor households in the village in 2015 found that among 227 poor households in the village, 18.75% of poor households were poverty-stricken due to schooling, and 66.83% of poor households, who enjoyed minimum living guarantee considered that the biggest difficulty they faced at present or in the last three years was the problem of schooling expenses for their children. In addition to the low education level of the poor households, the labor skills of the poor households are not satisfactory. Among the 227 poor households in the village, 37.69% have no working ability, 9.04% have lost working ability, 52.48% are the average labor force, and only 0.79% have certain working skills.

Sixthly, the subjective initiative of self-development is not strong, and there is a lack of positive understanding of industrial development and village governance. The combination of the above-mentioned factors has actually led to the overall conservative thinking of villagers in Puling Village. Lack of comparison with the external economic and social development, coupled with the lack of development conditions, the villagers of Puling Village, especially the poor villagers, do not have the subjective initiative to develop industry and participate in rural governance. Specifically, middle-aged and elderly villagers are more likely to rest on their laurels, lack a sense of innovation in production and life, and are less active in participating in village public affairs. According to the case interview data of the Puling Village Survey, "we are all afraid of being hungry and poor, and we dare not think about it, it does not matter if we have no money, as long as we have food", and the general public lacks the courage and fighting spirit to declare war on poverty.[11] One of the extreme cases of poor families in the village is a 58-year-old villager living at an altitude of 1000 m above sea level, who has never been out of the mountains until 2015, and has never even been to Zhuangxi Town (the seat of the town government), which is only 30 km away. All the family members lived in a thatched house, and slept on a broken cotton fiber bed, who were in extreme poverty. In addition, the first secretary in the village summarized the current situation where the lack of innovation and change in Puling Village as the lack of three types of people: the guide, the leader, and the knowledgeable person. The vast majority of farmers can't read newspapers and magazines or science and technology books,[12]who can't communicate with the outside world, can't get timely scientific and technological information and market information.

[11] It is understood that a villager in Puling Village family has three laborers, with 11 acres of land all used to plant corn, and then feed the pigs with corn. The family has annual net income of only 3,000 yuan. Other people's fields and corner plots are also used to plant a variety of crops, but nothing is large scale. The production is also for their own use. For example, people plant tea, only pick a season of bud tea. As long as the sales reach a few hundred yuan, they will be satisfied, as they simply did not think about the development ideas of scale, standardization, and specialization. It is completely dependence on the sky. After a year of diligent work, the villagers only had the average income of about 500 yuan per mu, and they can only achieve subsistence, let alone get rich.

[12] About this, I found in my field research that villagers work hard in the mountains every day. As the mountains are high and far, and the working time is generally more than 10 h a day. After returning home, they are so tired that they do not have the mood or time to watch TV. In addition, villagers almost never subscribe to newspapers, magazines, or books, so they do not know much information about the outside world.

Although they are experts in traditional planting and farming (planting corn, potatoes, sweet potatoes and scattered pig farming), they are the authentic "layman" in the development of modern agriculture. Andthere are basically no poor households in the village who understand the policy, science and technology, and the market in a real sense.

Seventhly, the frequency of disasters in mountainous areas and the lack of stability in village development environment. Changyang Tujia Autonomous County is one of the geological disaster-prone counties in Hubei Province because of its high slopes, steep mountains, deep river valleys, frequent neotectonic activities, abundant rainfall, and intensive human engineering activities. Geological disasters occur in many types and are widely distributed, high in frequency, and heavy in severity. Disaster is also one of the important causes for the poverty and return to poverty in Puling Village. Puling Village has adverse natural conditions. On July 19, 2016, a flood occurred in Puling Village, resulting in the house collapse involving 4 poor households in group 1 of Puling Village, including 16 victims and 16 damaged houses. Six main roads in the village were collapsed and the road surface was severely damaged, making it difficult for people to travel and the transportation was halted. Agricultural production and infrastructure were greatly damaged, and some of the poor households that had been "removed from the hat[13]" returned to poverty, while some of the poor households that had not been "removed from the hat" further increased their poverty level.[14]

5.2 Targeted Poverty Alleviation: Puling Becomes a Lucky Village

Under the national strategy of targeted poverty alleviation, Puling Village, which is described as the "ShibadongVillage" of Changyang Tujia Autonomous County, caught the express train of targeted poverty alleviation and achieved a magnificent transformation from poverty to wealth. In 2015, Puling Village ushered in a historic opportunity for poverty alleviation. Based on the experience of targeted identification of poor households in Bijie, Guizhou, the county Party committee and government of Changyang Tujia Autonomous County decided to implement a poverty baseline survey in 54 poor villages and impoverished villages across the county.

[13] Hat metaphorically means poverty. When it is recognized a poverty-stricken one, the one will wear a hat; while one is lifted out of poverty, the one will be taken off the hat. – Trans.

[14] *Report on the Work of Changyang Tujia Autonomous County in Combating Poverty*, February 2017.

5.2.1 Puling Became the "First Mover" in Changyang County for Targeted Poverty Alleviation

In the random sampling, Puling Village became the first pilot survey village among 54 poor villages and impoverished villages in the county. Changyang Tujia Autonomous County's targeted poverty alleviation kicked off in Puling. After determining the Puling Village as a sample village for targeted identification baseline survey, in June 2015, the main leading comrades of Changyang Tujia Autonomous County Party Committee led the team, and more than 30 county and town cadres were deployed to form nine research teams. It took them three trips into the Puling Village to conduct a one-month research, and wrote a main report "Puling Village Survey" and nine sub-reports which were distributed as a reference document by Hubei Provincial Party Committee and Yichang Municipal Committee. In Puling, the pilot, Changyang Tujia Autonomous County put forward the "four to look and four to calculate"as targeted identification methods and "one look, two calculation, three meeting, four evaluation" astargeted identification procedures. The Hubei Provincial Party Committee took the targeted identification practice of Puling Village as the experience of poverty alleviation work and called for a province-wide learning. According to the data of the Puling Village Survey, the poverty incidence rate of Puling Village in 2015 was 36.5%. In the process of implementing targeted identification work, the Party members and masses in Puling Villagewere very enthusiastic, confident, and actively involved in targeted poverty alleviation. The secretary of the village Party branch said, "Now Puling Village was included in the county's pilot targeted poverty alleviation, which is the greatest trust of the higher government to the village, so we do not care how much to sacrifice, we must do a good job!" In the meeting held by the villagers' representatives, the villagers generally reflected that "this time the work is real, and the working group has a discerning eye, whose work is convincing".

5.2.2 Birth of the "1156" Model

Based on the continuation of the "1321" model of supporting the whole village,[15] Changyang Tujia Autonomous County has determined the "1156" model for targeted poverty alleviation in poor villages based on the pilot project of targeted identification in Puling Village and the county-wide targeted identificationbaseline survey. The "1156" model, as a targeted poverty alleviation model of Changyang Tujia Autonomous County that integrates multiple resources and initiates multiple collaborations among poverty alleviation action subjects, fully combines the "Five Measures for Poverty Elimination[16]" concept of targeted poverty alleviation and grassroots

[15] The implementation of the whole village to promote the "1321" help model refers to a county-level leader leading more than three departments for two consecutive years to help a whole village.

[16] Regarding the question of "how to help," Xi Jinping has proposed five measures to be taken according to the specific conditions of poverty-stricken areas and impoverished populations:

Party building, and more comprehensively implements a multi-dimensional and comprehensive approach of aid and poverty alleviation for poor villages and poor population, which embodies the integration of poverty alleviation resources and the organization of poverty alleviation measures, as well as the concept of multi-dimensional anti-poverty for targeted poverty alleviation, which is of great practical significance for the formation of sustainability for poor villages and sustainable livelihoods poor households. The specific contents of the "1156" model are as follows: to build a strong rural Party organization, to build a solid bottom line for policies, to weave "five nets" for industrial development, and to implement "six measureson households" for targeted poverty alleviation. Under the guidance of "1156" model, Puling Village was positioned as a border poverty village by the county Party committee and the county government, and supported as a key village for targeted poverty alleviation, which was described by the village cadres as "a good opportunity rarely met in a hundred years".

In this poverty alleviation model, the town of DuzhenwanwherePuling is located formulated the *Changyang Tujia Autonomous County Duzhenwan Puling Village targeted poverty alleviation and targeted poverty eradication plan (2015 ~ 2017)*, which aims to further accelerate the pace of construction of Puling Village from poverty to prosperity, strengthen infrastructure construction, vigorously develop pillar industries, improve public service systems, improve production and living conditions, and keep pace with the town in 2016 to achieve the goal of poverty eradication. The general idea of the plan is: to enrich the people and strengthen the village as the goal, to take project construction as a carrier, to improve the infrastructure as the entry point, to develop the leading industries as the focus point, to enhance the endogenous power as the anchor point, to promote in-depth implementation of the "five mega projects", to promote the "boutique tea village, alpine medicinal material village, livable New Village" construction, so as to present the "cycle road in the mountains, gold industries everywhere, courtyard farm stays, quadruple income per capita, a townish living, harmony like a family" prosperous scenes, and to create a demonstration village for the county's targeted poverty alleviation and targeted poverty eradication.

It can be said that Puling Village has turned into a lucky one in the wave of targeted poverty alleviation. From the pilot village of Changyang County's targeted poverty alleviation identification to the village that county Party secretary is heldaccountablefor its poverty alleviation, Puling Village has become the "star" village in Changyang County's targeted poverty alleviation and poverty eradication action. With the resources from all sides and the attention of multiple subjects, the pace of poverty eradication in Puling Village has taken a new height and the industrial development has ushered in a new opportunity.

1.Boosting the economy to create more jobs for the disadvantaged.
2.Relocating those living under adverse natural conditions.
3.Providing eco-jobs for the poor.
4.Improving education in poor areas.
5.Improving social security for poverty alleviation.

5.3 Scale Planting: Puling Pressed the "Accelerator Key" of Tea Industry

5.3.1 The Unique Advantages of Industrial Development

Although Puling is located in the depths of the mountains, but the characteristics of high altitude also provide a unique advantage toPulingin developing high mountain organic tea and medicinal herb cultivation. As early as in the 1980s, the village built the first batch of tea plantations. However, farmers considered that the tea garden would reduce the land for cultivation of food crops,[17]and since tea was not well known then and the sales met difficulties and other problems, so in recent decades the enthusiasm of villagers who relied on the tea planting to make richhas been not high, and villagers did not focus on tea planting. However, the alpine tea garden in the mountains ofPuling Village at an altitude of 1000 ~ 1200 m has lush vegetation, pure air, sufficient sunshine, soil rich in zinc, selenium, and other trace elements, which is extremely favorable to the formation and accumulation of special beneficial nutrients for tea tree growth. All along, due to the lack of industrial capital investment and operation, Puling's organic tea is just like a "diamond in the rough", and has not had the opportunity to complete the transformation of commercialization.

5.3.2 New Practice of Scale Development of Tea Industry

Combined with the ecological advantages of high mountainous areas, in the planning, Puling Villagepositioned the industrial development of poverty alleviation asthe main development of tea, herbs, economic forestry and fruit, and established a poverty alleviation idea for industrial synergy development of "scaling up the tea and herbs, developing fruit trees and expanding livestock production, increasingbenefits from tourism and labor work". In the plan for industrial synergy development to get out of poverty, Puling Village firstly implemented the "four three-thousand" project, and intensive development of planting industry. The "four three-thousand" project refers to the completion of the belt distribution of "four bases,each covering three-thousand mu" within three years, namely three thousand mu of medicinal herbs, three thousand mu of tea plantations, three thousand mu of fruit trees, and three thousand mu of pasture.[18] Puling Village's development of three thousand mu of tea plantations

---

[17] I found in the interview with the villagers that, the villagers are worried about the adjustment of industrial structure. For example, in terms of tea planting to replace corn planting, a representative viewpoint of the villagers interviewed is: "planting tea produces tree leaves, and it is not food if cannot be sold; while planting corn is very reliable, even if it can not be sold, it can be kept as food, and at least it can solve the problem of food rations.".

[18] Three thousand mu of medicinal herbs refers to the area with altitude of more than 1,000 m above sea level. Based on the existing 336 mu of medicinal herbs, giving full play to the advantages of benign companion planting of medicinal herbs under the forest, vigorously expanding the scale of

is also aimed at giving full play to the advantages of the existing old tea plantations, making full use of the existing resource endowment, so as to accelerate the scale of agricultural development in the village. According to the plan, it is expected that by 2017, the planting area of village's efficient economic crop can reach 9260 mu. In order to promote the development of the whole village industry, Puling Villagetook an opportunity of integrating the policy of returning farmland to forest, planned to implement the return of 1000 mu of forest on the slopesthat exceeds 25 degrees, so as to combine the ecological protection and industrial development to achieve poverty alleviation and wealth.

In August 2015, the village established a plan to plant 2266 mu of new tea, involving 448 households and more than 1800 people; 734 mu of old tea gardens were renovated and planned to be implemented in two years. In addition to Group 1, the remaining seven villager groups in the village have the plan of building new tea gardens and renovating old tea gardens. In order to improve the enthusiasm of poor households and farmers to plant tea, Puling Village has adopted two approaches of policy subsidies and skills training. In terms of policy subsidies, Puling Village has given corresponding subsidies for tea seedling planting based on the policy of "giving awards instead of subsidies". In the new round of tea development subsidy policy implemented in 2018, the tea seedling subsidy was 1000 yuan / mu, of which 700 yuan / mu for planting, and if the acceptance rate of survival exceeded 85%, afurther subsidy of 300 yuan / mu would be provided; tea seeds subsidy was 100 yuan /mu, which was measured by 30 kg per mu; renovation subsidy for old tea garden was 200 yuan /mu. In terms of skills upgrading, Puling Village organized 100 industrial demonstration households, and representatives of poor households to visit Dayan Qianzhangkeng, Yidu Panwan, and Wufeng Yuyangguan and learn the tea industry development model.

In order to encourage the linkage between non-poor households and poor households for tea planting to form a large-scale effect, the "two committees" team ofPuling Villagemade rational use of special support funds to buy tea seedlings through open bidding;on the one hand, the tea seedlings will be distributed free of charge to the targeted poverty-stricken households; on the other hand, a certain number of tea seedlings will also be issued to the low-income households and farmers who are willing to develop the tea industry. In terms ofthe scope of planting, first of all, it

---

planting, newly developing 2,924 mu of medicinal herbs, reaching 3,260 mu, including 1,100 mu of new development of solanum in groups 1 and 6; the new development of 794 mu of fritillaria and 430 mu of Gastrodia elata in groups 1, 2, 3, 5, and 6; and the new development of 600 mu of papaya in group 6. Three thousand mu of tea garden refers to the construction target of completing 3000 mu of high standard, green, and organic tea garden below 1000 m above sea level, renovating 734 mu of old tea garden in group 2, 3, 4, 5, 6, 7, and 8, and newly developing 2266 mu of fine tea garden, to reach 3000 mu in total, and reaching an average household of more than 5 mu of tea garden in the industrial zone. Three thousand mu of fruit trees refers to the renovation of 800 mu of walnut base in 8 groups in the village, the new development of 700 mu of walnuts in group 2, 3, 4, 5, 6, 7, 8, the new development of 1000 mu of good chestnuts in group 6, 7, 8; the planting of special fruits in areas not suitable for herbs and tea planting, that is, the new development of 500 mu of plums in group 4, 5, 7, 8. Three thousand mu of pasture refers to the development of 3,000 mu of pasture in the village.

started from the tea planting to be scaled up in the village, and taking full account of the real needs of officially registered poverty-stricken households and non-status poor households in the village, so as to form alarge-scale industry in the village to achieve the common development of both non-poor households and poor households. In addition, in order to increase the support for poor households, Puling Village also arranged a certain percentage of the special poverty alleviation funds to purchase pesticides and fertilizers and distributed them to the officially registered poverty-stricken households, and helped poor families reduce their agricultural planting costs. In addition, Puling Village also focuses on strengthening the skills training for tea growers. In 2015, Puling Village carried out practical technical training of tea and other agricultural industriesfor 10 times benefiting 800 people.

"The people once have a backbone, they will do thing with extra motivation!" Under the scientific planning of the Party committee and the government, the initiative of free seedlings and fertilizer supply solved the worries of the poor households in the village to plant tea, and we gradually abandoned the outdated idea, i.e. planting tea is "planting leaves". Anaunt of poor household talked to the research team: "I have long wanted to develop tea, and also dug holessomewhere to plant seedlings.Now the state gives us free seedlings, so we have to seriously engage in the development, and it is not enough to just plant corn, as it is a hardworking job and I still can't earn some money, so it is not cost-effective".Providing pruning services for tea garden and carrying out the skill training for planting tea, it boosted the confidence of everyone in planting tea. Through the efforts of many parties, the development of tea in Puling Village has completed the transformation toward large-scale planting.

As of April 2019, the total area of tea planting in Puling Village is more than 3000 mu. In the village,centered around the four leading industries of tea, medicine, grass, and fruit,it has developed ecological alpine poverty alleviation industry, in which the scale planting of tea has become the backbone of industrial poverty alleviation, and it accelerated the pace of industrial development in Puling Village.

5.4 "Pu Red" Tea: "Business Card" of the Puling Poverty Alleviation Industry Modernization

The completion of large-scale planting is the first step of tea industry in Puling Village to alleviate poverty. "Sell out, sell well" is the key to turn the Puling Village tea into "golden leaf", which is inseparable from building the core competitiveness of Puling Village tea and managing the branding operations. This is precisely the most scarce external resources of Puling Village, which is deep in the mountains. In order to complete the modernization of the Puling tea industry, with the help of supporting departments and organizations at all levels as well as village cadres of the two committees, Puling Villagemade a big deal out of "making the tea sell a good price".

5.4.1 Quality Identification of "Selenium-Richness"

In 2017, through the detection by authoritative organization, the content of selenium was 5.8 unit in every 100 g tea of Puling Village. In March 2018, the technical committee of experts of Hubei Federation of Geographical Indication Products Enterprises specifically went to Puling Village to conduct a special research on the development of selenium tea industry and brand poverty alleviation, and Puling Village also joined the "industry technology innovation strategic alliance pilot base for national selenium-rich agricultural products". After the "selenium-rich" quality is recognized, Puling's high mountain organic tea has gained the core competitiveness to participate in the market, and the tea that villagers previously regarded as "tree leaves" has become the "golden leaf" that everyone spreads by word of mouth.

5.4.2 Leading Companies Come

As the saying goes, "wine is never afraid of deep alley". To facilitate the smooth promotion of high-quality tea, it needs to modernize the processing technology and product marketing. Fortunately, a fellow-villager who went out of the Puling Village, Xiao Dongyang, became an important matchmaker. Xiao Dongyang is the general manager of Hubei Dapu Agricultural Development Co. Ltd. (Hereinafter referred to as "Dapunong Company"). As early as 2013, he made a matchmaking support for Duzhenwan Town for his company.From 2013 to 2019, the company donated a total of 400,000 yuan to the primary and secondary schools in Machi, Duzhenwan Town. In the background of targeted poverty alleviation, Dapunong Company turned from "donations" to "investments".Since 2018, ithas begun to run a tea processing plant in Puling Village, and implemented the integration of agriculture, industry, and trade for targeted industry poverty alleviation. In the specific help, the Dapunong Company invested more than 7 million yuan to help Puling Village tea industry to expand the scale of planting, enhance the quality of tea processing, and make category segmentation according to different market demand. It successively created a "Pu Red" "high mountain wild green tea with selenium" In April 2019, the "revolutionary old area industrial poverty alleviation project" Pu Red tea processing base in Puling Village was successfully put into operation by the Dapunong company. The "Pu Red" tea brand won the gold medal at the 2019 Tea Expo in Wuhan, China. The company also in 2019 rated as "to help fight against poverty, Pu Red take the lead, as the excellent enterprise pioneer" by the "two committees" of Puling Village.

The introduction of the leading company has accelerated the modernization of the tea industry in Puling Village. Firstly, the interest linkage mechanism of Puling villagers getting rich through the industry has changed. Dapunong Company set up Pulingblack tea-specialized cooperative, to help some poor households get employed locally, and contribute to the diversification of the villagers' income structure in the form of recruiting workers, incorporating tea plantations as shares, etc. Secondly, it has enhanced the skills and confidence of the Puling villagers, so that their ability to develop and utilize local resources has been enhanced. As villagers said, "with the Dapunong Company'ssupport, tea income of our village is promising this year. They taught us to plant, helped us sell, and we are more confident with the tea industry!" Thirdly, the initiatives of the preferential price, preferential acquisition of tea completely address the concerns of poor households and non-poor households in growing tea together. A 63-year-old villager who suffered from poverty, Lv Xuepan,has picked new tea for half a month, with the average daily income of about 500 yuan. Compared with last year, the tea factory can increase the income of each household by about 2000 yuan in 2019. Fourthly, the completion of the tea processing plant can give full play to the advantages of tea that is exempted cyclical fluctuations asthe deep processing will help villagers effectively avoid the difficulties of price fluctuations of agricultural products. In 2019, the Dapunong Company completed the task of collecting 90,000 kg of fresh tea leaves, with a total cost of more than 300,000 yuan. With the further expansion of the production line of rough tea, the processing plant can purchase fresh tea leaves all year round, and the production capacity will be further expanded. According to the plan, in 2019, the company continues to build 100 mu of high-standard industrialized demonstration tea plantations in Puling, and place "Pu Red" brand as the core to form the industrial development model of one body with three wings, i.e. "agriculture + technology + finance + poverty alleviation", andconsolidate various foundations for the modernization of Puling Village industry.

5.5 Civilized Village at the City Level: The Achievements of Puling Industrial Poverty Alleviation in Strengthening Village and Enriching People

After experiencing the large-scale planting of tea and the enterprise operation of Hubei Dapunong Company, Puriling tea industry has gradually shown positive results of strengthening the village and enriching the people. As of July 2019, Puling Village has built 3800 mu of high mountain tea, 4100 mu of Chinese herbal medicine, in addition to the development of 3000 mu of small alpine fruits, 5000 mu of fallow ecological livestock area by returning the grain plots to pasture. The "four three-thousand" goals set for that year have been achieved.

The development of tea industry, not only let the modern agriculture ofPuling Village have a "backbone", also let Puling Villagehave a "engine"for building a well-off society. As the then "ShibadongVillage" in Changyang, Puling Village firmly grasped the main line of industrial poverty alleviation, and gradually completed the upgrade of infrastructure, living environment, production conditions, rural governance, and good life expectations. From the pilot village of targeted poverty alleviation identification in 2015 to the village with all the poor households lifted out of poverty, and collective economic income of more than 200,000 yuan in 2019, the former remote village situated in the deep mountains with occasional cooking smoke was rated as Yichang civilized village. Only industry can gather population, and only industry can gather people. Puling Village combined thetargeted poverty alleviation project with the project development of tea industry, etc., focused on the goal of "gathering people for local employment and building a beautiful home", and promoted the synergistic development of industry and infrastructure. Since 2015, Puling Village has paved 53 km of rural roads with concrete, repaired and expanded the roads by 50 km; renovated and realized the full coverage of the rural power grid; newly established 12 centralized water supply pools, laid nearly 100,000 m of pipeline networks, and newly established 3 communication base stations, renovated 200 households of rural dilapidated houses, relocated 64 households and 216 people for poverty alleviation. The whole village has also established four demonstration areas of Xueshanping, Yangshuwan, Shuijingwan, and Niejiaba for thanksgiving and poverty alleviation, forming a "four help model" of "help with spirit encouragement, help with policy publicity, helpwith industry motivation and help with experience sharing".

The huge changes in Puling are a sample of 39 key poverty-stricken villages in Changyang Tujia Autonomous County. In the former words of mouth from cadres and people of Puling, "the mountains are large with sparse population, and the mountains are like roofs, in the middle are three streams, three pings, and a dustpan", now have been replaced by "the large mountains with sparse populationbecoming a treasure land, high mountain herbs growing like ladder after ladder, Zhongshan fresh tea leaves turning green, new-style houses and buildings raised up one by one, the network cable delivering information, and the masses living in good happiness ".

References

Han, C. (2011). *The "Three Rural Issues" in China's Modernization Process* (Revised Edition). China Agricultural Press.

Hu, W., Huang, Z., & Peng, W. (2018). The mechanism of the role of industrial targeted poverty alleviation, realistic dilemmas and cracking paths. *Jianghuai Forum*, No. 5.

Lan, H., Zhang, Y., & Zhou, Z. (2017). Analysis and reflection on the model of industrial poverty alleviation in China. *China Development Observer*, No. 17.

Liang, Q., & Cai, J. (2017). Resource Endowment, Asset-Based Income and industrial Poverty Alleviation—A Multi-case Comparative Study. *Journal of Central South University (Social Science Edition)*, No. 4.

Ma, N. (2016). Research on Targeted Poverty Alleviation in Special Industries in Ethnic Regions—Taking Chinese Herbal Medicine Development Industry as an Example. *Journal of Central South University for Nationalities (Humanities and Social Sciences Edition)*, No. 1.

Wang, C., & Zheng, Y. (2017). Research on Industrial Poverty Alleviation in China since the 21st Century: A Genealogy of Research and Themes. *China Population, Resources and Environment, 6.*

Wang, W. (2019). The innovation of industrial paths for targeted poverty alleviation in rural areas from the perspective of rural revitalization. *Chongqing Social Science, 1.*

Zhang, L., et al. (2019). *Case Collection on Targeted Poverty Alleviation in Ethnic Minority Areas of China (2018).* China Economic Press.

Yafang Ning is an associate researcher at the Institute of Ethnology and Anthropology, Chinese Academy of Social Sciences, with research interests in forging a sense of community among the Chinese people, and the anti-poverty in ethnic areas.

Chapter 6
Big Changes in a Small Village: A Study on Rural Development and Targeted Poverty Alleviation in Si'ergou Village, Qinghai Province

Hong Wang

Abstract Poverty-stricken villages are the basic units of China's poverty alleviation policies, and are also at the forefront of the country's battle against poverty. Through a study of Si'ergou Village in Dongchuan Town, Menyuan Hui Autonomous County, Haibei Tibetan Autonomous Prefecture, Qinghai Province, from 2016 to 2019, this paper examines the significant changes that have taken place in social security, rural development, and poverty alleviation industries and business in this semi-agricultural and semi-pastoral village on a plateau. The examination of the poverty alleviation practice of the village ecological breeding industry focuses mainly on a series of issues arising from the contradiction between the concept and practice of industrial poverty alleviation. These issues include the conflict between the policy environment and project management, the imbalance between administration and market, the technical and economic issues of the project, and the benefit sharing and interest conflict.

Keywords Poverty alleviation business development · Targeted poverty alleviation · Rural development · Si'ergou Village

Located at the foot of Daban Mountain, and to the south bank of the Haomen River, Si'ergou Village is a semi-agricultural and semi-pastoral natural village in Dongchuan Town, Menyuan Hui Autonomous County, Haibei Tibetan Autonomous Prefecture, Qinghai Province. This village is nestled by mountains and waters, and inhabited by multiple ethnic groups. The Si'ergou River, a tributary of the Haomen River, flows from south to north, passing through the houses, farmlands, and grasslands of the village. The river valley is open and flat. Upstream the Si'ergou River is the Naoshan mountain area with high mountainous woodlands and grasslands. Si'ergou Village is beautiful and tranquil throughout the four seasons. In summer,

H. Wang (✉)
Institute of Quantitative and Technical Economics, Chinese Academy of Social Sciences, Beijing, China

Case Studies of Targeted Poverty Reduction and Alleviation in 100 Villages, International Research on Poverty Reduction, https://doi.org/10.1007/978-981-95-0549-4_6

the golden rapeseed flowers, purple potato flowers, and colorful wildflowers on the plateau will add a touch of color and fragrance to this place, creating a captivating atmosphere.

Like many other multi-ethnic villages in the area, Si'ergou Village primarily developed in size after the land reform and population migration after 1949. From 2016 to 2019, the research team conducted several years of investigations into the targeted poverty alleviation and targeted poverty eradication efforts in Si'ergou Village. This period also witnessed the development and changes in social security, rural development, and poverty alleviation industries in this village. These big changes are of historical significance for the village, and have benefited the villagers at large.

6.1 The Intensive Promotion of Social Security and Poverty Alleviation

Si'ergou Village is a provincially designated key poverty-stricken village located in the deep high mountainous region of Qinghai Province. In recent years, the country has provided unprecedented support and assistance to the poverty-stricken population in the village, with an aim to fundamentally change the poor people's situation and the environment they lived in, and at the same time build up their self-development capabilities.

In 2016, 45 households (152 individuals in total) were registered as poverty-stricken population, and the poverty rate and poverty incidence were 18% and 14%, respectively. The figures were all higher than the local average. In terms of basic living indicators for measuring the level of poverty, such as per capita arable land, average household farming machinery, housing conditions, average household food expenditure, and transportation conditions, Si'ergou Village was above the survival level, and the villagers had both food and shelter.

Disease, disability, and lack of labor force and incapacity to generate income are the main poverty-causing factors for the poor households in Si'ergou Village. According to the List of Poverty Alleviation Targets in Qinghai Province submitted by this village at the end of 2016, only 3 of all the 45 poverty-stricken households were caused by the lack of labor force, and only 1 was caused by lack of skills. The other 41 households fell into the illness- or disability-caused poverty. The result was testified by the investigation of the village and households. There is a significant difference in the health rates between the poor and non-poor populations. The higher prevalence of illness, total medical expenses, and out-of-pocket expenses imposed a heavier burden on poverty-stricken households. There is a significant disparity exists in per capita living consumption expenditure between the poor and non-poor households, mainly in terms of medical expenses. Illness and disability have reduced the labor forces in poverty-stricken households, undermining their ability to generate income through local farming and out-of-town work. Moreover, the poverty-stricken population are generally low-skilled, so the poor and non-poor households differ significantly in the number and structure of labor force, days of out-of-town work, and daily income, etc. All affected the income-generating capacity of the poor labor. The slow increase in income and the rising cost of household expenses have resulted in poverty that features low income and high expenditure.

To achieve real poverty eradication requires distinguishing two different groups of poverty-stricken individuals. For those who lack the conditions to lift themselves out of poverty through their own efforts and market returns, it is necessary to provide them with risk protection and social security guarantees. Therefore, social security is an important component of targeted poverty alleviation. China has promptly implemented relevant policies and given corresponding subsidies and assistance to those who meet the conditions for rural subsistence allowances, medical assistance, temporary assistance, housing assistance, etc. In 2016, the total amount of state assistance and support received by villagers in Si'ergou Village was 1,346,506 yuan, which greatly reduced the economic pressure on the villagers. Specifically, the country has issued 210,000 yuan of rural subsistence allowances, 43,000 yuan of five guarantees, 9600 yuan of disability subsidies, 50,000 yuan of medical assistance for serious illnesses, 7000 yuan of temporary assistance, and 7200 yuan of subsidies for children in difficult situations. A total of 126,000 yuan was distributed as pensions to villagers aged 60 and above, while elderly individuals aged 70 and above received an old-age allowance of 36,000 yuan. The reimbursement rate of medical expenses for villagers reached 28%. Moreover, priority was given to the renovation of dilapidated houses for those eligible beneficiaries in agricultural and pastoral areas. In 2016, a total of 177,000 yuan was provided for the renovation of dilapidated houses for a total of 9 households in the village. These social security policies have provided tangible benefits to villagers and greatly reduced their economic pressures.

6.2 Building Beautiful Countryside: Significant Improvement of the Living Environment

Si'ergou Village is 13 km away from the town government, 35 km away from the county, 40 km away from the Menyuan High-speed Railway Station, and 1.5 km away from the nearest bus station. The remoteness made it difficult for the villagers to enjoy convenient living and housing conditions that were only available in towns. However, in recent years, governments at all levels have actively integrated funds from various sources to carry out poverty alleviation with infrastructure reaching each household in the village. Hence, the living conditions in the village have been greatly improved. Since 2016, the local government has integrated funds from a series of projects, such as the collaborative construction project of the Party, government, military, and enterprises, the comprehensive project of village appearance enhancement, and the Highland Beautiful Village project, to build the Si'ergou Village into beautiful countryside. This project involved a large number of infrastructure projects, including the construction of roads, hydropower, cultural squares, etc. Besides, a total of 11.6 km of road were built, and the treatment of hazardous rock mass as well as river channel regulation was completed, coupled with two bridge culverts constructed. In 2017, the Development and Reform Bureau of Menyuan County approved an investment of 13.26 million yuan in construction funds for the building of the Highland Beautiful Countryside Ecological Square of the Si'ergou Village. The project constructed ecological gardens of 5000 square meters, wooden pavilions of 36 square meters, horticultural forests of 400 square meters, a plaza of 1000 square meters, and 40 solar streetlights. Additionally, a sports square was built, which included a garden area of 1500 square meters, a basketball court of 800 square meters, a set of fitness equipment and basketball stands, and 20 solar streetlights. When the project was completed, the village's appearance realized radical changes. Today, Si'ergou Village has become a "most beautiful village" characterized by pastoral beauty, village charm, and quality of life.

With the construction of various public facilities in Si'ergou Village, the daily cultural, entertainment, and leisure activities of the villagers were enriched increasingly. The newly built village cultural square has become the main venue for villagers to relax, entertain, and engage in social activities. The office building of the villager's committee is built to the north side of the village square, with a construction area of 220 square meters. Its construction began in March 2015 and was completed in December 2016. The spacious and bright building has blue tiles and white walls. In front of the office building, on the village cultural square, there are basketball stands for young people, and the elderly chat and bask in the sun leisurely. Villagers engage in daily activities on the square, so their spare time activities become richer and healthier. In the village kindergarten, children enjoy happy times under the guidance of teachers from the early childhood education center. The Happy Courtyard next to the kindergarten allows the seven "Five Guarantees elderly people" who are collectively housed in the village to spend their twilight years in peace.

6.3 Start-Up and Operation of Industrial Projects for Poverty Alleviation

The approach of poverty alleviation by developing industries and businesses is undertaken for poverty-stricken villagers who have either full or partial labor capabilities but have difficulty in generating income due to their conditions and the level of local economy. In Si'ergou Village, the development idea of the industrial projects for poverty alleviation is to leverage the advantages of the highland pasture resources in order to drive the development of large-scale animal husbandry industries. The investigation and research between 2016 and 2019 witnessed the process from the establishment to the operation of the Si'ergou Village Enterprise Ecological Breeding Cooperative out of nothing, which is the village's first government-led collective industrial poverty alleviation project.

Si'ergou Village enjoys favorable environmental, resource, and location advantages for the development of highland animal husbandry. Located at the foot of Daban Mountain, the village is far from industrial pollution sources with clean air and quality water. The village enjoys a relatively warm climate, fertile soil, and abundant water resources, providing conditions for producing green agricultural products. The grassland spans 13 km on both sides of the Si'ergou River, with a natural grassland area of approximately 40,630 mu.[1] This natural, pollution-free, and pristine highland pasture is uncontracted under collective ownership. The grass is of high yield, rich in nutritional value, strong in palatability, and producing livestock with high-quality meat. Therefore, it is a great place to develop a forage base as well as semi-pastured feeding and semi-confined breeding industries. To address the shortage of natural grass during winter and spring seasons, Si'ergou Village grows about 2500 mu of pasture annually, with an average yield of 1800 kg of fresh grass per mu, totaling approximately 4500 tons of fresh grass per year. Over the years, villagers have roughly achieved a sound balance between natural grasslands, pasture planting, and cattle and sheep breeding. According to village officials and skilled breeders, with such a large area of grassland, in a way of semi-confined breeding, the grassland can accommodate over 5000 cattle and over 10,000 sheep without jeopardizing the ecological balance. At present, the livestock inventory of the village has not yet reached the limit, which leaves ample room for the development of large-scale farming. In addition, the upgrading of infrastructure in recent years has greatly changed the production conditions of the village and provided necessary conditions for the exchange of commodities and information between the village and the outside world. Furthermore, Menyuan County, where the village is located, is an important production base for livestock products such as beef and mutton, milk, and other specialties in Qinghai Province, which provides a sound market environment for the development of the special breeding industry in Si'ergou Village. The villagers of Si'ergou have also long been engaged in animal husbandry, and many of them have experience in family or larger-scale breeding operations.

Developing animal husbandry is an important source of income for rural households. According to the villagers and village officials, the cost of raising a Simmental beef cattle, including the calf, feed, and labor, is around 4000 yuan. The cost of raising a sheep is around 400 yuan. The selling price of cattle is around 15,000–16,000 yuan, with an average of 15,500 yuan, while the selling price of sheep is around 600–1000 yuan, with an average of around 900 yuan. Cattle are usually ready for sale after 2 years, while sheep can be sold after 1 year. Therefore, the income from one beef cattle could reach around 5000 yuan per year, and the income from one sheep could reach around 500 yuan.

However, the breeding industry in Si'ergou Village is still featured by traditional family-based scattered production, with a simple product structure, small scale, low added value, vulnerable to risk, and weak foundation, making it difficult for the poor population to increase income in more ways. In order to improve the income-generating capacity of villagers and help them lift themselves out of poverty, in

[1] Mu, a unit of area (=0.0667 hectares). – Trans.

November 2015, the stationed First Secretary was sent to the village. After multiple consultations among the villager's committee and the village Party committee and some Party members, the decision was made to fully utilize the advantages of Si'ergou Village to develop special breeding industry in accordance with the local conditions and promote poverty alleviation through creating new economic activity. After discussion, the villager's committee decided to establish a specialized breeding cooperative, with a breeding leader who also serves as the village director recommended and elected by the village to be the chairman of the cooperative.

On March 1, 2016, the Specialized Ecological Breeding Cooperative in Si'ergou Village was officially established. The cooperative's development plan was reported to the Dongchuan Township Government and received strong support. In the first half of 2016, the Dongchuan Township Government decided to support Si'ergou Village in implementing an industrial project under the targeted poverty alleviation plan, with the Si'ergou Village Specialized Ecological Breeding Cooperative as the main implementing body. In June 2016, the Dongchuan Township Government of Menyuan County formulated *the Plan for Implementing the 2016 Targeted Poverty Alleviation Industrial Support Project in Si'ergou Village.* The project was supervised by the Dongchuan Township Government, applied by the Si'ergou villager's committee, and was led by the town governor. The plan provided detailed designs for the project's construction conditions, goals and contents, investment estimates, benefit analysis, operation mechanism, and organization management. The site of the poverty alleviation project is in Dadonggou Ditch Beach of Si'ergou Village, Dongchuan Town, which is at a higher altitude. The project plan is to adopt the form of "Cooperative + Poverty-stricken households" in investing poverty alleviation funds in the village cooperative, which is responsible for developing the planting and animal breeding industries in stages.

The investment and dividend distribution arrangements of the cooperative are reviewed and approved by the Poverty Alleviation Bureau of Menyuan County and Dongchuan Township Government. The cooperative signed an agreement with the villager's committee. Taking the form of "Cooperative + Poverty-stricken households", and following personal wishes of the poverty-stricken households, the poverty alleviation funds (6400 yuan per person in Tibetan areas) for the targeted poverty alleviation households are invested in the village enterprise, the Specialized Ecological Breeding Cooperative. On the principle of "enjoy the profits, and not bear the losses", there will be a dividend of 10% proportion of the injected capital to be offered at the end of the year, regardless of the profitability of the project. When the dividend is paid, the cooperative will hand over the dividend funds to the township government which will deliver the money to the targeted poverty alleviation households.

The total amount of actual investment for the project construction is 3,267,200 yuan, including the poverty alleviation funds, 947,200 yuan allocated to Menyuan County. The cooperative utilized the special poverty alleviation funds as guarantee funds to apply for a loan of 1.8 million yuan from the Agricultural Bank of Menyuan County. The Haibei Tibetan Autonomous Prefecture Ethnic and Religious Affairs Committee provided 330,000 yuan as development funds, and the contact support units provided 30,000 yuan as well as the county-level subsidy funds 60,000 yuan.

The non-poor members of the cooperative contributed 100,000 yuan in shares. A total of 42 poverty-stricken households with 148 poor individuals (excluding those covered by subsistence allowances) benefited from this project.

The fixed investment in project construction reached more than 2 million yuan, accounting for over 60% of the total investment. The cooperative built an ecological farm in Dadonggou Ditch Beach, covering an area of 30.05 mu, with a total construction area of 4632 square meters. There are four livestock farming sheds, each with an infrastructure investment of 190,000 yuan, taking up a total area of 2184 square meters. The construction cost of the four sheds was nearly 800,000 yuan, and that of the 700-m perimeter wall reached up to 700,000 yuan. A grass storage shed covering 585 square meters and 8 accessory offices were also constructed. After the infrastructure of the farming base was completed in 2017, supporting infrastructure such as water and electricity supply gradually came into place. The ecological farm is located in the deep mountains of Si'ergou Village, so an investment was made to build a 3-km-long gravel road leading to the farming site. In 2018, the power supply department connected over 3 km of electricity lines from the village to the farming site. The drinking water comes from a well, which was drilled and supplied within the farming site with an investment of over 3000 yuan by the cooperative. The cooperative also installed monitors mostly used for calf production.

The cooperative officially started in 2016. In an interview with the cooperative Chairman and concurrent Village Director, we knew that the cooperative's production and operation activities ran normally from 2016 to the first half of 2019. In 2016, the cooperative purchased sheep, and 1200 lambs were fattened for market. The average sale income from each lamb was about 860 yuan, with a total income of 1.09 million yuan. The variable costs, including labor and feed, amounted to 230,000 yuan, while the cost of purchasing the lambs was approximately 550,000 yuan. In 2016, the village enterprise of Menyuan County, the Specialized Ecological Breeding Cooperative paid a dividend of 94,720 yuan to 42 households, benefiting a total of 148 poor individuals in Si'ergou Village, and the average dividend was 640 yuan per person. Non-poor households also received a dividend of 10,000 yuan based on 10% of their investment shares. The total dividend of the above items reached 104,720 yuan. The cooperative did not incur any bank loan interest in 2016, and the income excluding fixed asset depreciation was around 200,000 yuan.

In 2017 and 2018, the cooperative adjusted the structure of livestock breeds, and kept the normal operation as usual, but the income decreased year by year. From 2017 to 2018, the cooperative purchased more than 70 Simmental beef cattle with more than 20 calves to be reproduced, and raised more than 200 sheep. In October 2018, 700 large ewes were purchased, and more than 500 lambs were reproduced. More than 50 beef cattle and 200 sheep were sold from 2017 to 2018, generating sales revenue of approximately 1.21 million yuan. The total cost of purchasing, breeding, and reproducing cattle and sheep was around 424,000 yuan, and the variable costs, including labor and feed, amounted to 460,000 yuan. The cooperative paid a dividend of 209,440 yuan to poor households and non-poor villagers who had made share investments. After repaying a bank loan of 600,000 yuan, the remaining 1.2 million yuan loan incurred an interest income of 100,800 yuan. The total cost amounted to 1.19 million yuan. From 2017 to 2018, taking into account the loan interest and depreciation excluding fixed assets, the cooperative incurred a loss of approximately 20,000 yuan. The net income in 2017 was around 100,000 yuan, while in 2018, there was a loss of around 80,000 yuan.

The proportion of cattle and sheep farming was further adjusted in 2019, with more than 30 cattle and 600 sheep. Since the costs of purchasing or reproducing and breeding the calves and lambs have already been included in the costs of the years 2017–2018, there is no need to double count in 2019. However, even after deducting the remaining interest of 50,000 yuan on the 600,000 yuan loan, the labor and feed costs of 230,000 yuan, and the dividends to be paid, the profitability of cooperative remained less positive in 2019. After the loan was paid off, the cooperative faced difficulty in maintaining working capital.

6.4 Industry Poverty Alleviation: The Inherent Contradiction Between the Philosophy and Practice

In recent years, the implementation of the poverty alleviation project in Si'ergou Village is more like an unprecedented experiment of industrial development. In the process of project implementation, the organizers, implementers, and participants have directly or indirectly experienced the conflicts arising from the inherent contradiction between the philosophy and practice of industry poverty alleviation. This conflict has had an impact on various aspects involved in the poverty alleviation projects, presenting practical challenges and difficulties to the implementation of the industrial poverty alleviation model and even hampering the sustainable development of the projects.

Objectively, there exist certain inherent contradictions between the philosophy and practice of industry poverty alleviation. The goal is to lift people out of poverty, and the means was industrial development. "Industrialization" implies the significant role of the market economy in resource allocation. However, the measures of industry poverty alleviation per se are part of social policies. Governments at all levels formulate social policies, exercise administrative means, carry out institutional arrangements, and allocate public resources to enhance the self-development capacity of poverty-stricken groups and improve the economic development environment in economically disadvantaged areas. Therefore, in the process of industry poverty alleviation, it is necessary to resolve the contradictions between market power and administrative policies. On the one hand, the government should respect the market power, and on the other hand, properly use administrative power. The government should not take over everything or even take replace of others, but instead should provide sufficient public services of professional skills, promote more rural households engagement, coordinate cooperation between villagers, and cultivate villagers' self-development capabilities.

Supported by the national industry poverty alleviation policies, the design of operational mechanism for the poverty alleviation project in Si'ergou Village is systematic and complete, and the investment sources are also guaranteed. However, due to the inherent contradiction between the philosophy and practice of industry poverty alleviation itself, the project has encountered some conflicts and problems during its actual operation. The main manifestations are as follows.

6.4.1 The Contradiction Between Policy Environment and Project Management

The industry poverty alleviation project in Si'ergou Village was implemented in a favorable environment. With strong support from the central government, Qinghai Province has formulated comprehensive and targeted industry poverty alleviation policies and built a comprehensive industry-based poverty alleviation system from the county, village to households. Substantial financial resources have been invested in poverty alleviation, and made outstanding cases as a reference for studying such as the Lage'ri Village in Ningxiu Township, Zeku County. The Dongchuan Township Government, as the organizer and coordinator of the project, has formulated an implementation plan for industry poverty alleviation, which stipulates the implementation plan and operation mechanism of the project, the poverty alleviation funds and the dividend-sharing methods of shares investment, etc. The government has given full support to Si'ergou Village in carrying out the industry poverty alleviation project.

However, a favorable policy support environment does not offset the practical difficulties in project implementation and management. As the grassroots management institution for the Si'ergou Village industry poverty alleviation projects, the Dongchuan Township Government expressed that there are significant challenges in government management during the project implementation. It is the primary responsibility of the Dongchuan Township Government to ensure the security of poverty alleviation funds for poverty-stricken households and the distribution of dividend funds on schedule, and further to achieve the expected poverty alleviation targets for poverty-stricken households. For this reason, the Dongchuan Township Government scrutinized the project plan prior to implementation, and coordinated government poverty alleviation funds. After multiple discussions, the government injected poverty alleviation funds into the cooperative and then utilized these funds as leverage to attract commercial loans from local agricultural banks, and grant the cooperative free-interest treatment in the first year. Even so, during this process, the town government encountered practical difficulties. The cooperative in Si'ergou Village was just started and did not own any high valuable assets as collateral then, so it could not implement the procedure of evaluation and notarization, which means the invested funds cannot be guaranteed due to the lack of effective collateral. Additionally, as a newly established cooperative, its organizers and operators have no experience in large-scale production and market operation. Besides, in order to encourage the development of the village collective cooperative, the Dongchuan Town has applied the principle of "sharing both benefits and risks" to the investment and profit sharing. Therefore, it involves certain economic risks. In this regard, Dongchuan Township Government clearly expressed its concern about the risk of the project.

6.4.2 Contradiction Due to the Imbalance Between Administrative Power and Market Power

Industry poverty alleviation not only requires the country to formulate various policies, exercise administrative means, implement institutional arrangements, and allocate public resources, but also the market economy to play an important role in resource allocation, so as to properly regulate the balance between administrative and market power. During the investigation and research of the village, it is found that in the process of implementing industry poverty alleviation projects, the administrative power of the government far exceeds the market power, and there is a significant imbalance contradictions between the two.

The local government worked actively and conscientiously during the project implementation, but it also took on responsibilities beyond its capacity. The Dongchuan Township Government has coordinated and managed to provide interest-free or low-interest commercial loans for the project despite the high pressure when the village cooperative lacked higher-value effective collateral assets. The village industry poverty alleviation project has been heavily dependent on government support in terms of investment, fixed asset construction, working capital, and profitability. The total investment of the project was up to 3,267,200 yuan of which a commercial loan of 1.8 million yuan came from the local Agricultural Bank, only accounting for 55% of the total investment. The local government allowed the cooperative to use poverty alleviation funds as collateral for the commercial loan, and the loan was interest-free in the first year. The remaining investment came from poverty alleviation funds for poverty-stricken households, county subsidies, and support funds from supporting departments and organizations. In the construction and operation of cooperative, most of the fixed asset investment was covered by government support funds, and the interest-free commercial loan in the first year provided the cooperative with all the working capital in need. In terms of profitability, although the cooperative made some profits in 2016 and 2017, this was achieved without considering the depreciation of fixed assets, and the income and profits of the cooperative significantly declined since 2017. Taking the depreciation of fixed assets into consideration, the cooperative may not be truly profitable even in the first year. During the cooperative operation, the Secretary of the Menyuan County Party Committee took two field trips to Si'ergou Village, and approved highly of the role of the cooperative in poverty alleviation. However, he also found the financial difficulties encountered in development and then provided Si'ergou Village with 300,000 yuan of poverty alleviation premium for its production and operation. The

Chairman of the cooperative believed that this fund was an important help in time of need. However, it also reflects the fact that the project of poverty alleviation through industry in Si'ergou Village is overly dependent on government support.

In order to support the market-oriented operation of industry poverty alleviation projects, it is necessary to select, design, and operate the projects in accordance with market rules at the beginning of the project cultivation. In terms of profitability, according to the information provided by the chairman of the cooperative, during the 3 years from 2016 to 2018, regardless of fixed asset investments, the situation of the cooperative changed from 200,000 yuan to 100,000 yuan and finally to a loss of over 80,000 yuan, along with the shrinking production scale and declining business profitability continuously. The cooperative had to face a lack of cash flow and no profit accumulation. According to the loan contract between the cooperative and the bank, 2019 was the final year for loan repayment. However, the cooperative lacked the ability to repay the loan in full and on time. As breeding, especially larger-scale breeding, requires large amounts of working capital for the purchase of calves and lambs, the cooperative cannot maintain or expand its scale of production after repaying the loan. The cooperative fails to realize real market-oriented operations and lacks market competitiveness as well as sustainability.

6.4.3 The Technical and Economic Problems of the Project Behind the Changes of Chairman's Mindset

During the implementation of the industry poverty alleviation project in Si'ergou Village from 2016 to 2018, the attitude of the cooperative chairman toward the project changed significantly. In late 2016 and February 2017, during the first two visits of field trips, when the cooperative breeding project was at the start-up stage, the chairman was highly ambitious about its development prospects. During another field trip in July 2017, the infrastructure of the breeding farm was basically completed, and supporting infrastructure such as water and electricity lines was about to be completed in sequence. The chairman of the cooperative confidently showed the research team around the breeding sheds, grass storage sheds, office space, and other facilities, and presented the breeding plans of the cooperative. He believed that the village's 40,000 mu of high-quality resources could boost the income of the villagers, especially those in poverty. The cooperative also provided two employment opportunities for the villagers, which brought them real income. However, during the field trip in July 2018, the chairman led the researchers to have a guided tour to the breeding sheds in investigating the beef cattle and the breeding operation, and expressed concern about the shortage of working capital and hoped that the government could provide financial assistance. In just 3 years passing, the chairman's full confidence turned into deep concern.

Behind this change of mentality showing diminished confidence and increasing concern, there lie the inherent flaws in the project that existed even before its initiation. Without scientific analysis of its technical and economic conditions and rational project design, the poverty alleviation project failed to make good use of the funds. Normally, agriculture and animal husbandry industry projects often have the characteristics of high fixed investment, high demand for working capital, low return on investment, and a long investment payback period, which poses a significant challenge for the market-oriented project in poverty alleviation industry. Generally speaking, when allocating funds for investment, it is necessary to fully consider the unique characteristics of the breeding projects, appropriately allocate the proportion of investment in fixed assets, scientific estimation, and meet the working capital requirements of the project, so as to ensure the normal operation of project. Along with the production and operation, it is important to properly configure the scale and structure of products. With the market demand taken into account, it should be ensured that the sales income can secure sufficient capital inflow and a certain profit can be obtained while meeting the cash flow demand. In the actual operation, the initial investment plan, product plan, and revenue estimation will have to change to a certain degree, and need to be adjusted timely according to the market and operational conditions.

The survey in this village has revealed some questions in the development of the cooperative's breeding base. The cooperative has only conducted basic investment and cost estimation, product design, and profitability analysis. There was a lack of proper technical and economic analysis for the project, with insufficient consideration of depreciation costs of fixed investments and the failure to rational plan the relationship between fixed investments and working capital. There were also no rational adjustments to the product scale in accordance with the management and market situation, resulting in suboptimal utilization of funds. The cooperative's production scale, cash inflows, and profitability did not reach the level required to operate the project normally, thus adversely affecting its proper functioning. According to the Chairman, the fixed asset investment in the construction of the breeding base amounted to over 2 million yuan. The construction investment of only four sheds reached 0.8 million yuan and the construction cost of a 700-m fence was up to 0.7 million yuan. In addition, there were expenses for building roads to the base, feed storage and processing factories, dormitories, and the purchase of motorcycles, etc. The proportion of fixed asset investment was too high, accounting for over 60% of the total investment, which severely affected the sound operation of project funds. Since the funds were mainly used for the construction of fixed assets, there was very little liquidity left in the cooperative's account. Additionally, after the project was launched, the product design changed, and the previously planned poultry farming was not carried out, and the Tibetan sheep farm was changed to Hu sheep[2] farm. The scale of farming was also reduced. Without sufficient product size, there is no adequate cash income for the cooperative to reach the cash inflow and income levels that make the project function properly.

[2] A kind of sheep raised in Zhejiang Province. – Trans.

From the case of Si'ergou Village, it is evident that local governments and grassroots administrative departments must have a comprehensive understanding of the technical and economic characteristics of the agriculture and husbandry industries when implementing poverty alleviation projects, particularly those related to agriculture and animal husbandry. It is necessary to make technical and economic analysis of project costs and benefits to optimize the utilization of funds. For projects with a high proportion of fixed asset investment and large liquidity demands, it is necessary to rationally allocate the proportion of fixed asset investment and scientifically estimate and guarantee the amount of liquidity needed for the project. To ensure the smooth implementation of poverty alleviation projects, the government should provide arrangement in advance of the technical training and training on enterprise management for capable people who play a leading role in poverty alleviation, which will enable them to acquire the skills needed for industrialized operation management and allow them to configure the scale and structure of products according to market demand during the production. In cases where there are some changes in the initial investment plan, product plan, and income estimation during the project operation, timely adjustments should be made in accordance with market and business situation.

6.4.4 The Balance Between Benefit Sharing and Interest Conflict

The implementation of the industry poverty alleviation project in Si'ergou Village faces the inevitable challenge from balancing the conflicts of interest and the benefit sharing between participants and non-participants, as well as those internal conflicts among participants. The project has received financial support from the government and the coordination and organization that various departments made in full swing. It has also obtained interest-free loans from the commercial banks. At the village level, the cooperative has also been granted the priority right to use the village collective grasslands by default. These preferential policies and resource allocations result in tilted interests in favor of participating villagers. However, this can also mean a certain degree of unfairness in benefit sharing for other villagers. On our way to the cooperative's farming base, we encountered a woman hitchhiking to feed the cattle in her own breeding shed located in the grasslands. She expressed her dissatisfaction by stating that as she had a family-run farm, so she could not join the cooperative to enjoy any benefit or preference.

The benefit sharing among project participants is set fairly through the profit-sharing mechanism reviewed and approved by the Poverty Alleviation Bureau of Menyuan County and Dongchuan Township Government. The cooperative and the villager's committee signed an agreement based on the principle of "enjoy the profits, and not bear the losses", which was to distribute dividends at the end of the year and protect the villagers from losses. Regardless of the profitability of the project, a dividend of 10% of the injected capital amount will be distributed to the households at the end of the year. When it is time to distribute the dividends, the cooperative will turn in the money for distribution to the township government which will then give the money to the poverty alleviation households. From 2016 to 2018, the poverty-stricken households who invested in the cooperative received the expected dividends on schedule and in full. However, the cooperative's benefit-sharing mechanism is currently faced with two difficulties. First, when the industry poverty alleviation project underperforms, experiences a decline in profitability, or incurs losses, the interests of the villager shareholders will be also affected, which is also a loss of government support funding. Second, at present, the Party Secretary of the village has limited knowledge of the specific management situation of the cooperative which has a low participation rate of poverty-stricken villagers. The operation of the cooperative should be improved to be more transparent and standardized.

Another important purpose of the industry poverty alleviation project is to enable poverty-stricken households to actively participate in industry development, so that they can gain production and business experience, and improve their income-generating and increasing capabilities, which is another benefit-sharing mechanism. In practical terms, local capable people or larger households take the lead in implementing the poverty alleviation project with more advantages and capabilities in terms of market, technology, and products compared to ordinary villagers. Participating in the national industry poverty alleviation project has provided them with greater advantages and capabilities, which is difficult for individual villagers to acquire through learning. For poverty-stricken villagers, although the dividend mechanism ensures their economic benefits, they still lack an effective participation mechanism that allows them to gain production and business experiences and enhance their income-generating and income-increasing capabilities through learning. In this regard, the government should adhere to the principles of fairness and justice, allocate public resources reasonably, provide learning and practice opportunities for poverty-stricken villagers, and establish a cooperation mechanism that genuinely involves households, promotes co-progress through learning, and facilitates benefit sharing. This will enable poverty-stricken villagers to not only share economic benefits but also enjoy opportunities for learning and improvement.

References

Chen, L., & Huo, X. (2006). Exploring the Development Paths and System Construction of Green Agriculture in China: The Case of Menyuan Basin in Qinghai. *Development Research*, No. 4.

Dawa, C. (2017). A Study on the Consistency and Differences of Different Cultures in Multi-ethnic Mixed Villages: A Sample Survey of Interlocking Residential Villages in the Farming and Pastoral Areas of Qinghai Province. *Qinghai-Tibet Plateau Forum*, No. 4.

Liang, C. (2015). The Operation Mechanism of Industrial Poverty Alleviation Projects and The Role of Local Government. *Journal of Beijing University of Technology (Social Science Edition)*, No. 5.

Ma, B., & Zhu, C. (2018). Research on Targeted Poverty Alleviation in Ethnic Autonomous Regions of Qinghai Province—An Investigation Based on Haibei Tibetan Autonomous Prefecture. *Climbing*, No. 1.

Shen, H. (2014). Research on the Construction of Industrial Poverty Alleviation Mechanism in Tibetan Areas of Qinghai. *Ningxia Social Science*, No. 4.

Wang, C. (2015). Research on Rural Development and Poverty Alleviation from the Perspective of Social Governance. *Journal of the Party School of the CPC Fujian Provincial Committee*, No. 3.

Yuan, E., & Peng, B. (2010). Analysis of the Income Situation of Rural Residents in Qinghai Province Since the Reform and Opening Up. *Science and Technology Information*, No. 15.

Zuo, T. (2018). Institutional Design and Path Choices for Stable Poverty Eradication. *Guangming Daily*, September 25.

Hong Wang , Associate Research Fellow at the Institute of Quantitative & Technical Economics of the Chinese Academy of Social Sciences. Her major research interests are technical economics and circular economics.

Chapter 7
A Taihang Mountain Village's Road to Tourism and Cultural Prosperity: Practice of Poverty Eradication in Luotuowan Village, Fuping, Hebei

Yuejin Wang and Jing Li

Abstract This paper examines the path of poverty alleviation in a deep mountain village in the Yanshan-Taihang Mountains under the jurisdiction of Fuping County, Hebei Province. Through observation of the process of poverty alleviation in Luotuowan Village from 2017 to 2020, the author finds that the prosperity experience of Luotuowan Village is to turn its disadvantaged environment into an advantageous tourism resources, thus injecting vitality into this dying mountain village and forming a prosperity pattern with the synergy of tourism culture and other industries. The big change in Luotuowan Village has explored a new model based on the synergy of development-oriented and targeted poverty alleviation. The paper also considers how to increase the participation of young migrant workers returning to their hometowns and the relative poverty in the future.

Keywords Targeted poverty alleviation · A moderate prosperity · Cultural revival in village · Luotuowan village

Most of the poor villages in China are located in mountainous areas with harsh geographical conditions, and poor mountain villages are the main battlefield for poverty alleviation. Luotuowan Village is such a poverty-stricken village in deep Taihang Mountains. December 30, 2012, is a historic day for Luotuowan Village. Early in the morning of that day, Xi Jinping, General Secretary of CPC, came to Luotuowan Village deep in the snow-capped mountains. During this research, General Secretary Xi suggested that "to help people in need to get out of poverty and get rich, we should carry out targeted work and investigate their situation one

Y. Wang
Huzhou University, Huzhou, China

J. Li (✉)
Rural Development Institute, Chinese Academy of Social Sciences, Beijing, China

Case Studies of Targeted Poverty Reduction and Alleviation in 100 Villages, International Research on Poverty Reduction, https://doi.org/10.1007/978-981-95-0549-4_7

by one",[1] which provided the basis for Chinese poverty alleviation to shift from development-oriented to targeted poverty alleviation, and also pointed out the direction for the poverty alleviation in Luotuowan Village. Since then, Luotuowan Village has embarked on an endeavor to make a significant change through poverty alleviation. 8 years later, the previous poverty-stricken mountainous village has become a tourist destination. And Luotuowan Village has been transformed into a new model for the nationwide poverty alleviation in China.

7.1 Basic Situation of Luotuowan and the Causes of Poverty

"Nine Mountains half-and-half with water and arable land, Luotuowan is located in the high mountains and deep in the ravine", the villagers use a short phrase to describe the situation of Luotuowan. The natural village of Luotuowan is located in the west of Fuping County, deep in the Taihang Mountains and to the west of Wutai Mountain. It is an administrative village under Longquanguan Town, about 5.4 km away from Longquanguan Town. It became a village during the Hongwu Period of Ming Dynasty out of the commercial road at the Weihe River Wharf, and was a small village where the ancient imperial road of the Qing Dynasty must be passed by the Kangxi Emperor on his five western pilgrimages to Mount Wutai, the Yongzheng Emperor on his one way to liturgy, the Qianlong Emperor on his six visits to the holy places, and the Jiaqing Emperor on his one visit to offer incense. When Kangxi passed through Fuping on his private visit to Wutai Mountain, he trapped in this big ravine and finally rode a camel in the village out of the big ravine to Wutai Mountain, so the village got the name Luotuowan[2] Village.

The administrative village of Luotuowan has 9 natural villages, including Luotuowan, Wayao, Liaodaobei, Muqiao, Caishuta, Zhuxingta, Yangshuta, Qingshitanggou, and canglianggou. Now, the villagers mainly live in two natural villages, Luotuowan and Wayao. Fuping County, where Luotuowan is located, is a typical mountainous and poverty-stricken county, which belongs to the national contiguous extremely poor area. It is also the combined area including old revolutionary base areas, the mountainous area and the poverty-stricken area. The Shanxi-Chahar-Hebei border area, to which it belongs, is the first enemy's rear area for anti-Japanese base created by the Chinese Communist Party and the Eighth Route Army.[3] Nie Rongzhen[4] formed the deepest bonds with the people here. He later said in a deep tone at a meeting of cadres: "It is true that Fuping is poor and many people eat

[1] Speech at the Inspection of Poverty Alleviation and Development Work in Fuping County, Hebei Province (December 29 and 30, 2012), "Being a Jiao Yulu-style County Party Secretary," Central Literature Publishing House, 2015, p. 17.

[2] English translation of Luotuowan is Camel Bay. – Trans.

[3] The army was led by the Chinese Communist Party during the War of Resistance Against Japan. – Trans.

[4] A renowned PLA marshal. – Trans.

leaves to get by. The impression that Fuping is poor made me feel a strong sympathy for the people of Fuping and often think about how to improve their lives and ease their burdens".[5] Fuping has been rated as a national poverty-stricken county since the country's "87" poverty alleviation program.[6] According to data from the Fuping County Poverty Alleviation Office, there were 164 poor villages out of 209 administrative villages in the county in 2012, accounting for 78.5 percent; the population of officially registered poverty-stricken members at the beginning of 2014 was 108, 100, accounting for 47.0 percent of the total population (total population 229,800). The poverty level of Fuping was high, and the economic indicators ranked back in the provincial and municipal rankings, far below the national, provincial, and city averages.

Fuping is poor, and Luotuowan (hereinafter referred to as the administrative village) is even poorer. The average altitude of Luotuowan is 1510 m, and the geographical location of Luotuowan is high in the mountains and deep in the ditches, and the terrain is precipitous and harsh. There was only one small mountain road from Longquanguan Town to Luotuowan Village and it was impassable for any vehicle, so villagers had to take several hours to go to Longquanguan Town on foot, which made the Luotuowan Village rarely known to local people. Moreover, the population of Luotuowan Village is extremely scattered, with 245 households in 9 natural villages, the farthest of which is 7 km away from the central village, and the smallest of which has only 4 households with 8 people.

The natural environment of high mountains and deep ditches is the main cause to the villagers' poverty. Gu Runjin, the former village CPC secretary of Luotuowan, has been leading the village to fight against poverty since 1995. According to Gu Runjin, in 2000, the Fuping County Animal Husbandry Bureau imported 100 milch goats from Shanxi Province to Luotuowan, and each of the 20 households in the village was given five goats. When the villagers were ready to make a big effort, the country started to implement the project of returning farmland to forest, and Luotuowan was included in the forest area, so the villagers had to sell the milch goats. After that, Gu Runjin encouraged the villagers to take advantage of the forest land to plant fast-growing forests, but as a result, the soil in the mountains was so infertile that the fast-growing forests could not grow at all. The last hope was to plant potatoes. "Luotuowan's potatoes are small with high nutritional value, delicious taste, and could be sold at a good price in the county, but it did not last long, due to the lack of technical guidance, there was low yield of potatoes, and potatoes were too small, and soon there was no way to sell".

In the eyes of the old secretary, Luotuowan has resource, because it is located to the west of Wutai Mountain, near the Tianshengqiao waterfall which has become a large-scale Tianshengqiao scenic area. Luotuowan is so close through the Luotuowan oxygen bar forest in the high altitude area directly to the Tianshengqiao waterfall that most tourists to Wutai Mountain will also tend to the Tianshengqiao waterfall. If some

[5] Nie Rongzhen, Memoirs of Nie Rongzhen, PLA Press, 1983, p.123.

[6] "87" means the seven-year program to help 80 million people out of poverty, from 1994 to 2000. – Trans.

tourists would like to Luotuowan tourism, then the tourism industry in Luotuowan will naturally grow up. Nevertheless, this requires the overall development of the village with huge amount of money to invest, and especially the road access is the primary problem, which makes entrepreneurs discouraged when they want to engage in tourism development.

After several struggles against poverty, the villagers of Luotuowan still have "one mu of land per capita, growing a little bit of corn, drinking some porridge and hoping to eat rice". Luotuowan has a small amount of continuous land and insufficient arable land resources. The "nine mountains half-and-half with water and arable land" means that aside from narrow lands to be irrigated, there are only "barren field" made out of stone blocks piled on the along the ridges of the mountain. Inside the Luotuowan Village, in a way of rough planting, agriculture planting has been involved with potatoes and corn crop predominantly which also serves for both people and animal with insignificant income. In 2012, there were 608 people in the village, 428 of whom were poor, and the main income of the villagers came from farming and working outside the village, with an annual per capita income of less than 900 yuan.

The result of increased poverty is a loss of labor, as young people leave, leaving the elderly and sick in the village. With long-term labor drain, Luotuowan has become an almost empty village. More and more young people began to count the economic accounts of inputs and outputs, and in 2012 there were only 200 people left in the village, the oldest of whom was 83 years old and the youngest 42 years old. Due to their low education and lack of skills for career advancement, most of the villagers who work outside the village have to get trapped in the urban poverty group, and it is difficult to rely on their income from working outside the village to give back to their hometown.

In the last two days in 2012, the widely known poverty-stricken village of Luotuowan finally encountered the turn of destiny. On December 30, 2012, General Secretary Xi Jinping braved the cold to visit the village at an altitude of 1512 m. During this visit, Xi Jinping said, "The most arduous and heavy task of building a well-off society is in the rural areas, especially in the poor areas. Without the prosperity in the rural areas, especially in the poor areas, there will be no prosperous society built in all aspects".[7] Moreover, he also put forward four principles for poverty alleviation and development work: to suit local conditions, to make scientific planning, to give targeted guidance, and to take advantage of the situation.

Soon after the General Secretary's visit to Fuping County, Fuping became a new landmark and sample for poverty alleviation in China, and Luotuowan Village was given a chance to change its fate. Fuping County was identified as a pilot county for regional development and poverty alleviation in the Yanshan-Taihang Mountains Area, and the State Council Leading Group Office of Poverty Alleviation and Development set up a coordination group for the Fuping pilot project in the Yanshan-Taihang Mountains Area. Hebei Province set up a leading group for poverty alleviation for Fuping. National ministries identified Fuping as a special support object,

[7] Xi Jinping: "No prosperity in poor areas, no prosperous society built in all respects", Xinhuanet, http://www.xinhuanet.com/, 29 December 2012.

which also approved Fuping as an economic development zone at the provincial level, and thus made an investment of 16 million RMB into the infrastructure. In 2013 alone, Fuping received 1.261 billion yuan in special funds from all levels, seven times the local revenue.

In 2013, under the guidance of the State Council Leading Group Office of Poverty Alleviation and Development, Fuping County completed the "Regional Development and Poverty Alleviation Implementation Plan for Fuping County in Yanshan-Taihang Mountains Area" on the basis of the county conditions, and set the goal of "three years to see great results, five years to stabilize poverty, eight years to build a moderately prosperous society". Since 2013, Fuping County has taken a holistic approach to promote economic and social development into consideration through poverty alleviation campaign, insisting on taking two steps to eradicate poverty and build a moderately prosperous society at the same time, and promoting poverty eradication and county development in an integrated manner. Fuping County proposed six major goals: first, to establish the Yantai Area regional development and poverty alleviation pilot, and to be the first to achieve the Yantai Area planning goals in implementing policies, innovating mechanism and institutions, in order to play a demonstration role in the Yantai Area. Second, to build the production and processing supply base for green and safe agricultural and sideline products. Third, to build a science and technology-oriented advanced manufacturing base. Fourth, to establish a well-known tourist destination in northern China. Fifth, to form an important logistics node in North China. Sixth, to build a demonstration zone for ecological development in the Beijing-Tianjin-Hebei metropolitan area.

7.2 Exploration of the Road to Poverty Alleviation and Prosperity

After General Secretary Xi's visit to Luotuowan, Fuping County included Luotuowan Village in the Yantai Area Regional Development and Poverty Alleviation Pilot Project, which solved the problem of Luotuowan's access road at first by building a new asphalt road more than 6 m wide which connects the national highway 382 from Fuping County to Shanxi Province in the north. After the road was paved, there were visitors coming here one after another. According to Gu Runjin's recollection, "there were new people coming almost every day when some were to invest in the construction while some were to investigate the project. Usually they drove to Luotuowan in the morning and drove away at night after taking a short tour, and there were countless cars with car plates of various areas, but no team was willing to stay for some days".

Further south to the Luotuo[8] Village, there are some villages such as Liaodaobei, Caishuta, etc., at the altitude close to 2300 m. The Liaodaobei Village is a natural village in the air which is located deep in the Taihang Mountains and is surrounded

8 Seems like Luotuo is a misspell word of Luotuowan, or the abbreviation. – Trans.

by primeval forest, which looks like a fairyland. There are more than 2000 kinds of vegetation and hundreds of medicinal herbs in the mountains, and it is called a natural oxygen bar. The Secretary General Xi Jinping's visit adds more fame to the Luotuowan Village. To develop tourism in Luotuowan and get rich is the common dream of villagers. "So many people come to have a tour, and if they stay here for a day, having two or three meals here, then the whole Luotuowan villagers' income will boost up". Some villagers began to run an agritainment business with the mentality of giving a try.

However, from 2013 to 2016, the 3 years saw Luotuowan's agritainment underdeveloped. Many people come for a tour, but not many want to stay in the homestay. And there are many people driving cars with dried food, so people are rarely seen to have dinner here. Why that happens? First, the villagers' business is of lower standard with insufficient equipment, which cannot attract tourists to stay overnight; second, the local villagers' cooking does not fit the taste of outside tourists, without varieties, and specialties.

In order to make Luotuowan Village a tourist destination, Fuping County has carried out a radical transformation and upgrading project for Luotuowan Village since 2015, inviting the China New Rural Planning and Design Institute to carry out a unified planning and transformation of Luotuowan's residential houses, and to advance the design and construction in accordance with the local traditional residential characteristics, in combination with the wishes of the household owners, household by household. According to the introductions from cadres stationed in the village, at first the people were resistant, as some of them felt that their white walls were good enough, why should they turn the white walls into adobe-colored walls, but when the people saw that the shabby and low adobe houses of others had turned into Taihang-style houses featuring green bricks, gray tiles, and adobe-yellow walls, they all joined the transformation and upgrading of their houses one after another. Today, there are rows and rows of neat and tidy featured houses, so you can not only experience the traditional and ancient atmosphere, but also overlook the surrounding mountains around the village with dense vegetation from afar, making people forget all worries and enjoy nature almost instantly. In 2018, the state included Luotuowan Village in the fifth batch of Chinese traditional ancient villages nationwide.

With the completion of the renovation of residential houses, the number of Luotuowan agritainment farmhouses has grown from 2 in 2015 to 13 in 2018. In 2019, a professional team from Beijing came here to build a special B&B tailored for Luotuowan, and Fuping County Gujiatai Luotuowan Tourism Development Limited Liability Company rented the villagers' houses to develop a unified high-standard for Luotuowan B&B ecotourism, which has been open since May 1, 2019. Since then, Luotuowan Village has cultural activities almost every weekend. In today's Luotuowan Village, the village traffic, public facilities, and villagers' morale have been greatly improved, full of vitality and hope, becoming a beautiful home for people to live and work in peace and happiness. There are mountain specialties shop, tea house outlooking mountains, Luotuowan New Year pictures, folklore skills workshop, wineries, Tofu Workshop, new B&B of primitive simplicity, food street carrying fragrance seen all over the place, which turns a once poverty-stricken mountain village into a well-known tourist attraction. In 2019, Luotuowan Village was awarded as the most beautiful leisure village in China.

On December 30, 2012, General Secretary Xi Jinping came to Luotuowan Village in Fuping County who visited Tang Rongbin's house and sat on the bed to talk with his family. Many tourists come to Luotuowan to visit the must-see attraction in Luotuowan, the Luotuowan No. 1 courtyard, the home address of Tang Rongbin, where still kept the same layout when General Secretary Xi Jinping came here. Everyday, there will be visitors one after another just for the purpose of getting a glimpse of the Luotuowan No. 1 courtyard. Tang Rongbin recalled that the iron pot on the stove was still steaming when General Secretary came in. The General Secretary uncovered the pot and saw steamed buns, corn cakes, sweet potatoes, potatoes, and pumpkins inside. Tang Rongbin's wife took out a piece of steamed potato from the pot and handed it to the general secretary. The General Secretary took a piece and put it in his mouth: "It tastes good!" He also asked his fellows to taste it. Then, the General Secretary sat on the bed and chatted with Tang Rongbin's family members about their family life. What impressed Tang most was that the General Secretary urged him to improve the education of his young grandson by saying that hope lies in the next generation so the next generation must be educated at first in order to lead a good life. Today, Tang Rongbin's Luotuowan No. 1 is rented by the village and become a tourist attraction, and his family moved into a new house renovated by the government in 2015, with thermal insulation on the exterior walls and floor heating in the house, which makes it warm in winter and comfortable to live in. Tang Rongbin used to do occasional day-work and farming, and he couldn't earn much money during a whole year. Now he has pensions, minimum living guarantee, with contracted land under the company cooperation, earning 1000 yuan per year from each mu[9] of land, and he can also work in the company to earn a salary. Furthermore, his land is transferred into the stock, so when the benefits are yielded, he can also enjoy 50–50 share dividends from the stock.

Another house that General Secretary Xi Jinping visited is of Tang Zongxiu who got out of poverty in 2017 with quite a lot of income from land transfer, share dividends, etc. On the May 1, 2019, a guest house tourism project developed by Fuyu Investment Company opened a business formally. The old couple, Tang Zongxiu and her husband, actively applied for jobs and were employed to do the house sanitation, take care of the flowers and plants, and earn more than 2000 RMB/month per person. "The company provides three meals a day, so we can eat in the company. The stewed vegetables, rice, noodles are served variously everyday, more preferable than eating at home!" In the past, some villagers were idle every day, but now they all have jobs, and it is hard to see idle people in the village. Fuyu Investment Company alone has employed more than 30 people from Luotuowan and more than 60 people from surrounding villages.

In 2018, when I came to Luotuowan for research, Luotuowan was doing the finishing work of demolishing old houses and building new ones, and various pipes

---

[9] 1 mu equals 1/15 hectare. –Trans.

were being laid under the village streets. Although there were tourists visiting the village every day, they left in a hurry after touring the No.1 courtyard. At that time, I stayed in a guesthouse, although the facilities inside were good enough, but low-end ones to me, which cost me 100 yuan per night. As there were few people checked in, they prepared meals less than usual, and I ate a bowl of egg noodles and left 20 yuan for the housekeeper who said 10 yuan was OK. Now again, the villagers' guesthouses are rent to Fuyu Investment Company. In front of the counter, the check-in procedures made me wait more than half an hour, because there were so many guests to check out and check in that people have to queue with only two clerks at the counter who were very busy with their stuff. The price of guesthouse charged per day ranges from 200 to 500. After checking in the small courtyard room, I found a variety of facilities in the house, which is the equal level as that of hotels in Fuping County. With higher level of services, the price also goes up. After checking in the guesthouse, I walked around the streets of Luotuowan, where there is a tofu workshop and an aromatic snack street. When I entered the tofu workshop, several guests of tables were already eating, and I picked up the menu and ordered two dishes and a bowl of congee costing a total of 50 yuan. While eating and watching tourists coming in and out, I felt the taste of Taihang Mountains, and the once poverty-stricken ravine of Luotuowan became a forever memory. Another change in Luotuowan is that more people from Fuping County come to work in the village. In 2018, I made a four-day research into the village and all the contacts were villagers. Now, the contacts when I checked in the guesthouse were salesmen whose home is in the county and commute to Luotuowan company to work. Luotuowan villagers told me that quite a lot of people outside come to work here, and they live in the Luotuowan staff dormitory and eat in the Luotuowan canteen. Luotuowan is now a veritable tourist destination, and many villagers work in the Fuyu company.

7.3 Young People Return to Their Hometowns to Inject Vitality to Luotuowan

By building up a leading tourism industry, Luotuowan Village has achieved poverty eradication. In the view of Liu Huage, the first secretary stationed in the village, the tourism industry is now doing great and has completely driven the villagers out of poverty and into prosperity, while Luotuowan Village does not stop at the tourism industry. The village task force dispatched by the province used the poverty alleviation funds to introduce a professional company to raise broiler chickens, but there was no available land in the village. The village Party branch and the village task force changed their ideas and opened a chicken farm in Pingyang town to start an "enclave economy". The chicken farm was put into operation in April 2019, and thus the village collectively earns more than 200,000 yuan per year. With tourism development as the driving force, projects such as shiitake mushrooms and alpine apple planting are also being promoted.

In May 2018, Luotuowan also set up a collective enterprise, Luotuowan Industrial Development Co., which identified the road map for developing tourism as a leading driver with special breeding and photovoltaic industry in a coordinated development. The year of 2019 saw benefits from it, and villagers took away the dividends. In 2019, Luotuowan also established the Luotuowan Bazaar e-commerce platform, selling more than 4000 pounds of tomatoes, 2000 pounds of apples, and 3000 pounds of black fungus, helping villagers solve the marketing problem with their agricultural products. With the development of various industries, the average disposable income of a villager increased from 950 yuan in 2012 to 13,620 yuan in 2019; the annual income of the village collective is more than 400,000 yuan.

I learned that now Luotuowan Village is not worried about the lack of industrial projects, but the lack of human resources to do industrial projects because most of the young people are migrant workers, only a few young people returned to their hometowns in recent years, but the number is limited. Attracting young people to return to their hometowns is a major issue in Luotuowan Village, but of course there are also some young people who are enthusiastically returning to their hometowns to start their own businesses. One of them is Ren Erhong.

Born in 1978 in Luotuowan, Ren Erhong was the same age as China's reform and opening up. At that time, Luotuowan was very poor, and every household had adobe houses with newspapers pasted on the windows, and later changed from newspapers to plastic sheets. When the wind blew, the window would whistle. It is harder in winter since the temperature in quite low indoors. In 2000, Ren Erhong was demobilized from the army and went to Beijing to work. This is her first time to big city. Seeing so many high buildings and large mansions in her eyes, Ren Erhong felt dazed. Living in a rented house, with elevator linking directly to the door, and enjoying air conditioning in summer, heating in winter, Ren Erhong is no longer be bothered by the weather. On one occasion, Ren Erhong and her colleagues went to Mentougou to tour, and lived in a farmhouse. Then, Ren Erhong had the idea: "the hometown scenery is not worse than here, if my house at hometown is built well, I will live comfortably, and open a farmhouse will also have a stable income. It is the best, isn't it?" Since then, she has been attentive to the development of Luotuowan. However, after many years passing away, there was no big change in the village, and people still lived in adobe houses. In the end of 2012, General Secretary Xi Jinping came to Luotuowan Village and eventually started the great changes in Luotuowan Village. During 2015 Spring Festival, Ren Erhong returned to the village, found that the road connecting the village was about to be repaired, and when she learned that the village was going to build a beautiful countryside, and the old houses were demolished to build new residential houses, Ren Erhong resigned her job in Beijing and returned to the village in May of that year in order to start her business in guesthouse. On May 1, 2017, the guesthouse was open, and it was the first agritainment in the village since the building of beautiful countryside. It is called "Sixth Courtyard Inn". Ren Erhong's guesthouse has two stories, with a construction area of 300 square meters, providing six rooms with independent bathrooms, water provision, and sewer facilities. Wing-room sets up a kitchen as well as a restaurant. Ren Erhong spent a total of more than 100,000 yuan in building this guesthouse, accounting for about 1/3 of all construction funds, the rest of which are subsidized by financial funds. Since then, the net income of Ren Erhong's guesthouse is about 40,000 yuan per year.

Seeing her brother's business in Luotuowan getting bigger and bigger, Ren Yonghua, who was working in Beijing, received a letter from the villager's committee to mobilize young people to return to their hometown, and she made her determination to return hometown and started their own business without hesitation. Today, while working in the village's guesthouse company, Ren Yonghua helps her brother manage the Luotuowan mini-mart. She selects branded goods, and the quality of the goods here is no less than that of the big supermarkets in the city. During the peak tourist season, the small store is full of customers. When asked why she decided to return hometown and pursue development here, Ren Yonghua told me that she always felt like she was wandering in a foreign country without roots, and her children had to go to school but it was hard to find a school in Beijing without Hukou,[10] so she came back as she saw that Luotuowan was developing and there were many job opportunities. Ren Yonghua, born in 1982, came to Beijing to work in 2000, and she did jobs such as cashier in supermarket and promotion specialist in shopping mall. She planned to return to Luotuowan in 2021 for her child's schooling, but because she saw that Luotuowan was developing and there were many job opportunities, she returned to Luotuowan in 2019 and is currently working in a guesthouse company with a monthly salary of 2000 yuan. Although she earned less compared in Beijing, the expenditure was less too, barely nothing. In Beijing, she earned 6000 yuan a month, but subtract the rent, only 2000 yuan left. And that was overtime pay, unlike working at Luotuowan, where I have the freedom to work near my home while taking care of the children, neither will be affected anyway. The only thing that makes Ren Yonghua dissatisfied about working in Luotuowan is that in Beijing, the company pays "five insurances and one fund",[11] while working for Luotuowan guesthouse company, she didn't have five insurances and one fund to be paid by the company. "If this problem is to be solved, I believe there will be more young people returning to their hometowns. As you can see, the old-aged people working in the guesthouse company earn 2000 yuan per month, while the young people like us also earn 2000 yuan outside and work more than here. Although many young people did not want to go hometown, if the 'five insurances and one fund' problem could be solved here, it surely be more young people coming back to the hometown. After all, this is home, who does not want to make contribution in developing the hometown?".

Today, about 100 young people have returned to the village to start their own business. Some of them are planning to open restaurants, some are engaged in special breeding, some are doing e-commerce, and some are opening guesthouses. With young people, the whole village looks more lively and more younger. The village work team, of course, also includes young people. Agriculture Department of Hebei

---

[10] A Beijing local residence permit. – Trans.

[11] According to Chinese Labour law and Labour Contract Law, China's social security system consists of five mandatory insurance schemes, which include Pension (Endowment Insurance), Medical Insurance, Unemployment Insurance, Maternity Insurance, Work Injury Insurance, as well as the Housing Provident Fund. Generally speaking, we called "Five Insurances and One Fund" in China. – Trans.

Province dispatched three staff members to station in the village, and two grassroots cadres to take exercise. Most of them are young people who not only bring the cultural atmosphere of the big city, but also attract young people outside back to Luotuowan Village. In 2018, the resident work team member Tang Chaonan was stationed in the village who is born in 1990s. Youth is written all over her young face. Yet, when talking about her work in the village, she knows exactly how many streets, doors, and people in Luotuowan; anyone whose family is short of rice or noodles, anyone whose family member is sick or hospitalized, anyone whose family is anxious for their children's schooling, and anyone whose family needs help with anything, can call for Tang's help.

"In the past, there was no way out of the mountains working in the fields, so only the old people were left in the village, and many courtyards were empty. Now there are industries in the county and the village has jobs to do, so many young people are coming back here for these jobs, and the more they work, the more energetic they are!" In a recent meeting of the village Party members, Tang Chaonan found that the young CPC[12] members contributed many good ideas for the development of Luotuowan, "special agriculture needs complementary development, taking advantage of the high altitude, we plant ice grapes which do not exist in other places", "planting herbs is also a good project", "Establishing an animal park to keep the tourists who bring their children to play here". Listening to their discussions, we can tell that the young people of Luotuowan are united together and setting off again toward a better tomorrow with great vigor.

7.4 Folk Culture Enriches Villagers' Lives

Rural culture is an important part of rural life. How well a place develops in rural areas depends not only on material life, but also on cultural life, and poverty eradication in rural areas is not only material poverty eradication, but also cultural poverty eradication. Before the poverty eradication, Luotuowan was located in a deep ravine in the Taihang Mountains, where many villagers did not even have a TV set, let alone the internet. And for poor households who had to worry about the next meal after eating the last one, there was no way to inherit and develop rural culture. Since the fight against poverty, with the overall improvement of the infrastructure of Luotuowan Village and the increase of villagers' income, the promotion of folk culture has come to the forefront.

Liu Huage, the first secretary in the village, said that previously the governance of Luotuowan Village was loose, and there were no village rules and regulations, but we started with Party building, actively playing the leading role of Party members, and organizing cultural activities for villagers in various forms. The villagers' motivation is gradually stimulated, and hearts and minds of the villagers make changes from "scattered" state to "gathered" state, and thus people are more united and exerting

[12] CPC refers to Communist Party of China, and "Party" is the abbreviation for CPC. –Trans.

more strength. There is an old opera stage in the center of Luotuowan Village, which was built in the 1980s. After the General Secretary came, the village rebuilt the old stage, and now there are cultural performances on the Luotuowan stage every weekend, and the village also organizes cultural performances very often such as yangko[13] dance, square dance, Shan'ge,[14] and operas, which greatly enrich the cultural life of villagers and tourists on leisure and holidays.

Combining the folk culture and tourism in Luotuowan Village will not only enrich the daily lives of villagers, but also bring wealth. On January 2, 2020, a folklore activity under the theme of "Folklore Luotuowan and New Year in a Small Village" was held in Luotuowan, with folklore culture experience as the main theme and a variety of interactive forms to integrate folklore culture, folklore performance, and New Year fair. It is a unique folk culture tour with various interactive forms that integrate folk culture, folk performances, and New Year's Eve fair into one, and various experience activities are well prepared. The folk artists and the folk arts and crafts workshops bring tiger shoes, embroidery, paper-cutting, clay sculpture, and other handicrafts, by turning the villagers' old household crafts into commodities that can be sold, helping the villagers get rid of poverty and get rich.

Visitors can not only enjoy the natural scenery of Taihang Mountains, but also experience the traditional folk culture. It also arranged a series of "Intangible Cultural Heritage" folk activities for visitors by inviting craft artisans who show their various folk delicacies and handicrafts in a live demo, such as paper-cut for window decoration, making shoe mats, making handmade shoes, writing couplets, painting Chinese New Year paintings, grinding bean curd by hand, making special flower bun, pressing hele noodles, flying kites, and so on. According to Liu Huage, these traditional cultures will disappear if they are not explored properly. Before, villagers had a certain heritage of these traditional crafts, but Luotuowan was so poor that young people worked outside, and these traditional crafts would disappear. As for now, these crafts will not only enrich people's lives but also make money, so those young people coming back to home start to learn crafts.

Today's Luotuowan folk culture has gone to the network platform, Tik Tok, Kuaishou, and other network platforms began to promote Luotuowan public account, and the village youth Tang Chaonan is currently responsible for live broadcast, who makes Luotuowan more well known. Many people can learn about Luotuowan through live broadcast, but also through villagers' live program of a variety of handicraft production, so that viewers can both watch the program and place orders to buy the folk crafts of Luotuowan. The live broadcast is just open for a few months, and many online orders have already been received. The live webcast will promote the folk crafts and souvenirs of Luotuowan in the national market. Tang Chaonan intends to train a few university students coming back to Luotuowan Village to expand the webcast market. Although these university students originally thought to pursue development out of Luotuowan Village through examinations, now they see the changes in the development of Luotuowan Village, and they want to return

[13] A popular rural folk dance. – Trans.

[14] Its literal meaning is mountain songs. – Trans.

home to start a business. They possess an advantage over the villagers in webcasting, they are "post-90 s" who grew up with the network development, and they are full of confidence in starting their own network business for the construction of their hometown. The production of traditional handicrafts also depend on the village's elderly. To Tang Chaonan's surprise, when doing live webcast, the villagers are very cooperative, and they act very naturally in front of webcast camera.

7.5 Conclusions and Questions

From the end of 2012 to 2020, in just eight years, Luotuowan has transformed from a deeply poverty-stricken village situated deep in the Taihang Mountains to a popular tourist destination, which reflects the implementation of the national strategy of combining overall mountain development and targeted poverty alleviation. It also witnessed step-by-step exploration of poverty alleviation and prosperity for all the Luotuowan Villagers. In this process, tourism has become the leading industry to lead the development of Luotuowan Village. The overall facilities of the village are upgraded at first, and then the follow-up traditional folk culture as well as the promotion of the overall image of the village follows. Prosperity through tourism has not only lifted Luotuowan Village out of poverty, but also enabled the villagers to achieve well-off. The villagers can earn part of their income from land transfer, from renting out guesthouses, plus pensions. They can also earn money from working in tourism companies. Now, there is no idle people leaning against the wall and basking in the sunshine on the street. The villagers are working really hard on the road to prosperity, and the cultural activities of the village are also increased. The villagers are no longer materially poor, neither spiritually poor, and it has become a matter of concern for the villagers to show their traditional crafts and inherit the traditional folk culture.

I came to Luotuowan Village several times from 2017 to 2020, and found that the change of the overall environment of the village is the key factor for the villagers to get rid of poverty and become rich. The environment changed, so does the people. Before the changes, there are "passively longing for national assistance, expecting government grants and claiming for poverty reduction funds" in the attitude of villagers toward the poverty eradication. After the environment changes, people change the attitude and work hard to win prosperity. Plus, the environment changes bring young people back. Luotuowan Village, once about to disappear from history, is now full of vitality again.

During my visits to villagers, I also found that although villagers are leading a well-off life, some of them are still living in a tight balance due to illness. The people with "three highs"[15] and cardiovascular diseases still account for a large proportion of population in Luotuowan, especially the middle-aged and elderly. Although the residents of Luotuowan Village have various health and medical guarantees, such as basic

[15] It refers to the high index of blood lipids, blood sugar, and blood pressure. – Trans.

medical insurance, major medical insurance, and medical assistance. Especially, there is a medical protection net for special groups. However, these guarantees can hardly cover the various expenses of patients with major, serious, or chronic diseases. There are some villagers, especially those who suffer from cardiovascular and cerebrovascular diseases, taking a lot of drugs purchased by their children outside. These drugs cannot be bought locally and are not covered by the medical insurance, while the drugs included in the medical insurance list are not effective, so without the help of their children, these people's income is difficult to offset the expenses of buying drugs. Some people with serious illnesses are bedridden for a long time. Although the government has a protection net guarantee for such villagers, such a patient needs someone to take care of at home, so one person who gets sick will cause two people out of work. As time goes by, the income gap between sick villagers and others will be enlarging. In view of the situation of Luotuowan, the long-term support for people who return to poverty due to disability and illness is a big problem that needs to be solved urgently, which may be the main direction to solve the relative poverty problem after the national poverty eradication and prosperity campaign is completed.

References

Excerpts from Xi Jinping's Discourses on Poverty Alleviation, edited by the Institute of Party History and Documentation of the Central Committee of the Communist Party of China, Central Literature Publishing House, 2018.

Li, J., & Wang, Y. (2015). Analysis of the Relationship Between Health and Farmers' Subjective Well-Being: A Survey Based on 1000 Farm Households in Five Provinces (Districts) Across China. *China Rural Economy*, No. 10.

Propaganda Department of the Central Committee of the Communist Party of China (CPC). (2016). *Readings from General Secretary Xi Jinping's Series of Important Speeches*. People's Publishing House.

Tang, X. W., & Li, J. (2017). Deepening Research on Xi Jinping's Thought on Precise Poverty Alleviation in Practice. *China Rural Economy*, No. 9.

Xi, J. (2015). *Being a Jiao Yulu-Style County Party Secretary*. Central Literature Publishing House.

Yuejin Wang , lecture at Huzhou University, with research interests in finance and poverty studies.

Jing Li , researcher at Rural Development Institute of Chinese Academy of Social Sciences, with research interests covering poverty and well-being, rural finance.

Chapter 8
Study on the Sustainability Mechanism of Poverty Alleviation Through Relocation: Based on the Investigation and Research of Chixi Village in Fujian Province

Xin Li, Shaoju Wang, and Yu Geng

Abstract This paper examines the history of poverty alleviation through relocation in Chixi Village which is known as the "first village in China to alleviate poverty". Since the 1980s, Chixi Village has undergone the three phases of poverty alleviation and development: "blood transfusion–blood exchange–blood production". Through the implementation of the relocation project and follow-up measures, Chixi Village has crossed the "spatial poverty trap" and enabled the villagers not only to relocate, but also to stabilize, settle down their families, and become well-off, which realized "sustainable livelihood".

Keywords Poverty alleviation through relocation · Spatial poverty · Sustainable development · Chixi Village

Chixi Village is a She[1] administrative village in Panxi Town, Fuding City, Ningde City, Fujian Province, and is called as "the first village in China to alleviate poverty". The officials and masses of Chixi Village have gone through 10 years of "blood transfusion" poverty alleviation on site, 10 years of "blood exchange" poverty alleviation through relocation, and 10 years of "blood production" through "tourism + industries". By adjusting measures to local conditions, and making efforts in a targeted way, it ultimately goes on the way to poverty eradication and prosperity. In 2015,

[1] One of the ethnic minority group in China. –Trans.

X. Li
Fujian Academy of Social Sciences, Fuzhou, China

S. Wang
Publicity Department, Ningde Municipal Party Committee, Ningde City, China

Y. Geng (✉)
Institute of Sociology, Fujian Academy of Social Sciences, Fuzhou, China

Case Studies of Targeted Poverty Reduction and Alleviation in 100 Villages, International Research on Poverty Reduction, https://doi.org/10.1007/978-981-95-0549-4_8

the poverty alleviation and development work of Chixi Village received the approval of General Secretary Xi Jinping, and on February 19, 2016, General Secretary Xi Jinping also communicated with the villagers of Chixi Village through the Video Link provided by People's Daily Online. On December 7, 2015, then Vice Premier Wang Yang visited Chixi Village and took it as one of the typical examples of the "Ningde Model" of targeted poverty alleviation.

8.1 The History of "Blood Transfusion" of Poverty Alleviation in Chixi Village (1984–1993)

In the 1980s, Ningde was identified by the State Council as one of the 18 contiguous poor areas in the country, with 6 of 9 counties in the region designated as national poverty-stricken counties and 52 of the 120 townships listed as provincial poverty-stricken townships. The per capita net income in the region was less than 160 yuan. There were 770,000 living around the minimum subsistence line, accounting for one-third of the population in rural areas. The village of Chixi was a typical poor village in Ningde, with steep hills, dangerous slopes, curved streams, narrow land, remote villages, and poor people. The village's 14 natural villages are scattered in the remote nooks and crannies of the mighty mountains to the west of Taimu Mountain, surrounded by the Jiuli Creek and the Xiashan Creek. The only road out of the village was the narrow path coiled between the mountains, and the distance of round trip is 100 li.[2] To go from the village to the market town, you had to walk on the rugged mountain road, and all the production and living materials that villagers needed had to rely on shoulder carry. The people and goods in and out of village were very difficult. The village had only 500 acres of unproductive rice fields, most rice yield of which were used to pay taxes in public grain and pay for the collective purchased grain. The only staple food originated from the per capita 0.5 mu[3] of barren farmland for growing sweet potatoes, and 1/3 of the households had to dig wild vegetables to feed themselves. Although the people in the natural village under the mountain had some traditional side businesses, limited to the inconvenience of transportation, information blockage, people could only be engaged in some bamboo raft transport of firewood pieces, and made some moso bamboo processing products to support the family. Xiashanxi is one of the most harsh environment and difficult living conditions. It is a She village hanging halfway up the mountain, with 18 households living in six nooks and crannies, respectively Gangwei, Yangtoukeng, Shibitou, Shuijingmian, Daqianxia, and Zhangchouwan. It is obvious that the living conditions are very harsh by just saying these village names above; houses standing on the cliff edge, with only the sound of unseen creek reverberated at the bottom of cliff. There is a folk song that says: "In the old days, mountain stream flowed down a poor village, with high mountains, risky road, and rare footprints. In the morning, people went outdoor to

[2] Chinese unit, 1 Li equals 500 m. – Trans.

[3] 1 mu equals 1/15 hectare. –Trans.

get firewood in exchange for oil and salt, and in the evening, people could finally return home with the sunset in the west".

With the development of the market economy and the establishment of the national public service system, villagers need to strengthen their bonds with the outside world. It forms a contrary relationship between "high mountains and long roads" and outside communication: villagers had to buy daily necessities for months' needs in reserve, in case that they couldn't find a place to buy a lighter; It took hours to carry chemical fertilizers and farm chemicals to the top of mountains; it was hard to go outside to work especially do a part-time job nearby; it was difficult to get medical treatment in time; children from high mountain villages had to walk for 1 or 2 h to go to the elementary school at the center of village. The harsh geographical environment makes it difficult to provide public goods such as medical care and education. In the early days, the village of Xiashanxi hired a private teacher from a neighboring village, Shen Chaolian, who was paid 10 yuan a month to teach kids only up to the third grade of elementary education, and the fourth grade students had to continue their education at Chixi Primary School. Speaking of the schooling in the past, Li Naisong, a villager remembers it well, saying "When I was in the fourth grade, I had to walk 15 li on rugged mountain road to Chixi at dawn in the morning to go to class, and travel the same distance home in the evening. I couldn't care less about the wild cat calls and jumping monkeys on the way, but later the more I thought about it, the more scared I felt afterwards……" Xiashanxi is far from the township health center, lack of medical care and medicine. Once suffering from an emergency, the condition of patient will worsen at the least, and it is at the mercy of God at the most. The three brothers of Lei Wenjin's family, due to the lack of medical care, had even no more money to hire a doctor. After the death of the eldest brother, the two young brothers also died because of the disease that cannot be treated, who died one after another, finally it became a homeless household. Li Xianru, head of the Xiashanxi villagers group, said: "Our village has neither a single paddy field nor a large piece of farmland, and the staple food, sweet potatoes, is grown on the rocky edge of the rocky corners of Douliqiu[4] and Meimaoqiu.[5] The only economic income is from cutting wood and carrying bamboo that are sold in the market outside the mountains. It costs half a day to cut bamboo, half a day to carry and transport, just for the price of one yuan per hundred pounds of bamboo. While carrying a hundred pounds of bamboo on one's shoulder and walking on the curved and bumpy mountain road, which needs more strength than shouldering three hundred pounds on the flat road. People get up early and work late in the night in exchange for a little bit of money. I was able to save up a little with this income, and got married when I was 23. Poor couples love each other more often than not, and a year later my beloved Lei Juhua was pregnant. When my wife went into labor, she suddenly started bleeding and fell into a coma. Relatives and neighbors got down on their knees and prayed for the safety of the mother and child. When the 3-pound baby boy silently came to the world, she never woke up. Everyone cried out, calling out to the heavens and the

[4] It literally means bamboo hat mound. – Trans.

[5] It literally means eyebrow mound. – Trans.

earth, in great pain. If only there had been doctors or medicine in the village, if only the mountain hadn't been in the way, and if only the health center was closer, my beloved's life would not end so soon!".

In 1984, Wang Shaoju, then deputy director of the Fuding County Party Committee Office and head of the news section (report team leader), came to Xiashanxi, a village submerged in deep forests, and saw with his own eyes the hardships and dilemmas of the villagers who had no food to eat and no clothes to cover their bodies, which shocked him so much that he wrote an article entitled "The hope for poor village – to carry out special policies in solving poverty and getting rich", and sent it to the editorial office of People's Daily. On June 24, 1984, the front page of People's Daily published a letter reflecting the poor condition of the She natural village of Xiashanxi in Chixi and a commentator's article "Caring for the poor areas", which aroused great concern from the Party Central Committee and strong reactions from all over the country. On September 29, 1984, the CPC Central Committee and the State Council issued *the Notice on Helping Poverty-stricken Areas to Change the Appearance as Soon as Possible*, and the nationwide work of poverty alleviation has begun since then.

In June 1984, Fuding County Party Secretary Zhou Yiwu, who had just taken office, held discussions on poverty problems in Chixi Village. He agreed on a poverty alleviation program, and led the heads of the departments of agriculture, food, forestry, supply and marketing, animal husbandry, civil affairs, and old areas, in bringing relief money, rice, fish, meat, clothes, cotton quilts, and other supplies to the poor households, along the rugged mountain road to the Xiashanxi. They went from house to house, visiting the poor and sending warm regards to them by giving rice, fish, meat, and other supplies, and the giving quota was set according to the population of each household. The animal husbandry department sent more than 60 goat pups and 50 long-haired breeding rabbits; the forestry department sent more than 3000 fir tree seedlings and 2000 fruit seedlings; and the agriculture and medicine departments sent medicinal seeds and planting methods. After the issuance of *the Notice on Helping Poverty-stricken Areas to Change the Appearance as Soon as Possible* by the CPC Central Committee and the State Council, Fuding County's Party and government leaders again led the heads of poverty alleviation, food, education, family planning, and other relevant departments into the mountains to "take the pulse". In view of the fact that there is no paddy field in Xiashanxi and it is difficult to produce grain, and the small amount of sweet potatoes that the farmland planted could not feed themselves, the county governor made decision and declared on the spot that a special policy would be implemented to exempt all the people from paying requisitioned grain and selling premium priced grain from the summer of that year, which must remain unchanged for 5 years. The next year, Chixi administrative village also enjoyed this policy.

Compared with most villages that were still in the stage of resource extraction at that time, Chixi Village had already received resource input and subsidies in many aspects from the government, which not only enjoyed exemption from paying agricultural taxes, but also various assistance programs in industry, education, medical care, etc. However, the purely "imported" poverty alleviation can hardly change the plight of Chixi Village, as "the local land and water cannot feed the people living here". Because the village was too barren, coupled with the drought and low rainfall, more than half of the cedar seedlings died in less than a year, and those that survived did not grow tall enough to become good materials, and a large number of peach and plum trees were crowded on narrow farmland such as Meimaoqiu[6] and Douliqiu,[7] which could produce a few fruits, but before the harvest, they were stolen by wild monkeys. The goat pups were raised separately in some households, but because the thatch in the mountains was too coarse and hard to eat, the mouths of the goats generally blistered with blood after gnawing and then became septic and festered, leading to more than 60 goat pups dead before growing up. Many long-haired rabbits also died of disease or bites by wild dogs due to the lack of feeding techniques. The villagers planted a batch of highly adaptable rhizome herbs, which were expected to be harvested, but were bitten by ruthless wild boars. "It's this thatch that cuts our face and hands, and goats can't eat it. If eat it, goats will get 'rotten mouth disease' 'rotten ear disease'. Saplings are in the same situation, as the mountain is too barren to grow roots, even though we plant them year after year". The both private teacher and "barefoot doctor" hired from a neighboring village a few years ago were so poorly paid that he had trouble even getting a date, and eventually resigned and went to work outside the mountains. "The annual per capita income is only 120 yuan, so where to find a girl who would marry a man in the village?" "The bones cannot grow flesh", which cannot change the face of "poverty and blankness[8]". By 1993, the village's per capita net income was less than 500 yuan, and some of the She people who had been lifted out of poverty soon fell back into poverty due to natural disasters and lack of momentum going, so generally the She people were still very poor. According to statistics, in 1993, there were still 41 poor She households in the village, accounting for 31% of the total She households. Ten years of "blood transfusion" to help the poor, the results are very little.

8.2 The History of "Blood Exchange" in Chixi Village (1994–2003)

In August 1994, 22 households with 88 compatriots from the She ethnic group in Xiashanxi were included in the first batch of whole village relocation projects in Fujian Province, and they moved to Chang'an New Street, where is the central village of Chixi in April 1995. On May 26 1995, the project of power station was completed, which was the largest poverty alleviation project in the history of Chixi Village, and also the key project in turning around the fate of Chixi people. During the construction, villagers of Chixi had to be migrant workers to increase their income, while after the completion of the power station, the pace of poverty alleviation and

[6] It literally means eyebrow mound. – Trans.

[7] It literally means bamboo hat mound. – Trans.

[8] Blankness refers to the cultural state of being blank, and blindness to sciences. – Trans.

development, and the poverty elimination and getting rich in Chixi Village was accelerated. Since 1994, a total of 12 natural villages with more than 350 households have been relocated to the center of the village through the welfare project, and Chang'an New Street has been extended as well, and the size of the center of Chixi village has reached more than 1520 people today. One after another, the She people in the mountains have moved from dilapidated thatched huts to spacious and bright brick houses, and the per capita housing area has increased from 8.5 square meters to 40 square meters, eventually saying goodbye to the poor mountains (Table 8.1).

The biggest resistance to the migration and relocation project of Chixi Village is the villagers' concept. The village of Xiashanxi has no water and no soil, "the local land and water cannot feed the people living here". In the face of this situation, Huang Guolai, then secretary of the CPC Party branch of Chixi Village, had the idea of building a road from the village to connect to the gravel road of the hydropower station, and then to gather the 14 scattered natural villages. Xu Wengui, then secretary of the CPC Party Committee of Panxi Town, came up with an idea that the method of relocating migrants from the hydropower station could be "transplanted" to Chixi. When the two ideas collided, the word "relocation" came out of their mouths, and they were in agreement with each other. So, in the case of "blood transfusion" is ineffective, the village of Xiashanxi is ready to relocate the entire village, so that to achieve an off-site "blood production". The news of the relocation spread to the villagers, like a drop of water immediately boiling up in a frying pan, with waves of discussion higher and higher. "Relocation of the whole village? How is that possible?" "It's hard for the old and young to adapt to a strange place!" "What are we going to do down the mountain? Then the sky is not our sky, the land is not our land, and there is no place to bury us after we die!" "Our ancestors settled here 300 years ago, and we are used to the mountain life, so we don't want to go anywhere!" "We will be rich or poor by fate. If we are poor, then we have to suffer". Relocation met the "anti-relocation", so the county, town, and village leaders agreed to "exchange the blood" but it must first change the mind. The old traditions, old ideas, and fatalism have to be completely reversed, in order to successfully carry out the relocation work. So, the officials split up to do ideological work from door to door. Their first consultation aim is the villagers' group leader Li Xianru. Li Xianru said: "I originally did not want to move, because generation after generation of our family had their lives like this for hundreds and decades of years, so let's suffer the bitterness of life like before! Later, the secretary of the village CPC Party branch came my home, and told me something that poked the most painful part of my heart. I worked so hard to marry a wife, and it was even hard to pray for a son who was born but she passed away soon after giving birth. If we lived in an easily accessible place, not in this mountain nook, then her life would not have ended so early …… if we do not respond to the government's call to relocate, not to mention the poor life of all villagers, there will be a second and third woman as miserable as my wife!" Li Xianru's heartfelt and true words moved many villagers.

In 1994, new migrant residents were arranged in the two brick buildings of uniform standards accommodating 22 households (11 households on each side of the planning line), and the sand, cement, hollow bricks, and other building materials were all

Table 8.1 History of poverty alleviation in Chixi Village through relocation

Year	Number of relocated households	Number of relocated people	Preferential policies
1994	22 (Xiashanxi)	88	320,000 yuan of building subsidies provided by CPC Party Committee, government, and all people from all walks of life
1995	28	124	CPC Party Committee and government offer 3000 yuan of subsidies to each household; village provides some bonus for the construction of foundation and renders some reductions on various fees
1997–2007	208	992	Village provides some bonus for the construction of foundation and renders some reductions on various fees
2008	5	20	Subsidy of 2500 yuan for everyone
2011	11	43	Subsidy of 2500 yuan for everyone; and those who have family planning will get 2500 yuan plus per person; and those of ethnic minorities will get 600 yuan per person furthermore
2012	29	106	10,000 yuan for each household or 3000 yuan for one person; those of ethnic minorities, family planning, households enjoying the five guarantees, households enjoying minimum living guarantee, and identified poverty-stricken households will get subsidies ranging from 600 to 15,000 yuan
2013	6	18	
2014	4	19	10,000 yuan for each household or 3000 yuan for one person; those of ethnic minorities, village from old revolutionary base areas, family planning, households enjoying the five guarantees, households enjoying minimum living guarantee, and identified poverty-stricken households will get subsidies ranging from 600 to 15,000 yuan
2015	31	107	

provided by the villagers' committee and the village's Party committee of Chixi Village, as well as the county government from the assistance at a higher level. The villagers of Xiashanxi Village only brought 80 sticks of wood from the mountains, whose children were transferred to Chixi Primary School, and even the graveyard about which the old people were concerned and the town and village also took it into consideration: the graves could be moved to the mountain areas behind the Chixi Village. The new buildings were completed one after another within more than half a year, and on May 4, 1995, all the villagers of Xiashanxi Village moved into the new buildings.

Originally, there was no street around the site of Chixi administrative village. With 22 households and 88 people joining the village, a new street was planned and gradually constructed in a neat and symmetrical way along both sides of the 15-m-wide road, which was named "Chang'an New Street" with the meaning of "Long Live Long and Safe". As the town and village leaders planned, a new street with cement pavement was paved, which looks flat and hard. There are mostly small three-story buildings with uniform standards, of which the first floor is a store and the second and third floors are apartments. Each unit is 3.8 m wide and 12 ~ 15 m deep, and connected to each other, leaving no space in between. The two communities, She-Han, get along well and lives are more and more flourishing. The resident population has increased dramatically from the original scattered 93 households with more than 400 people to the present 356 households with more than 1580 people, accounting for more than 86% of the total population of the village. The four purely She natural villages of Banshan, Xiaoxi, Qiuzhai, and Dongpingli and the mixed She-Han natural villages of Paitou, Xidong, Qiganli, and Chixiping have been relocated out of the mountains, down the mountains or migrated elsewhere in three phases one after another. Han villagers previously living in small places scattered in Chixi, such as Kenglinong, Chixidian, and Qigandou, also gathered on both sides of Chang'an New Street, and even the Nanbing She natural village in Dujia Administrative Village was relocated here.

In the new environment, those migrant villagers had to face the process of livelihood reconstitution and restoration. Before relocation, most of the resettled villagers lived in mountain villages, mainly farming in the fields or working in the woods in the mountains, and the survival skills they mastered were mainly simple agricultural farming, forest harvesting, and other primary technologies, with a high degree of dependence on agricultural production and mountain forest work for survival. Plus the isolation to the outside world and rare external exchanges, people lacked the knowledge of the new technologies as well as new achievements.

In the process of poverty alleviation and resettlement project, the resettled villagers will inevitably compare the income level and living condition before and after the resettlement, and when the change value is lower than the expected value, they will feel unfairly treated, and thus become discontented, or in more serious cases, frustrated, angry, or it even grows destructiveness. The input of large amount of resources without supporting procedures will only stimulate some villagers to over-imagine their rights and narrow down their obligations as a matter of course, and more and more people will talk about their rights but not obligations. Finally, it formed a weird but realistic logic chain of public goods in rural areas: a lot of resources invested in public goods by the government → develop the villager dependency on government → more dependent on government's investment → government needs to put in more resources without shaping a democratic political culture. And the government finds out that the input of resources becomes a negative force that undermines village governance, and the more resources are input, the more the people's mentality of "passively longing for national assistance, expecting government grants and claiming for poverty reduction funds" grows. After the relocation of Chixi Village, some villagers became rich which exerted bad feelings. Some of them squandered a lot of money, some of them worshiped God and built temples, some of them gambled together, became addicted to alcoholic and caused trouble, and some of them even provoked conflicts between family names and clans …… In the past few years, Chixi Village saw chaos for a time. A typical example is: born in Chixiping, the natural village of Chixi Village, Wu Jingxi, an able villager, who served in his early years as a clerk, accountant of the Chixi administrative village, and later passed the entrance examination of civil officials, and therefore transferred to work at the government office of Xiapu county, and he is responsible for Yangjiaxi scenic tourism development in that county. Considering that Yangjiaxi scenic Jiuli Creek is the downstream of Chixi Jiuli Creek, will it be possible to carry out the interaction between the two Creeks? Wu Jingxi, who had his heart set on the economic development of his hometown, made acquaintance with the chairman of Wanbohua Tourism Company through a good friend of him, and invited the chairman to visit and investigate the mountains and waters of Chixi and Huli. Once the chairman saw the beautiful landscape of Chixi, he made a decision to invest in the tourism development of Chixi Village. However, a few villagers had conservative thinking, old-fashioned ideas, while some people only cared about the immediate small profits, in terms of taking land acquisition as the opportunity to salt price for land compensation, and even after the land was transferred to you, you still have to hire me again to dig out; if you engage in infrastructure construction, you must hire me to do building construction …… all of which eventually forced the chairman to give up Chixi and moved to the neighboring village, Wubei Village, to develop outdoor development.

8.3 The History of "Blood Production" Poverty Alleviation in Chixi Village (2003 to Present)

It needs perseverance and takes long time to achieve long-term goals of targeted poverty alleviation and elimination. After "blood transfusion" and "blood exchange", with the support of the CPC's poverty alleviation policy, the officials and people carried forward the spirit of tenacious struggle and the spirit of dripping water to wear away the stone, and made efforts to adapt to local conditions, so as to "produce blood". They have established the development idea of "building an ecological village and letting tourism to make people rich", vigorously developed special industries, and promoted the combination of targeted poverty alleviation and customs change, and the combination of targeted poverty alleviation and the construction of grassroots organizations, which realized the magnificent transformation from a far-famed poor village to a well-off village.

8.3.1 Combination of Targeted Poverty Alleviation and Development of Tea Industry

Industry development is the fundamental solution to achieve relocation, stability, and prosperity. To be effective and sustainable, industrial poverty alleviation needs the coordination of the local villagers who lived in the village community to achieve economic production, social relations, and cultural values generated and circulated within the village. Take the white tea industry as an example, Chixi Village has invested in infrastructure as equity, and cooperated with several enterprises to build the She Village White Tea Experience Museum so as to sell Chixi souvenir tea, with sales more than 5 million yuan. The villagers have increased their income from dividends of participation in business and labor work, with nearly 180 households earning more than 100,000 yuan a year, accounting for 44% of the village. Du Ying, a native of Chixi, born in 1990, graduated from Guangxi Yulin Normal University and could have applied for a job as a teacher, but he gave up the opportunity to work in the city and returned with both his classmate and girlfriend Chen Chunping to the village where he was born and raised up. He saw the villagers of almost every family grow tea, but there was no processing plant, so villagers only sold raw tea leaves without realizing any the added value. While the first batch of spring tea leaves can sell a good price, the following two or three batches cannot sell a good price. Even the price of tea green is not enough for the cost of tea leaves picking work, directly affecting the economic income of tea farmers. Seeing all above in his eyes, he undertook a small tea factory run by his father, and determined to make it bigger and stronger. Du Ying registered his own company, created the "Shangyixi" brand, and made business in combination of both online and offline sales with his "the first bucket of gold" over 100,000 yuan. The village Party branch took Du Ying as a promising seedling for "blood production", and the village secretary visited his company whenever he could, and enthusiastically helped him to solve specific problems. He happened to meet a good policy for graduate start-ups by the national government: Du Ying can get a living allowance of 300 yuan per month, business start subsidy of 3000 yuan in one payment, and tax exempt for 3 years. Within 3 years, he can get a subsidy of 6000 yuan for the house rent each year. The Human Resources and Social Security Bureau of Fuding City has given Du Ying a business fund of 120,000 yuan for 2 years and an interest-bearing loan of 100,000 yuan. In order to expand the processing site, Du Ying also needed a low-interest loan of 100,000 yuan from the Agricultural Bank of China, and Du Jiazhu, secretary of the general branch of the village CPC Party, guaranteed it for him without saying a word, and made decision with Wu Yiguo, the then villager's committee director, to spare a piece of place covering 400 square meters to expand his processing factory, which is a dream coming true for him. At the beginning of 2016, Du Ying expanded his production again, in addition to purchasing high-end equipment such as automatic dryers, and with the support of the town and village, he transferred more than 400 square meters of land, built a new standardized factory, and successfully passed QS quality certification. Through the base cooperation construction and forming a business community with some villagers, the company operates more than 30 acres of ecological tea garden base and more than 600 square meters of white tea experience garden, driving a group of villagers together to get rich. Du Ying's dream, with the support from the favorable policies, is gradually realized. Today, there are more than 30 college and university graduates like Du Ying who enjoyed policy support to return to the hometown for a start-up and employment. They went to the city to learn knowledge and skills, and came back to sow the seeds of knowledge on the fields of hope, so that it lets the villagers have visible and tangible benefits. They are bold to break with the old tradition, dare to break the old industrial development model, and explore the new era of "e-business poverty alleviation", which endows the villagers with a real sense of gain.

8.3.2 *Combining Targeted Poverty Alleviation and Ecological Tourism*

"Lucid waters and lush mountains are invaluable assets". In August 1988, after inspecting Fuding, Comrade Xi Jinping left a message: "You can get rich by focusing on the mountains, keep them under control and insist on them for 10, 15 or 20 years, and our mountains will be 'banks'". Today, a copy of the Fuding Newsletter, which is based on the recording of his speech, is placed in the display room of the village history of Chixi Village. The development of leisure agriculture and rural tourism is a new way to promote agricultural efficiency and peasants' employment and income, a new engine to promote the construction of beautiful villages and integrated development of urban and rural areas, and a new platform to enrich tourism resources and improve the happiness index of residents. Chixi Village is rich in tourism resources, with 35 single units of various types of tourism resources, which is an important part of the Taimushan Scenic Spot, mainly found with tourism resources such as the Jiuli Creek waterside scenic belt, the canyon-type waterside scenery of the Xiashan Creek river section, as well as the Dujiabao ancient dwelling group and the natural idyllic scenery, further forming a tourism resource layout featuring Jiuli Creek and Xiaoshan Creek as bonds with the characteristics of She culture and poverty alleviation work as tourism resources, which is of high tourism development value.

With the development of tourism in the surrounding area, the horizons of the villagers in Chixi have been broadened and the ideas have been changed too. After the village officials and villagers made up their minds to choose ecological tourism as a foundation to develop their village, tourism companies re-entered. Since 2005, based on ecology, relying on the Taimushan scenic area, and using the Jiuli Creek tourism resources, Chixi Village has introduced tourism companies and professional cooperatives such as Wanbohua, Fenglin Gardening, and Gengleyuan, to invest more than 78 million yuan in the development and construction of tourist attractions with She characteristics, and is committed to developing scenic area-dependent rural tourism.

Now, it has built bamboo rafting, canyon sports park, real CS[9] field base, camping fun, among other tourism projects, to develop the special rural tours such as ancient country roads, Dujia ancient fortress, and rural scenery. There are also series of experience tour products to be developed, such as butterfly ping, "colorful farm", rare seedlings and flowers viewing, selected fruits and vegetables picking, water-side fishing village sightseeing experience and tea picking, spring bamboo shoots digging, agricultural labor experience, among other things.

It is necessary to comprehensively upgrade the infrastructure like transportation to develop rural tourism. From 2010 to 2012, the government renovated and upgraded the Tongchengguan Highway, reducing the travel time from 2 to 1 h from Chixi to the national and provincial roads; to speed up the integration of Chixi into the Taimushan scenic area, the nearly 10-km tourist road connecting Chixi Village to the Taimushan scenic area was rerouted, with a new 3.62-km line from Longting to Dujia and a 6-km line from Dujia to Chixi, thus opened to traffic of the "last kilometer" to the Taimushan scenic area. In November 2013, with the support of and great significance attached by the Ningde Municipal CPC Committee, the construction of a tourist road from Yangjiaxi Scenic Area to Chixi Village was launched, and the Yangchi Road was opened to traffic, shortening the travel time from Chixi Village to the expressway to 20 min, thus realizing "Taimushan–Chixi–Yangjiaxi" tourism integration development. At the same time, through the provincial poverty alleviation support for the whole village with department point-to-point assistance, earmarked funds to support, Chixi Village infrastructure supportive facilities continue to improve. At present, the Ministry of Water Resources has completed the small watershed management project, with the new flood control dike for the two streams flowing around the village, a landscape belt along the stream, and the village water system transformation. It achieved the combination of ring roads, embankment, greenway, and slow road, which now gives Chixi Village more color to the beautiful landscape of "A village in the scenery, the scenery in the village, close to the mountains and near the water". Relying on the opportunity of the Provincial Department of Ethnic and Religious Affairs to help the whole village to promote poverty alleviation and development, and listed as a pilot village for the protection and development of minority villages with ethnic characteristics, the village carried out the façade renovation, She style shopping street, greening and beautification, and Shexiangshanshui[10] wooden house repair projects. All measures are committed to creating a village with characteristics of the She ethnic group in Eastern Fujian. In addition, with the introduction of tourism enterprises, there are 3 parking lots, 2 visitor service centers, 3 ecological leisure mountain villas and tourist public toilets, and other tourism service facilities having been built in the scenic area. Based on the new positioning, Chixi Village is improving and upgrading the scenic spot and tourism-related supporting facilities, and steps up the integration into the big tourism pattern of Ningde.

The development of tourism has led to the development of farm restaurants, farm accommodation, tourism products, labor services, mountain agriculture, and other

[9] Counter-Strike, a PC game popular in China. – Trans.

[10] Literally means She countryside landscape. – Trans.

extended industries, broadening the villagers' path to increase income, and enhancing the "blood-production" function of stable income for villagers, which benefit the villagers directly or indirectly from tourism. "Over the years, under the leadership of the Party, the officials and the people have been working together, and we have seen radical changes here, as the village has become more and more beautiful with more and more tourists coming here, and our lives are getting better and better". Zhong Limei, president of the Women's Federation of Chixi Village, said happily, "I renovated the remaining four rooms at home and converted them into guesthouses, so I can receive tourists during the tourist season, and have income more than several tens of thousands of yuan within a year. Now I earn money at home so easy". In recent years, nearly 200 people have been employed in the tourism industry in Chixi Village, earning a wage income of about 6 million yuan. In addition, more than 400 temporary workers are employed during the peak season whose wages reach 130–150 yuan per day. There are 36 specialty stores (including snack stores), 12 agritainment farm stays, and more than 400 accommodation beds. In 2019, Chixi Village received 270,000 visitors, and the income from tourism-related industries exceeded 21.6 million yuan, accounting for half of the village's industrial income. In addition, Chixi Village also introduced leading agricultural enterprises such as "Pin Pin Xiang" and "Zhong He Food" to come to fruition and build bases, and transferred 1070 mu[11] of arable land in the village, so that people can receive an annual rent income of 500 yuan per mu, and can also increase their income by working in companies and cooperatives. The people can receive an annual rent of 500 yuan per mu, and can increase their income by working in companies and cooperatives. Also, driven by tourism, the village also set up Chixi Ecological Industry Development Co., Ltd., to tap the collective assets of the village and enhance the blood-production function of the village collective economy in the form of outsourcing fish ponds, renting out land, gaining land shares in tourism enterprises, and collecting public service fees through making cooperation in village infrastructure investment.

8.3.3 Combining Targeted Poverty Alleviation and Social Tradition Transformation

To build a moderately prosperous society in all aspects requires the material and spiritual unity. Poverty is not socialism, and distorted development of only material things is not socialism either. Comrade Xi Jinping pointed out that true socialism cannot be understood only as a highly developed productive force, but must also have a highly developed spiritual civilization, "on the one hand, to let the people live a relatively affluent life, on the other hand, to improve the people's ideological and moral level and scientific and cultural level, which is the real meaning of getting rid of poverty and getting rich". Some villagers benefit from the poverty alleviation policy with their economic income increasing day by day, but due to their mistakes

[11] 1 mu equals 1/15 hectare. –Trans.

such as keeping up with the Joneses and showing off their wealth, wasting money, playing poker and gambling, participation in superstition activities, they quickly return to poverty. It is necessary to achieve both stout wallets and rich head, as rural civilization is the foundation for sustainable prosperity. Only by strengthening the construction of spiritual civilization while promoting poverty alleviation and material wealth in the poor areas, we can successfully realize "full granary", "sufficient food and clothing", "knowing etiquette", and "knowing honor and shame" step by step.

The officials and people in Chixi Village are sober-minded and proactive, and they are determined to break the slack thinking of "being poor but free", "passively longing for national assistance, expecting government grants and claiming for poverty reduction funds" as well as complaining to God. They turn their idea of "Let me get out of poverty" to "I want to get out of poverty". In the spirit of commitment, and through tenacious struggle, they innovate the prosperity. At the same time, the village consistently promotes the transformation of traditions and a new style of rural civilization. To solve the problems such as the dirty, disorderly, and poor village environment, the inharmonious community and conflicting neighbors, the fighting, gambling, and superstition, Chixi Village held a CPC village Party meeting, the villager congress to divide the work responsibilities for Party members and officials, and widely published on the LED display of the village. The village organized regular sanitation work, and guided villagers to gradually restrain themselves to form good health habits; organized women to form "anti-gambling alliance", and respected elders to set up a persuasion team;set up a police room to intensify the investigation and punishment of gamblers and counter the bad tendency of gambling in the border areas; built a "lawsuit-free village" demonstration site with the Fuding People's Court to timely manage and solve conflicts between people and people, people and tour companies; actively improved the cultural facilities such as people's assembly room, villager book house and peasant fitness project, and carried forward the good moral virtues such as civilized manners, respect for the elderly and children, and national unity, and write the specific norms into the village rules and regulations to gather positive energy for development.

There is a young man in the village in his early twenties, who was strong and hardworking. He got up early to do farm work and back to home very late, and could endure any hardship. With laborious work to make a fortune, he not only got out of poverty, but also saved a sum of money to get married. Unexpectedly, 2 years later, 1 day, he felt weakness in his arms and legs, even difficult to walk. Gradually, his face turned yellow and thin, and he was sleepless at night. One late night, after he felt drowsy and just slept, suddenly he saw a buffalo goring his abdomen, and then it pains him hard to bear, frightening him to wake up in a cold sweat, which turned out to be a nightmare. And he had three nightmares in consecutive 3 nights, driving him in a trance and talk nonsense. His parents resorted to the gods for fortune telling. According to the "Psychic" guidance: he offended the Bull Demon King, so it needs to hold religious rites for 3 days and three nights to honor the gods to keep safe. His father inquired about Daisen barefoot in a neighboring county who can "drive away the gods and ghosts", and cost at great expense to invite whom to home to hold religious rites for 3 days and three nights to honor the gods. All variety of expenses reached six or seven thousand Yuan and it did not get better since his abdominal pain became more acute. In order to cure their son's disease, the parents even used the money to marry their daughter-in-law, called out friends and relatives to the temple to burn incense and worship Buddha, praying for Buddha's blessing. As a result, the money was spent out, and the disease became more and more serious. Later, the village officials learned of this, and came with a village doctor and arranged a door-to-door diagnosis for him. After detailed questioning of the symptoms, finally it came to light: this simple-minded and honest young man, with youth and strength, without tiredness, often didn't have meals and directly went to the field to work. When he felt so hungry that had to come home to have a full meal, and he wouldn't stop eating until the stomach was full and even had swelling pain. Such a poor diet habit, he got serious stomach problems. Dreaming of bull goring belly is because: 1 day this young man was plowing the field, and the old buffalo was slack in work because it was not fed yet, which he could not help but make it a beating, but what he did not expect was the buffalo turned its head and glared at him. Suddenly, his heart thumped, an inexplicable sense of regret rushed to his heart, and from then on he became unhappy …… the root cause of his disease in dreaming the buffalo was found therefore. He was sent to the health center in the town and his gastroscopy report came out—gastric ulcer. The doctor prescribed the medicine, and he followed the medical advice for paying attention to diet in a scientific way. Within no more than six months, his stomach disease was cured, and he is energetic and well again to work. After this incident, the villagers deeply realize that superstitious beliefs in gods and spirits are useless, and that the cure for poverty must focus on the root cause of ignorance.

8.3.4 Combining Targeted Poverty Alleviation and Grassroots Organization Construction

Comrade Xi Jinping pointed out that there are only two fundamental things to get rid of poverty: the leadership of the CPC and the power of the people. Chixi Village strengthens the construction of the village organization with the Party branch as the core, and strives to play a leading role in poverty alleviation. Selecting the members and strengthening the village team of "villagers' committee and the village's Party committee", and sending two first secretary in the village from the province and the city, as well as selecting two excellent college students to serve as village officials in the village, are to enhance the overall level of the village "two committees[12]", and the team capacity of seeking policies, attracting projects, and introducing funds. The village Party branch always adheres to the Party's mass line and the fine style of work— "get it done now"—strives to implement the "six must" mass work method, improves various systems of villagers' self-governance and democratic management, guarantees villagers' participation in decision-making and supervision

[12] I.e. villagers' committee and the village's Party committee. – Trans.

of major issues at the village level, and implements organizational target management and arranges backbone officials posts and their responsibilities. The village breaks down each key project of poverty alleviation into subtasks for various organizations and backbone officials through open commitment, supervision acceptance, and implementation with the team's fighting power and leading capacity intensified.

Chixi Village leads the villagers in getting rid of poverty and rich through the strong guidance of the Party branch. Under the guidance of the Party branch of Chixi Village, seven professional cooperatives of the village were established to develop 300 mu of well-known fruits, 100 mu of precious seedlings, 900 mu of Camellia oleifera, and 80 mu of freshwater breeding base in the mode of "company + cooperative + base + villager" to promote the development of modern special agriculture and comprehensive development of mountain agriculture. At the same time, 12 Party branch members play a leading role, with their own practice of getting rich, to guide the poor people to develop freshwater breeding, rare seedlings, well-known fruits and vegetables, and other special breeding and planting, helping 30 households of the She people to get on the road to poverty eradication and prosperity.

Chixi Village makes efforts to cultivate officials from ethnic minority groups and makes close the relationship between the She-Han people. Chixi Village implements the policy of "three priorities" for ethnic minorities (priority implementation of the relocation welfare projects for ethnic minority, priority support for ethnic minority entrepreneurship and employment, and priority training of ethnic minority officials). Through election of the village organization in 2020, She young talents with "three haves and three brings[13]" are actively recommended to hold posts in the village "two committees", and establish a 30-member "big hand holding small hand" resident work team and volunteer team, which is composed of outstanding She young people, and excellent university graduates, etc., to participate in poverty alleviation practices in the village. By strengthening the team building, actively changing the work style, promoting the rapport between officials and the She-Han ethnic people, accurately grasping the thought dynamics of the She-Han ethnic people, timely understanding their suggestions and demands, poverty alleviation work can find the entry point to achieve accurate poverty alleviation.

8.4 Conclusion

General Secretary Xi Jinping spoke highly of Chixi Village's experience in poverty alleviation and poverty eradication, "Over the past 30 years, with the support of the Party's poverty alleviation policy, the officials and people of Ningde Chixi She Village have struggled hard and striven tenaciously against poverty, like dripping water to wear away the stone and working long and hard to achieve the final success, to build a

[13] "Three haves and three brings" means to have the ideas and convictions and spirit of devotion, and bring hope; to have business brain and capability of prosperity, and bring development; to have good virtues and heart of justice, and bring harmony. – Trans.

widely known poor village into a well-off village"; "'China's first village of poverty alleviation' is very highly deemed, which is also really concentrated reflection of the Ningde people as well as the Chixi Village's painstaking efforts and sweat. As I said in Ningde, we should work like dripping water to wear away the stone, working long and hard to achieve the final success, and weak birds need to fly first. All you have done it. Your practice also confirms our current approach, that is, poverty alleviation work should be tailored to local conditions and make targeted efforts".

The practice of Chixi Village illustrates that to establish a sound sustainable mechanism for the targeted poverty alleviation and relocation to alleviate poverty, we must effectively implement the people-centered development ideology, and make it the starting and ending points of economic development to enhance people's welfare, promote all-round human development, and steadily advance in the direction of common prosperity; we must deepen reform and opening up, constantly improve the policy system and long-term mechanism for poverty alleviation and development; we must adhere to the practical approach, and find the right way to implement targeted policies; we must give full play to the main role of the poor people in targeted poverty alleviation and targeted poverty eradication, and "Poverty alleviation needs to increase people's confidence first", "Poverty alleviation must help people acquire knowledge and skills"; we must make achievements like the dripping water to wear away the stone and work long and hard to achieve the final success. General Secretary Xi Jinping's strategic thought on poverty alleviation has established the basic principles and aim of struggle for the poverty alleviation work in Fujian and Chixi Village. Fujian and Chixi Village will always take "getting rid of poverty" as the main line of work, and adhere to the work blueprint to the end, make officials work one term after another, unite and lead the people to make unremitting efforts and struggle, and integrate poverty alleviation and development into the overall situation in which grasp, plan and promote poverty alleviation and development in the overall situation.

References

Chen, Q.-G., & Cheng, K. (2011). Poverty Alleviation in Ethnic Areas from the Perspective of Spatial Poverty Theory. *Journal of Central South University for Nationalities (Humanities and Social Sciences Edition)*, No. 1.

Gao, C. Y., Wu, W. Q., & He, D. H. (2016). Study on Sustainable Livelihoods of Farmers in Poverty-Relief Resettlement Areas. *Journal of the Party School of the CPC Fujian Provincial Committee*, No. 9.

Jalan, J., & Ravallion, M. (1997). *Spatial Poverty Traps*. The World Bank, Development Research Group.

Li, B., & Zuo, S. (2016). Encountering Relocation: An Exploration of the Logic of Implementing Poverty Alleviation Migration Relocation Policy from the Perspective of Targeted Poverty Alleviation—Taking Wang village in Southern Shaanxi as an Example. *Journal of China Agricultural University (Social Science Edition)*, No. 2.

Li, C., Liu, W., Feng, W., & Li, S. (2013). The Impact of Migrant Relocation on Farmers' Livelihood Strategies: An Investigation Based on Ankang Area in Southern Shaanxi Province. *China Rural Observer*, No. 6.

Li, P., & Wang, X. (2013). Migration, Poverty Alleviation and Ecological Civilization Construction: A Research Report on Ecological Migration in Ningxia. Ningxia Social Science, No. 3.

Li, X., Ye, J., Zhang, X., Tang, L., & Zuo, S. (2004). Report on Poverty in Rural China. *Journal of China Agricultural University (Social Science Edition)*, No. 1.

Shan, Z., Fan, C., & Cai, X. (2020). The village is beautiful, the day is good. *Fujian Daily*, July 2.

Wang, H., Fu, S., Zhang, W. (2017). The Evolutionary Characteristics of China's Easy Poverty Alleviation and Relocation Policy—A Quantitative Analysis Based on Policy Texts. *Journal of the National School of Administration*, No. 3.

Wang, G., Wu, X., & Lei, S. (2017). Light up the journey to wealth with faith. *Fujian Daily*, February 19.

Wang, X. (2016). Changes and Innovations in the Approach of Relocating Poverty Alleviation in Easy-to-Relocate Areas. *Reform*, No. 8.

Xi, J. (2014). Escaping Poverty. Fujian People's Publishing House.

[U.S.] Yan, Y. (2006). *The Transformation of Private Life* (Gong Xiaoxia, Trans.). Shanghai Bookstore Press.

Yang, F. (2008). Relocation and Cultural Adaptation: The Case of Relocated Migrants in Yongren County, Yunnan Province. Guizhou Ethnic Studies, No. 6.

Zhang, X., & Feng, Z. (2008). Spatial correlation and regional convergence of GDP per capita in China: 1978–2003. Quarterly Journal of Economics, No. 2.

Xin Li , former Vice President and Researcher at Fujian Academy of Social Sciences, whose research interests are applied sociology and social development.

Shaoju Wang , former Vice Minister of the Publicity Department of Ningde Municipal Party Committee, Chief Editor of Min Dong Daily, and senior journalist, whose research interests are rural construction and rural poverty reduction.

Yu Geng , Associate Researcher at the Institute of Sociology, Fujian Academy of Social Sciences, whose research interests are rural sociology and cultural sociology.

Chapter 9
It is Hard to Leave Homeland: Relocation and Under-Forest Farming in Jingyang Village, Guangxi

Sumei Fang

Abstract Jingyang Village in Xianan Township, Huanjiang Maonan Autonomous County, Guangxi, has the typical characteristics of a deeply impoverished village in the stony desertification area of Yunnan, Guangxi, and Guizhou provinces. Since 1980s, the local government and people have struggled against poverty, and gradually explored a path combining the poverty alleviation and development and the relocation of poor people. The people of Jingyang Village have actively participated in all stages of relocation and have seen remarkable changes in their production and living conditions. However, many of them have not been cut off from their homeland. While implementing the relocation, the officials and people of Jingyang Village and the supporting organizations have made use of the advantages of mountainous resources to develop the unique under-forest hog breeding industry, which has become an effective way to transform the industry of Jingyang Village and formed a new breeding industry epitomizing "one village, one product". In the face of some limitations of under-forest farming, the officials of the "two committees (Villagers' committee and the village's Party committee. – Trans.)" of Jingyang Village also explored the development of rural leisure tourism, so that the "stone mountain" becomes "gold mountain", thus enabling Jingyang Village to achieve a leap from poverty eradication to prosperity. The story of Jingyang Village is a microcosm of thousands of poverty-stricken mountain villages in China that get rid of poverty and develop toward revitalization.

Keywords Poverty alleviation · Industrial transformation · Under-forest farming · Jingyang Village

In the contiguous area of Guangxi, Guizhou, and Yunnan provinces, there is a large area with typical karst terrain, which is called Yunnan-Guangxi-Guizhou-stony desertification area. It is also one of the 14 contiguous poor areas as a whole, as well as the most populous area in the new round of national poverty alleviation and development

S. Fang (✉)
Institute of Ethnology and Anthropology, Chinese Academy of Social Sciences, Beijing, China

Case Studies of Targeted Poverty Reduction and Alleviation in 100 Villages, International Research on Poverty Reduction, https://doi.org/10.1007/978-981-95-0549-4_9

battle field. For a long time, the unique geographical environment and natural conditions have become a major factor affecting local economic and social development. In order to lift millions of people out of poverty who lived in the Boulder Mountain area, where water and land are scarce, transportation is difficult and it is short of resources, Yunnan, Guangxi, and Guizhou provinces have implemented a series of poverty alleviation models, among which relocation has been widely implemented and achieved remarkable results. At the same time, the relocation has also brought about a series of problems in terms of livelihood changes, social organization restructuring, and ethnic relations reconciliation. In particular, the change of livelihood is an important aspect that determines the ultimate effectiveness of relocation. While vigorously implementing the ecological relocation, Jingyang Village in Huanjiang Maonan Autonomous County of Guangxi has taken a path to develop new rural industries by taking advantage of mountainous resources, which provides a case of certain significance for the research and practice of targeted poverty alleviation and rural revitalization in the stony desertification area of Yunnan, Guangxi, and Guizhou provinces.

9.1 Poor Maonan Village Deep in the Mountains

In the northwest of Guangxi Zhuang Autonomous Region and the southern border of Guizhou Province, there is a beautiful river bay of Dagou River-Jingyang Bay. Adjacent to Jingyang Bay, Jingyang Village is an administrative village in Xianan Township, Huanjiang Maonan Autonomous County, where more than 98% of the residents are Maonan people. Jingyang Village is 12 km away from the township government and 72 km away from the county, with a total area of 27 square kilometers. The village is surrounded by mountains, with the lowest altitude 425 m, the highest altitude 780 m, and the area of rocky mountains accounts for 83.5% of the total area of the village. According to incomplete statistics, during the half century from the 1950s to the end of the 1990s, the population size of Jingyang was maintained at 600–700 people. After entering the twenty-first century, the population size of Jingyang has changed dramatically due to the construction of the Xiaqiao Power Station on the Dagou River and the relocation for poverty alleviation. By the end of 2016, the household population of Jingyang Village has been reduced to 105 households with 297 people, of which, 175 are male, 122 are female, and 193 are laborers. They live scattered in 22 cave fields deep in the folds of the mountains, divided into 13 villager groups.

Jingyang Village is located in the Boulder Mountain area, where arable land is scarce, with arable land of more than 1100–1300 mu[1] for a long time, accounting for only about 17% of the land area. These arable lands are mainly dry lands such as steep slopes, rocky hills, and rocky seams, with thin and infertile soils of poor water retention and subject to soil erosion. It can only be planted with dry land crops such

[1] 1 mu equals 1/15 hectare. –Trans.

as corn, sweet potatoes and soybeans, and the annual yield is low as always. Although there is the Dagou River flowing through the village, the majority of villagers can hardly use the river for irrigation due to the high mountains and deep valleys, and it is very difficult for people and animals to drink water. With the implementation of policy on returning the grain plots to forestry since the twenty-first century, the total area of arable land in Jingyang Village has reduced to 433 mu from 1700 mu as of 2014. Except for some subsidies for returning the grain plots to forestry, most of the young and strong laborers will go out to work to maintain their livelihood.

For a long time, the economic development of Jingyang Village was very slow and the people's life was extremely difficult. According to the statistics in April 1982, the total annual income of the whole village was 27,288 yuan, with an average of less than 35 yuan per person; the average annual grain sales of the village were 16,000 kg. There were 124 households and 786 people in the village, including 651 people without cotton clothes, 313 people without quilts, and 669 people without mosquito nets. There were 107 tile houses with 297 rooms and 26 straw houses with 42 rooms. There were 111 households with 457 people and 266 head of livestock without solving the drinking water problem.[2] In 2009, the national per capita net income of villagers reached 5153 yuan, but the per capita net income of Jingyang Village was only 1256 yuan. In 2011, the village's per capita income was 1669 yuan, far below the target of 5000 yuan set in the 12th Five-Year Plan for poverty alleviation put forward by the Guangxi Zhuang Autonomous Region. By the end of 2015, there were 56 poor households and 149 people in the village, including 25 poor households and 66 people with working ability and willingness to work in the new stage of poverty alleviation, among whom there were 116 people enjoying minimum living guarantee, 13 disabled people, 6 people enjoying the five guarantees, 5 households without labors, and 9 households impoverished by long-term illnesses. The average net income of poor households in 2015 was 2800 yuan. Difficulties in road access, water supply, schooling, and medical treatment restricted the people in Jingyang Village to improving their lives.

In short, before the implementation of targeted poverty alleviation, Jingyang Village showed the typical characteristics of deep poverty villages in the Yunnan, Guangxi, and Guizhou Stone Desertification Area: first, poor natural conditions, high mountains and deep valleys, lack of soil and water, homogeneous economic structure, and low production income; second, lack of infrastructure, serious difficulties in transportation, electricity, communication, medical care, education, drinking water, etc.; third, poor living conditions, living in straw houses, simple houses, and dangerous houses; fourth, the education level of the population is generally low, with a large proportion of illiterate and semi-literate in middle-aged and old-aged group. The cause of poverty in Jingyang Village is fundamentally the natural conditions in which the village is located, which constrains the development of traditional agriculture, directly affects the construction of infrastructure and effective supply of public

[2] *Investigation and Statistics Table of Economic Conditions of Maonan Area (1982)*, Huanjiang Maonan Autonomous County Archives, with record group number 80. The original records an average of 36 yuan per person, which was incorrectly calculated.

services, and the improvement of culture and education. Due to the scarcity of natural resources, the homogeneous economic structure, and the poor living environment, the shrinking population and brain drain, it is difficult for Jingyang Village to form a self-development mechanism and capacity. Under such conditions, without policy support and external assistance, Jingyang Village cannot realize the goal of overall poverty eradication.

9.2 The Practice of Relocation in Jingyang Village

In the mid-1980s, China started organized poverty alleviation work, and Huanjiang Maonan Autonomous County gradually worked out an innovative model combining relocation and poverty alleviation and development, and achieved remarkable results in poverty alleviation work. According to statistics, from 1993 to 2016, Huanjiang Maonan Autonomous County has expropriated 383,980 mu of land, set up 303 resettlement sites which were distributed in 50 administrative villages in 8 townships, and a total of 20,540 households and 93,858 people were resettled inside or outside the county, accounting for 24.83% of the county's total population of 378,000 people. Plus the independent relocated people, the proportion of the relocated to the total population of the county was even greater. As a result, Huanjiang has become the largest relocation populated county in Guangxi to alleviate poverty, and its migration phenomenon drew nationwide attention.[3] During the "13th Five-Year Plan" period, Huanjiang Maonan Autonomous County plans to invest 2.8 billion yuan to comprehensively implement the relocation project, involving 44,693 officially registered poverty-stricken people, and the relocation rate accounts for 53% of the county's poor households.

Lived in the Boulder Mountain area, the villagers of Jingyang have actively participated in all phases of the relocation activities. According to the interviews conducted by the research group, Jingyang Village originally had about 700 residents, and by the end of 2016, the village's household population was less than 300. Over the past ten years, the population relocated through the relocation activities is estimated to be around 350 people, accounting for nearly half of the total population of the village. After the work of targeted poverty alleviation and poverty eradication, 79 households and 223 people have registered for relocation in Jingyang Village, accounting for 75.24% and 75.08% of the village's household population of 105 households and 297 people, respectively. Among these villagers, some of them have already purchased land to build houses in other villages with better conditions in the township, either on their own initiative or by other means. According to the officials of the "two committees" of Jingyang Village, as of September 2017, only 20 households, accounting for 19.05% of the 105 households registered in the village, did not intend to relocate, and their once-dilapidated houses in the village had been renovated.

[3] Fang Sumei: *Relocation and Anti-poverty Practice in Ethnic Area – take Guangxi Huanjiang Maonan Autonomous County as an example*, Journal of southwest Minzu University, 2018 No.9.

These villagers are mostly bachelors and members of households enjoying the five guarantees, mainly because of the lack of funds, while a single person can only enjoy the policy subsidy for building 25 square meters, and this small area cannot be used to build a new house. In conclusion, through the implementation of relocation, the vast majority of households in Jingyang Village have migrated or plan to migrate to live in towns outside the village. Without any other measures, perhaps in the coming years, this small Maonan Village surrounded by mountains will become silent.

According to the investigation and analysis of the research group, under the current conditions, relocation is an effective way to solve the poverty problem of villagers in Boulder Mountain area. Villagers who have moved to new houses have made a qualitative leap in their living conditions, and their houses have become spacious and of higher quality. The industrial structure has changed, from the initially primary industry oriented development to the co-existence of primary, secondary and tertiary industries, and the number of people going out to work is constantly growing. Transportation and communication have become more convenient, and people have more rights in terms of network resources and information sharing. Basic public services, such as education, medical care, and health, have been greatly improved. Especially in terms of ideology, there is a gradual change from the original closed and conservative to the exchanges and openness to the outside world. It can be said that through the relocation, the poor relocated people in the Boulder Mountain area have solved their basic livelihood problems and gradually improved their lives from subsistence to well-off.

While recognizing the effectiveness of poverty alleviation and relocation in the Boulder Mountain area, we see that the relocation has also brought about a series of problems in terms of livelihood changes, social organization restructuring, and ethnic relations reconciliation. In particular, the change of livelihood is related to the ultimate effectiveness of relocation. After the people in Jingyang Village were relocated, because the area of newly transferred land was limited, each family only had a few of paddy fields or dry land of one or two mu, so working outside the home was still the main source of cash income. The relocation site for Jingyang Village is located in the Xianan Township, and the distance is more than 10 but less than 20 km from the Village to the site. Many villagers often go back to the village to cultivate the small arable land and raise some goats and pigs. As the saying goes, "it is hard to leave the homeland", and the mountains are still their homes of ancestors.

9.3 The Dream of Under-Forest Farming of the Capable Person Tan Daoyuan

In fact, Jingyang Village in the mountains is densely wooded, with a beautiful ecological environment and specific natural resource advantages. In 2000, Huanjiang Maonan Autonomous County began to implement the policy of return the grain plots to forestry. As of 2014, Jingyang Village had a total of 1320 mu of returned farmland, leaving dry land of only 433 mu for growing corn, soybeans, and sweet potatoes. After the return of farmland to forest, the villagers' economic sources mainly rely on subsidies for returning farmland to forest and growing ecological natural forest, family farming and working outside, which can meet the basic needs of living, but there is a big gap from the well-off standard, and about half of the residents in the village are not free from the state of poverty. Therefore, finding new economic growth points to realize industrial transformation has become the key to poverty management in Jingyang Village.

While implementing the relocation, how to use the advantages of mountainous resources to develop new rural industries has got the thinking of officials and people of Jingyang Village and the supporting organizations. Jingyang Village in the Boulder Mountain area has insurmountable shortcomings in natural conditions, with many mountains, little land, thin soil and lack of water, as well as poor infrastructure and backward public services, making it difficult to break through the limitations of traditional agricultural production. However, the village has nearly 40,000 mu of ecological public welfare forests and more than 1300 mu of fallow woodlands, which are suitable for vigorous development of the under-forest farming industry. To this end, the officials of the "two committees" of Jingyang Village have taken the lead.

Among them, Tan Daoyuan, who was born in 1980, can be regarded as a capable person to get rid of poverty and become rich in Jingyang Village. He graduated from junior high school, studied in a correspondence college for a few years, worked as a substitute teacher in the village, and also went out to work, and was elected as the deputy director of the villagers' committee in 2005 for two terms, and was elected as the director of the villagers' committee in 2011 for two terms. In order to lead the villagers out of poverty, he united the teammates of "two committees" to find projects and raise funds to build roads and water tanks, renovate dilapidated houses, and help the people in need. At the same time, he thought hard in hope of finding the direction of industrial development suitable for the natural environment and resource characteristics of Jingyang Village. Seeing that weeds were growing under the forest, after the mountainous area was returned to forest, he grew the dream of developing under-forest farming.

In 2010, Tan Daoyuan heard that wild boars are wild and suitable for free range, so he got a male boar and crossbred it with a local black sow. By relying on the unique advantage of under-forest resources, he raised the piglets under the forest in the mountains, supplemented by artificial feeding of pasture, corn flour, rice bran, and various vegetables. The feeding cycle is 15 ~ 18 months. Without fodder to digest, the pork is firm, tender but not greasy, only tasty, which meets people's demand for green, ecological meat products. Based on the market price of 25 yuan per catty[4] for live pigs, and 100–150 catties per pig, the income of each pig is more than 2500 yuan, and the net profit can reach 30% (about 750 yuan). After the experiment, Tan Daoyuan and the village officials think that the under-forest wild pig breeding can be the development direction of the emerging special breeding industry in Jingyang Village.

[4] A Chinese measure equal to 500 g. – Trans.

In 2012, Jingyang Village was listed as one of the 3000 poor villages in Guangxi Zhuang Autonomous Region to promote poverty alleviation and development in a holistic way. In order to help this impoverished mountain village to get rid of poverty as a whole, the Traffic Police Headquarters of the Public Security Department of the autonomous region became the one-to-one contact unit for poverty alleviation in Jingyang Village. In March 2013, the stationed work force and its first secretary were assigned to the village and started their work. Under the leadership of the higher government and according to actual situations of Jingyang Village, the "two committees" of Jingyang Village and the resident work team jointly researched and decided to develop the under-forest breeding industry and create the brand of "Jingyang Mountain Pig" to increase the villagers' income, make people rich, and build up the village as the development philosophy of Jingyang Village to get rid of poverty and build a new socialist village, and clearly put forward the goals and vision for the under-forest breeding industry of Jingyang Village in the next few years: to establish the under-forest breeding association; to give full play of the village "two committees" officials' and Party members' role in exemplary leadership, in pioneering the development, and promoting work in all areas by drawing upon the experience gained on key points; to mobilize poor villagers to participate in the breeding industry, to get rich through labor; to strengthen the collective economy, and increase villagers' income, to strive to complete the project goals of poverty alleviation and development of the village in a holistic way, and build a new socialist countryside. With the full support of the Regional Public Security Department's Traffic Police Headquarters, more than 800,000 yuan were raised in social support funds to establish three sow breeding bases, and the under-forest breeding industry in Jingyang Village began to take off.

The initial group of villagers engaged in under-forest mountain pig breeding are 10 households in Jingyang, of which village officials have played an active and exemplary leading role. As the pioneer and leader of under-forest farming, Tan Daoyuan, director of the villagers' committee, has established a sow breeding base and a mountain pig farm, which has not only driven villagers to develop under-forest farming, but also increased his family's income year by year. Around 2015, he and several villagers bought land in the Xianan community to build a new three-story building, with a family income of more than 100,000 yuan in 2016. With the expansion of under-forest farming in Jingyang Village, Tan Daoyuan led the cooperative to build a mountain pig slaughterhouse, vigorously expending the market of mountain pigs, and was responsible for transporting the live pigs (or pork) to be sold out of the mountains. In short, he plays a very important role in the under-forest farming industry in Jingyang Village. Tan Lianhan, secretary of the village Party branch, was also one of the earliest leaders of under-forest farming. He initially raised six sows to establish a breeding base, and lent piglets to those villagers in difficulties, and then paid him back after the pigs were sold to market. As of October 2016, the farm of secretary Tan Lianhan had 35 pigs in stock and had just sold 5 large pigs and 20 piglets. His family has five members, whose annual income from under-forest farming is about 20,000 yuan.

9.4 Establishment of a Professional Cooperative of Mountain Pig Breeding and the Creation of "Huan Xiang" Brand

The under-forest breeding of Jingyang Village brings new hope, which attracts villagers who worked outside to come back to engage in the under-forest breeding industry. In 2013, Xiaonan Township was identified as "whole township promotion" demonstration area in development and poverty alleviation by the autonomous county, and the construction and implementation began in 2014. Among the construction projects in the project area, the industry-driven project is of an important measure to increase the income of the people. In order to make more than 18,000 people in the township get rid of poverty and become rich in the process of "whole township promotion" and realize well-off together with the people of all ethnic groups in the whole county, the township government has formulated the township's industrial development plan during the "13th Five-Year Plan" period (focusing on the stage of poverty alleviation from 2016 to 2018), based on the special and in-depth research in each village and township, organizing discussion among general public and hiring experts to make suggestions. The guiding ideology is: to develop new special industries on the basis of stabilizing the traditional beef cattle industry, to accelerate the adjustment and upgrading of the township's industrial structure, to reasonably allocate spatial resources, to optimize the industrial layout, to improve industrial competitiveness, to accelerate the transformation of traditional agriculture to modern agriculture, and to promote the sustainable development of the township's economy and society.[5]The under-forest farming industry of Jingyang Village is included in the industrial development plan for the whole township during the "13th Five-Year Plan" period of Xianan Township, and the establishment of Jingyang Village Under-Forest Farming Professional Cooperative is proposed to focus on the development of mountain pig farming industry.

In accordance with the industrial development plan of Xianan Township, in order to make the under-forest farming industry develop soundly and sustainably, the "two committees" of Jingyang Village actively explored the practice and learned from enterprises the model of centralized operation, large-scale development and unified management, and organized villagers to establish the "Jingyang Mountain Pig Breeding Professional Cooperative" in 2013 which is led by Tan Daoyuan, the director of villagers' committee, served as the chairman of cooperative. In 2013, the village sold 368 wild boars, achieving revenue of 970,000 yuan, with profit of 360,000 yuan and per capita income of 947 yuan. It is an 311.74% increase compared with the same period in 2012 when the per capita income was 230 yuan. In 2014, the cooperative registered the "Huanxiang brand" ecological farming trademark and henceforth established its own brand. The membership of the cooperative increased from 21 households initially to 35 households at the beginning of 2017, and the business

[5] People's Government of Xianan Township: *Xianan Township "13th Five-Year" Industrial Development Plan*, January 18, 2016.

scope is the breeding and sale of mountain pigs, local poultry, and goats. The constitution of the cooperative stipulates: villagers must achieve local self-propagation, self-breeding, and "four unity", the latter of which namely is the use of under-forest cave fields to carry out unified free-range farming, and unified pasture, corn flour and other natural feeding materials, unified breeding period of 12 months or more, and unified external sales in the name of the cooperative. Any member who feeds chemical additives or counterfeits the cooperative's pigs will be expelled from the cooperative, whose share money of the cooperative will be deducted from 1000 to 5000 yuan according to the degree of adverse effects caused, so as to guarantee the natural and green quality of the pigs. From time to time, the cooperative organizes veterinarians and other technical personnel to carry out disease control and breeding technology teaching activities, organizes members of the cooperative to participate in breeding technology training, and gives financial assistance to members and sells mountain piglets to poor households on credit. As of 2015, 13 demonstration sites of under-forest economy have been established in Dongping Tun,[6] Dongpo Tun, Xiabijing Tun, and Dongyang Tun. The village has produced more than 300 pigs, with a farming income of more than 600,000 yuan, and the per capita income of the poor village has increased by more than 400 yuan.

While developing the mountain pig farming under the forest, some villagers, represented by Tan Liuhuai, the village family planning official (who was the director of villager's committee of the Women's Federation of Jingyang Village in 2017), tried to raise local chickens under the forest. Tan Liuhuai, who has a secondary school education, started to run a chicken farm in 2014 of which an investment of 50,000 yuan was mainly made in infrastructure construction, with a farm area more than 100 square meters. As of October 2016, the chicken farm was still being expanded at a later stage with another investment of 50,000–60,000 yuan. The farm began to yield income in 2015, with an annual income of 20,000–30,000 yuan. The sales channels are mainly of friends, relatives, acquaintances, and markets. The farm mainly hatches chicks and sells them to villagers for breeding. As of October 2016, Tan Liuhuai's farm had more than 300 chickens and ducks and more than 20 mountain pigs. Under her leadership, more than 20 households in the village have raised local chickens, with the farming scale ranging from more than 20, 30 to more than 100.

Since targeted poverty alleviation and poverty eradication was formally carried out, Huanjiang Maonan Autonomous County Veteran Cadre Bureau has made Jingyang Village the fixed-point assistance village. Through in-depth research and combined with the actual situation of Jingyang Village, the village resident work team formulated the *Measures for Poverty Alleviation in Jingyang Village* in March 2016. The focus of the measures is to actively seek and make full use of Party committees at all levels, government funds, policies, project support and support from backing units, caring enterprises and good-hearted people, vigorously develop and expand the forest breeding mountain pig industry, gradually improve the industrial chain, and continuously expand the scale to yield scale benefits. In building the "Jingyang mountain pig" eco-friendly and environment protection brand, the Xianan Township Party

[6] Tun is also a type of name for village in China. It literally means a station or garrison. – Trans.

Building Demonstration Project, Jingyang Village, under-forest breeding industry was really fulfilled in Jingyang Village, blossomed, and bore fruits. In growing the collective economy, and helping villagers increase income, the annual per capita income of poor villages will reach 5000 yuan by 2020, and achieve the goal of poverty alleviation and getting wealth. In accordance with the work measures, the resident work team in the village actively worked to help Jingyang Village further develop under-forest farming, such as raising funds to expand the breeding base of mountain pigs, standardizing the operation of Mountain Pig Breeding Cooperatives, etc. The first secretary, Qin Sirui, was also awarded in the work of poverty alleviation.

The family situation of the team leader (the leader of the villagers' group, male) in Shangnao Tun, Jingyang Village, shows the general situation of local poor households who were involved in under-forest farming. The leader is 50 years old and unmarried; the eldest brother is in his 40 s and unmarried; and the younger sister is 30 years old, migrant worker and unmarried. They lived together with their mother, and the brothers had registered independent permanent residence. In 2012, the old house was destroyed by fire, and the brothers built a new house of 120 square meters at a cost of 80,000 yuan, with a subsidy of 35,000 yuan (17,500 yuan/one person) and a subsidy of 20,000 yuan (for two people) from the civil affairs department, based on the quota for their family of two qualified persons to renovate dilapidated houses. In 2014, they applied for the relocation project for poverty alleviation. The team leader built the house together with his first brother, his mother, and his sister (because the construction area allowed for the unmarried is too small to build an independent house), and the unified construction area of house is 80 square meters, with the payment of 30,000 yuan for their residential land. The brothers borrowed money to buy the residential land and finished repayment in 2016. The younger brother is married and has a family of 4 people, and the sister-in-law is local in this town and has 2 children. They have lived other places with separate registered permanent residence, who also applied for relocation project. They also borrowed money, but we do not know if they have finished the repayment. They said they would sign up first and then find a way to solve the payment problem of the house construction. They were worried about the accident when lived deep in the mountains, and lived such a hard life that they decided to apply for the relocation for poverty alleviation. In 2011, the team leader got sick and asked for a doctor at the township health center, but because it was late and the road was treacherous, the doctor did not come so he had to charter a car to take him directly to the county hospital. There were only a few field plots in the resettlement site, and they did not know how much arable land they could share (buy), so they engaged in the under-forest mountain pig farming and joined the cooperative, raising only a few heads at the beginning, and each head could be sold for more than 1000–2000 yuan. In 2016, the family expanded their mountain pig farming scale to 20 heads, and they raised one cow furthermore. Since the work of targeted poverty alleviation, one cadre from the village resident work team has been responsible for helping the family and came to their house every month to work out a poverty alleviation plan with them. They planned to expand the scale of under-forest farming to 50 mountain pigs and 100 mountain chickens. The team leader is a little worried about the source of funds, as he said, "The plan is planned, but do not know whether I can achieve it". He also worried about the possibility that after the scale of mountain pig farming expanded, as more people raised more pigs, it will lead to the falling price.

All in all, after several years of development, the under-forest farming in Jingyang Village has become a new industry in the village and an important way for villagers to get rid of poverty and get rich, and the "Jingyang Mountain Pig" has gradually become a specialty brand of Maonanshan Township. By the end of 2016, the total assets of Jingyang Mountain Pig Breeding Cooperative were 3 million yuan, with more than 1300 pigs in stock, annual sales of 4.5 million yuan and annual dividends of 520,000 yuan. The brand of "Huanxiang" mountain pigs has gradually become popular, and the mountain pork of Jingyang Village is sold both inside and far beyond the region. The "blood-production" model of poverty alleviation characterized by "the two villager's committees' leadership + cooperative unified management + product unified marketing" in Jingyang Village has also been promoted in Huanjiang Maonan Autonomous County. Tan Daoyuan took the initiative to withdraw from the villager's committee election in the 2017, and served full-time as the chairman of the Jingyang Mountain Pig Breeding Professional Cooperative, who had determined to make every effort to promote the further development of the under-forest farming industry in Jingyang Village.

9.5 Limitations of Under-Forest Farming and the Future Development Plan

As of the end of 2019, the vast majority of farming households in Jingyang Village have realized relocation, but they are mainly settled around the township government and have not left their native villages, and agriculture is still their main source of livelihood and their dependence. Especially in the wave of rural revitalization, the industrial transformation in rural areas is undoubtedly of great significance. However, the industrial transformation of Jingyang Village also faces great dilemmas. Firstly, how to obtain the certification and protection of geographical indication products for the mountain pigs raised under the forest. In 2015, through the Huanjiang Maonan Autonomous County and Agricultural Bureau of Hechi City, the Jingyang mountain pigs were sent to the autonomous region to verify and obtain the green environmental protection mark. However, due to the limitation of production scale and sales, the popularity of Jingyang Mountain Pig needs to be improved. Secondly, how to scale up the farming of Jingyang Mountain Pigs in order to expand the influence of the brand. Due to the limitation of the biocapacity of forest land resources, the scale of special farming cannot be expanded indefinitely. If the scope of the cooperative is expanded to other villages, it is possible to expand the scale further. It may be necessary to learn from other mature experiences and follow the model of "company + farmer + base + farming". Thirdly, because of the long feeding cycle, more physical activities and low meat yield of mountain pigs, even though the meat is delicious, the cost of farming is very high, so it needs to invest a lot of money to expand the scale, which leads to no advantage in terms of price. The price of live pigs at the beginning of 2016 is 20 ~ 25 yuan per catty and the price of pork is 40 yuan per catty, which is much higher than that of domestic pigs. So it needs to increase market acceptance and put more efforts into management and market promotion. Fourthly, a single industry inevitably has its vulnerability and risk. Although under-forest farming can be developed into a new industry in Jingyang Village, there are relatively big limitations to driving all villagers to invest in under-forest farming, and we must seek diversified industrial development.

In order to break through the limitations of a single industrial structure, while developing under-forest farming, the "two committees" and the cooperative of Jingyang Village also plan to develop leisure tourism projects and strive to revitalize Jingyang Village. Jingyang Village is located in the road to Jingyang Bay from Xianan Township Government. Along the 14 km road from Xianan Township Government to Jingyang Bay, there are rising layers of mountain peaks, jungles and forests on the peaks, and lush trees and woods. The scenery is very beautiful, where Jingyang Village is situated. Moreover, Jingyang Village also has some unique natural and cultural landscapes. First of all, after the relocation of some villagers in Jingyang Village, the previous old houses are still preserved, most of which are traditional stilt houses of the Maonan ethnic group, which makes the ancient appearance of the village still exist. These dwellings mostly have brick, tile, wood and stone structure, and most of which have fallen into disrepair. If the traditional architectural features are preserved on the basis of maintenance and renovation, the charm of ethnic culture and the vitality of residential tourism will glow. Living in a village surrounded by mountains, heaven, earth, and people are integrated into one, which is very harmonious and comfortable. By staying in the village, visitors can also watch and appreciate the traditional cultural elements of the Maonan people, such as food, costumes, games, production, and legends, so as to acquire both material comforts and spiritual enjoyment. Secondly, there are two amazing caves in and around Jingyang Village that can be developed as tourism resources. One is located in the gap at the entrance to the village and was discovered at the end of 2016 when the upgrade and renovation project of the road toward the village was implemented. The caves are very large and deep, and there are fossils discovered. Village officials plan to develop it as a tourism resource for the village after the road renovation is completed. Another cave is located in the village and is said to be a sacred rock. With the renovation and upgrading of the road in Jingyang Village, hundreds of people have visited the cave every Spring Festival since 2017. Thirdly, there are nearly 40,000 mu of ecological public welfare forests in Jingyang Village, and the natural oxygen bar makes people feel relaxed and happy, making it a good place for urbanites to relax and recuperate. Fourthly, the scenery of Jingyang Bay is intoxicating and enchanting. In the past, since there was no road from Dongyang Tun to Jingyang Bay in Jingyang Village, which is about 4 km, villagers could only walk to and from the village, and it was difficult for outsiders to see and enjoy the scenery. In 2013, the approved plan of "the whole township program" for Xianan Township includes a project for the collective provision of water and agricultural irrigation in the area where township government is situated as well as in the adjoining villages and tuns, which plans to use the water from the Jingyang Bay, 14 km away from Xianan Township. The total investment of the project is estimated at 38.16 million yuan, which can solve the drinking water problem of 13,000 people living in and around Xiaonan Township. The water project was submitted to the National People's Congress as a motion in 2014 by the Huanjiang County People's Congress, and the motion was forwarded to the Supervision Office of Guangxi District People's Government. After all parties' investigation and research, the project got approval and was put into action. In 2016, the construction of the road from Dongyang Tun to Jingyang Bay started, and was completed and opened to traffic in 2018. In the 2 years since then, thousands of people have passed through Jingyang Village to visit Jingyang Bay for sightseeing.

The unique tourism resources of Jingyang Village have attracted the attention of village officials and villagers. If it is developed and constructed in a protective way, the whole village will have great potential for developing leisure tourism. Considering the fact that under-forest farming is limited in scale, the "two committees" of Jingyang Village and the village resident work team plan to develop leisure tourism projects and under-forest farming at the same time, in an effort to revitalize the economy of Jingyang Village. Especially with the opened whole traffic line connecting Xianan Township Government and Jingyang Bay, the traffic condition of Jingyang Village was promoted, and brought prospect of leisure tourism to be developed in Jingyang Village. Since 2017, the "two committees" of Jingyang Village and the backbone of the Mountain Pig Breeding Cooperative have organized several visits to tourist attractions in the county, hoping to learn useful experiences and measures, and apply them to the leisure tourism development project of Jingyang Village. They plan to establish a tourism cooperative in order to develop and operate independently, and promote the combination of Jingyang Bay and Jingyang Mountain Pigs, with ecological tourism and under-forest farming promoting mutual development. Of course, the leisure tourism project is still only in the conception stage for Jingyang Village. To really implement, it will face many difficulties and problems. If the independent development and operation is to be realized, since most of the population in Jingyang Village has been relocated, are they willing to come back and make investment? How to maintain their enthusiasm for development in Jingyang Village? The lack of talent is also reflected in the age structure. Currently, the resident population of Jingyang Village is only 130–150 people, mostly over 50 years old, and the number of young people is very small. In addition, although the road from Bochuan Village to Jingyang Village started to be upgraded and renovated at the end of 2016, with the cement roads built, the lane widened, guardrails fixed in some sections, and the treacherous section rerouted, it is still difficult for buses, SUVs, and large trucks to enter the village due to the narrow lane. Especially, it is very dangerous and difficult for two cars in opposite direction to pass by each other. The only way to travel to Jingyang Village is to arrange tour buses to enter the village from the township government site, and vehicles from other places have to park at the township government site or at the bottom of the mountain. Moreover, in terms of cooperation, management, distribution among other operational aspects, the difficulties that may be encountered cannot be ignored.

Generally speaking, the idea of revitalizing the village by the Party branch, villagers' committee, and cooperative of Jingyang Village is relatively clear, that is, while developing special breeding under the forest, developing rural leisure tourism to turn the stone mountain into a golden mountain, thus driving the villagers out of poverty and achieving the goal of building a well-off society for all. At present, the Maonan ethnic area including Jingyang Village has already achieved overall poverty eradication. We expect that the above-mentioned vision and initiatives of Jingyang Village will revive the village which has gradually become silent after relocation, and make the poor village in the big rock Mountain area realize the leap from poverty eradication to revitalization.

References

Guangxi Zhuang Autonomous Region Committee of the Chinese People's Political Consultative Conference, edited by One Hundred Years of Mao Nan Ethnic Facts, Guangxi Ethnic Publishing House (2013).

Guangxi Zhuang Autonomous Region Editorial Group: A Survey of the Social History of the Mulao and Maonan People in Guangxi, Guangxi Ethnic Publishing House (1987).

Huanjiang Maonan Autonomous County Federation of Social Science Circles, ed. Excellent Anthology of Huanjiang Development in the Era of World Heritage, Guangxi People's Publishing House (2016).

Huanjiang Maonan Autonomous County Local History Compilation Committee. (2002). Huanjiang Maonan Autonomous County History, Guangxi People's Publishing House.

Li, T. (2017). The Evolution and Characteristics of Poverty Alleviation Policies in Ethnic Areas since Reform and Opening Up. *Studies in Contemporary Chinese History*, No. 1.

Mao Nan Ethnic Compilation Committee, edited by Mao Nan Ethnic Compilation Committee, Guangxi People's Publishing House (2015).

Ye, J. (2016). A Review of the Current Situation of Poverty and Poverty Alleviation Models in the Stone Desertification Areas of Guangxi. *Journal of Guangxi Institute of Economic Management Officials*, No. 4.

Zeng, F., Zhang, H., & Duan, R. (2016). Major Needs for Innovation and Collaborative Development for Poverty Alleviation: Practice and Reflections on Poverty Alleviation in Huanjiang County, Guangxi Zhuang Autonomous Region. *Proceedings of the Chinese Academy of Sciences, 3.*

Sumei Fang is a researcher at the Institute of Ethnology and Anthropology, Chinese Academy of Social Sciences, whose main research interests include modern Chinese ethnic history and the development of ethnic regions in contemporary China.

Chapter 10
The Bitterness and Joy of Relocation for Poverty Alleviation: Observations on the Practice of Relocation for Poverty Alleviation in Shun'an Village, Guangxi

Yongsong Liao, Zongshuai Zhang, and Peng Wei

Abstract Shun'an Village is a key poor village in Du'an County, Guangxi. The per capita arable land area is small, and the young and strong labor force mostly goes out for work, so the resident population of the village is less than half of the total population. Although Shun'an Village is trying to carry out large-scale and cooperative farming, its industrial carrying capacity is limited due to the limitations of environment, soil productivity, transportation, and other objective factors. The relocation of villagers from the mountains to the outside world and from the village to the town has become an important way for Shun'an Village to achieve poverty alleviation. In the process of implementing the relocation policy, a small number of poor households in Shun'an Village are reluctant to relocate: some poor households have poor employability due to their old age or physical disability, and their lack of life skills in town concerns them that they will not be able to find a job after entering the town so that are unwilling to relocate; some poor households cannot adapt to town life in terms of lifestyle and values, and are also worried that the cost of living will rise after entering the town; some poor households are worried that there will be changes in policy, that their homestead will be taken back after relocation, that their living place will be distant from their farming land, and that their life in old age will not be guaranteed. In order to solve the above-mentioned worries of poor households, Guangxi Shun'an Village has developed some experiences and practices to be learned from the relocation of poor households.

Keywords Karst mountains · Relocation · Targeted poverty alleviation · Shun'an village

Y. Liao
Institute of Rural Development, Chinese Academy of Social Sciences, Beijing, China

Z. Zhang
Graduate School of Chinese Academy of Social Sciences, Beijing, China

P. Wei (✉)
Guangxi Investment Group, Nanning, China

Case Studies of Targeted Poverty Reduction and Alleviation in 100 Villages, International Research on Poverty Reduction, https://doi.org/10.1007/978-981-95-0549-4_10

10.1 The Basic Situation of shun'an Village and the Causes of Poverty

10.1.1 Natural Conditions

Shun'an Village is located in the western mountainous area of Guangxi, deep in the mountains in the 40 km north of Du'anyao Autonomous County.[1] It is a Zhuang village with a typical karst landscape. The village area is 8 square kilometers and consists of more than 50 rungh[2] fields. There are many karst regions in the village, which is a typical karst mountainous area. The mountains such as Luoshi and Cuiping can provide flat fields for planting crops. Shun'an Village is surrounded on all sides by mountains like Luoshi. The local people call this unique topography and landform "弄". "弄" means to open the door and see the mountains, which also explains the geographical conditions of this place—more mountains and less arable land. More than 80% of the area of Shun'an Village is limestone mountains, and the hilly slopes are dominated by red soil, with little arable land and infertile soil, which is called "nine piece of rock and one piece of soil". The total arable land area is 1654 mu[3] and forest area 13,616 mu. After 2005, with the development of national economy, the young and strong laborers went out for work, and it gradually returned the rocky desertification land to forest, which is now overgrown with shrubs and it is impassable. The part of this kind of land accounts for about 50% of the arable land when the household-responsibility system was initiated. In addition, the land expropriation was achieved for the construction of G72 river section of Lanzhou-Haikou Expressway, and the land still under cultivation was about 700 mu at that time. The current population of Shun'an Village is 1799, and the arable area per capita is less than 0.4 mu. The director of the county statistics bureau told us that when he was in school, his teacher once said, "You must study hard to go out for higher education and save one mu of land for the people of Du'an".

It is difficult to store water on the surface of the karst landscape, and the underground rivers are well developed, but the underground water is buried deep (generally 30–50 m from the surface), so it is quite difficult to develop and utilize. There is a local proverb going that "underground water is long, but the cattle on the ground die from thirst". The water resources are abundant in the valleys and hilly areas of the peaks and forests where there are rivers, while the water shortage is serious in the vast peaks and low-lying areas where there are no rivers, especially in the season of winter and spring. Therefore, the type of farming in Shun'an Village is mainly

[1] Du'anyao County is located in the key node of the southwest Guangxi sea route, the back garden of the capital Nanning and the south gate of Hechi City, with a subtropical monsoon climate, high north-west and low south-east topography, and is one of the most typical areas of karst landform (karst landform) development in China.

[2] Rungh, the Zhuang dialect, means the flat field between rock mountains. – Trans.

[3] 1 mu equals 1/15 hectare. – Trans.

dryland farming in the mountains, with no paddy fields. The drylands were interspersed with rocks and piles of stones, and there is almost no contiguous land of more than 1 mu. The crop is corn based, and it mainly depends on the rain irrigation; namely, villagers depend on Heaven for food. Shun'an Village has a mild climate, with little difference in temperature between the four seasons, abundant heat, and abundant rain. The frost-free period is more than 340 days, and the plant growth cycle is long, with double or triple cropping a year. Although the heat is sufficient, the mountains are so high and flat fields are so deep in the mountains with the lack of sunshine. Wind damage in the ravine often causes drought, flood, and wind disasters by turns. The arable land is mostly situated on the rocky fissure land, and there are many birds, animals, and insect pests. All kinds of unfavorable factors restrict the development of agriculture, and it is difficult to have stable and high food production.

10.1.2 Demographic Conditions

Shun'an village is mainly home to Zhuang people, and a small number of Yao people. There are 15 surnames such as Huang, Shi, Liang, and Wei. Affected by the topography, villagers live scattered, and there are more villager groups in the village than those in the administrative villages in the plains. In 2016, Shun'an Village had 27 villager groups, 444 households, and 1799 people, of whom there were 1788 Zhuang people and 11 Yao people. Near the village headquarters, there were 16 villager groups, 317 households, and 1274 people (including 12 households 57 people who were the spontaneous migrants from mountain to the center of the village, among whom there was a household 1 person enjoying the five guarantees with relatives' support). They live in a concentrated area, while the other 11 villager groups, 142 households, and 581 people (including 37 households 160 people who were the spontaneous migrants) live in the deep mountains. The number of households and population in each villager group is small. Among the 27 villager groups, there are 5 groups with a total number of less than 10 households: Nongwai, Babu, Nongmiao, Nongling, and Xiatang. These villager groups have poor transportation, serious contradictions between people and land, drinking water difficulties, and high incidence of poverty. The number of households in each group is less than 20 in 16 villager groups, such as Nongbang. And the number of households over 20 in only Gulao, Baitun, Xiashan, Jajin, Jajie, and Jiangban. The villager group with the largest number of households and population is Jiangban, and the Xiajiedui is the administrative center of Shun'an Village.

It is constrained by the above unfavorable regional environmental conditions; Shun'an Village is a key poverty village in Du'an County. At the beginning of 2015, through targeted identification, 209 households with 860 people were confirmed officially registered poverty-stricken households (member) with the village poverty incidence rate reaching 47.5%, matching the criterion of poverty-stricken village. In 2016, 179 households with 732 people were officially registered poverty-stricken households (member), and 98 households with 408 people enjoying minimum living guarantee, plus 19 households with 22 people enjoying the five guarantees. The collective assets of the village only include a two-story office building, a cultural and sports center, and a basketball court, of which the cultural and sports center as well as the basketball court are located in remote corners and have no use value for the time being, while the office building is used for daily operation of villagers' committee. In the absence of other assets, the collective economic income of Shun'an Village has been zero, which is a "shell village".

In terms of per capita arable land and other available land resources in Shun'an Village, there are too many people compared with little land resources. The village condition determines its basic economic and social pattern, i.e. food self-sufficiency and labor force going out for employment. Although the people of Shun'an Village grow corn twice a year, the small land area per capita and the poor land, coupled with the ecological restoration, plus the damages caused by wild monkeys in the mountains, all result in a very limited yield of corn, so the villagers cannot meet their needs by growing corn. The limited production of corn in Shun'an Village will not allow the corn to enter the market, but mainly for their own internal family consumption, including food consumption and family farming consumption. Family farming plays an important role in the livelihood of Shun'an villagers, and we also found that almost every household in Shun'an village raises chickens, pigs, and sheep. However, individual farming on a household basis is too costly to sell due to transportation conditions, so the role of family farming in increasing the villagers' economic income is also relatively limited. On the road from the county to the town, some cadres have been telling us a story about a villager raising pigs in the mountains: a villager raised three pigs and had to hire a few people to help carry his pigs outside. After selling the pigs, he had to buy drinks and meals for those who helped carry the pigs, and the cost of the meals was as much as the money he earned from selling one pig.

The income from farming is not enough for a family's expenses, so it is necessary to go out for work to increase income, which is the main income source of young and strong laborers of Shun'an Village. Among the 1084 laborers in the village, 570 people have to go out for work more than half a year; 200 people out for work less than half a year, including 100 whole families with 400 people; 79 people go to other provinces; 174 people go to other counties of Guangxi province; and 40 people will return home to engage in agriculture on a regular basis. Due to the large number of people going out for business, the resident population of the village is less than half of the total population, about 800 people. The male/female ratio in Shun'an Village is 110.7:100, which is similar to the national sex ratio in rural areas, i.e. the ratio of male to female is slightly imbalanced. However, due to the scattered villager groups, the villagers living in the mountains are restricted by the transportation conditions and economic income, and the imbalance between men and women is extremely serious in tuns[4] such as Nongwai, Jiajin, Nongdiao, and Fuxing. There are more than 40 "bachelors" in the village, and as the first secretary in the village said, there are

[4] Tun is also a type of name for village in China. It literally means a station or garrison. – Trans.

"four mores" in Shun'an village: more "bachelors" in the mountains, more wives to escape marriage, more people to study, and more people to work as teachers.

10.2 Policy Implementation of Relocation for Poverty Alleviation in shun'an Village

Although Shun'an Village has implemented industrial poverty alleviation and tried to carry out large-scale and cooperative farming, due to the restrictions of environment, soil productivity, traffic, and other objective conditions, the industrial carrying capacity of Shun'an Village is relatively limited and cannot carry too much capital, labor and equipment, and the large-scale farming still faces many challenges, such as water resources, capital, technology, talents, and other conditions restrictions. The first secretary of Shun'an Village believes that if large-scale chicken farming is carried out, the number of chicken will increase, and then the price of chicken will fall; if cattle raising is carried out, the initial cost is too high for start-uppers to afford; and if goats raising is carried out, the damage of goats to the environment will be too great since the large-scale farming will destroy the ecology that can hardly be restored; if pig farming is carried out, as the price of pigs fluctuates greatly, there will be no cost advantage over professional farms (households). Therefore, compared to industrial poverty alleviation, the implementation of the relocation policy to alleviate poverty and mobilize poor households to move out of the mountains and from the village to the town becomes an important way to achieve poverty alleviation in Shun'an Village.

Relocation and going out for work are the most important measures to get rid of poverty in Du'an County. In Du'an County, which is known as the "Stone Mountain Kingdom", the arable land, which is small as a bow or gourd, and even a straw hat can cover two pieces of land, is scattered in countless mountains and Runghs.[5] The contradiction between man and land is prominent. Although nine out of ten years will crop, it will be drought in spring and flood in summer, to have a grain at the cost of ten drops of sweat, and it still not be enough to get free from starvation. In 1993, according to the spirit of relocating some people in the poverty-stricken areas of Guangxi Zhuang Autonomous Region, Du'an villagers migrated out of the mountains once again on a large scale. At the end of 1998, when it was known as "the migration of the century", 30,000 people moved to Guangxi Huanjiang Maonan Autonomous County in a large scale. Du'an County is a large labor export county, and every year more than 100,000 people will go out for business, part of whom are workers and business people with skills, capital, and entrepreneurial aspirations, and they are very eager to live in the county. In 2005, Du'an County decided to deepen the "resettlement without land" model[6] based on this feature in combining

[5] Rungh, the Zhuang dialect, means the flat field between rock mountains. – Trans.

[6] Originally, for each group of poor households to be resettled, a large piece of residential land and arable land was needed, which was called "land resettlement". The "landless resettlement" means

poverty alleviation and urbanization construction, and built 6 relocation settlement sites on the barren land near the county, and hereby created a business incubator for migrant workers in town. In 2012, Du'an planned to spend seven years to acquire nearly 6000 mu of land to relocate all the people from Runghs, who live in remote and scattered tuns[7] with worse natural conditions, and those who lived in serious ecological degradation areas. There were 22,332 households with about 100,000 poverty-stricken population collectively relocated to Hongdu Village and Lantang Village of Chengjiang Town, or the An'yang community of An'yang Town with better transportation conditions and better location, which takes the advantage that radiates from these towns and receives benefits from supporting industries. In May 2015, Du'an poverty alleviation and ecological relocation and new township construction project - Hongdu poverty alleviation and ecological relocation park was initiated its first phase. This park covers an area of 16 square kilometers. Relying on the construction of the Hechi-Du'an Lingang Industrial Zone and the Du'an Poverty Alleviation Industrial Park, it planned to settle 100,000 people. The government's vision is that these 100,000 ecological resettlers will give a strong impetus to the urbanization of Du'an and steadily provide high-quality labor for the enterprises in the Hechi-Du'an Lingang Industrial Zone. During the "13th Five-Year Plan" period, Guangxi needs to relocate 1 million people to achieve alleviate poverty, and Du'an County needs to relocate 12,480 households with 52,414 people, including 2111 households with 9720 people in 2016, 8513 households with 35,899 people in 2017, and 1856 households with 6795 people in 2018.

The relocation project for poverty alleviation is a complicated system. The targeted poverty elimination headquarter at the county government is responsible for responding to the related policy consultations about relocation. The general goal of the policy is to allow the resettlers to "move out, live stable, be sustainable and get rich", and the original old houses will be demolished, the occupied land will be reclaimed and readjusted for utilization according to the principle of balancing the land increase and decrease in occupation after relocation, so as to achieve the goal that the total county's construction land will not be increased, the arable land area will be not reduced, and the quality of relocation project will be improved. On the issue of who will be supported to relocate, according to the regulations, the percentage of other villagers who need to relocate together with the officially registered poverty-stricken people will be controlled within 10% of the total scale of poverty-stricken population in all the townships. State-owned enterprise workers, cadres, teachers, and all kinds of technical personnel, cannot be listed as relocation population. Except the entire tun[8] relocation or impacts by geological disasters, the number of family members to be relocated must exceed 3 people. If there are less than 3 people to be relocated, they must join other households in their relocation.

---

that the government gives the relocated households a home base without compensation, but does not allocate arable land, and the relocated households raise their own funds to build houses and settle their living by engaging in secondary and tertiary industries.

[7] Tun is also a type of name for village in China. It literally means a station or garrison. – Trans.

[8] Tun is also a type of name for village in China. It literally means a station or garrison. – Trans.

The proportion of households with less than 2 people does not exceed 5%, and each household must have more than 1 labor force and without house in the original place of residence.

According to "Du'an Breakdown Table in Population for 'Ten Batches' of Targeted Poverty Alleviation", the relocated population of Shun'an Village is 440, including 94 households with 400 people from 9 villager groups who were collectively relocated in 2015 and 2017, including Babu, Nongling, Jiafan, Nongbang, Nongwai, Jiadong, Nongjiao, Nonglong, and Nongfeng. There are 48 officially registered poverty-stricken households with 215 people, 5 households enjoying the five guarantees with 6 people, 8 poor households with 35 people who had relocated of their own free will, 32 non-poor households with 141 people who had relocated of their own free will, and 1 non-poor household with 3 people who needed to relocate together with the officially registered poverty-stricken people. The total of 84 households with 356 people were planned to relocation (excluding those enjoying the five guarantees), of whom 45 households with 193 people were relocated completely in November 2017. In 2018, Shun'an Village relocated 8 tuns, involving 88 households, including 86 poverty-stricken households. In 2018, the work team supervised the implementation of all relocated households to move in, helped relocated households to apply for transitional living subsidies, and helped 35 poor households to improve materials for demolition of their old houses and also applied for demolition subsidies.

10.3 The Bitterness and Happiness in Relocating from shun'an Village

In the process of implementing the policy of relocation to alleviate poverty, there are cases that some poor households are unwilling to relocate because of their poor employability and lack of urban living skills due to their age or physical disabilities.

For example, when we visited a family in Jiadong Tun, Shun'an Village, we sat in the traditional wooden and stone house of the head of the family and praised the coolness and comfort of the old house, but the owner of the house did not say anything to us and was even rather cold to us, except for the hostess who said in Zhuang dialect and unrelated things that the monkeys came down from the mountains to eat the crops in the morning and they set off firecrackers to drive them to the mountains. The lady's husband never said a word to us, as he watched TV programs in front of the TV set at first, then went out to drive the sheep up the mountain, while his bachelor brother was lying in bed sleeping. When we walked out of this family's house, the boss of Fuxing Tourism Company, who was our guide, said to us, "This family is not willing to move out. As they heard you speak Mandarin and probably thought you went here to persuade them to move out, so they showed rather cold to you. If a local person speaking Zhuang had come, they would not have been like this, they would have been very enthusiastic".

The reason why they are reluctant to relocate is that, firstly, they are worried that they will not be able to find a job, they will not be able to adapt to urban life in terms of lifestyle and values, and the cost of living will increase after moving to the city. Secondly, they are worried that the policy will change. Lastly, because their old houses will be demolished, and the homestead will be returned (every household will be awarded more than 20,000 RMB), even as the relocated poor households still have arable land and land contracting rights, the distance between residence and arable land is far, so it is difficult to be employed in the village, and there will be no turning back, and no one will take care of them when they are old. The people who want to move to the outside world are those who have the ability to work and adapt, and also have seen the world outside (for example, they have done small business and have business acumen), but often these people are not poor. For example, the teacher of the village elementary school, who has an old mother and a collapsed house, wants to be relocated, but because his family are not a officially registered poverty-stricken household, he can only be relocated with the whole tun where some households do not want to relocate, so he has to rebuild his house in the village; some village heads also want to relocate, but they cannot enjoy the policy of relocation because they are not officially registered poverty-stricken households. Liang Jun, the "post 1990s" deputy director of Shun'an Village, returned to the village to engage in side business after he became a veteran with stronger economic strength. Liang Jun told us that his future plan is to leave Shun'an Village to work outside. He said his parents will get old, his brother will need to go outside to get married, and if he cannot take advantage of the time while he is young in pursuing his career outside, the future days for him will be difficult.

As for those villagers who are really poor and live in remote mountains, they often do not want to move out, and then it is necessary for the first secretary in the village to climb a long mountain road to do ideological mobilization. Through the discussion, the first secretary of Shun'an village told us that people who live in the deep mountains and are old-aged are generally unwilling to move out because they consider that their life is already like this and they will not get used to the life after moving out. The best reason to convince them to relocate is not to tell them how their life will be better after they move out, but to persuade them from the perspective of thinking about their children's future, which is often the most effective strategy. When people in the mountains think about themselves, they usually do not have a strong desire to relocate, but if they are told how good it will be for their children after moving out, such as receiving better education and finding a marriage partner more easily, they will have a stronger will to relocate for the sake of their children. When the first secretary in the village persuades and convinces the poor households to relocate, besides explaining the national policy, the intention, and benefits of relocation, he also takes into account various factors in tradition, custom, and belief. For example, one household was unwilling to relocate because they thought it was inauspicious to move out this year through fortune telling and divination, then the first secretary in the village would talk to a feng shui master to resolve this "inauspicious" through the feng shui master's magic, and let the feng shui master tell the household that it was okay to move this year. The importance that rural people attach to their homes and feng shui locations is a national psychological structure with a long history of accumulation, which cannot be simply criticized as "feudal superstition", compared to the simple mobilization method; this mobilization method reflects the respect for villagers' customs and psychological habits.

However, in Shun'an Village there is also a household who is unwilling to relocate whatever the first secretary do his work. Our research team visited this household. We climbed the mountain road for half an hour, panting at the gap, and over the gap we could see this family in the mountain nest. This family has been living here for five generations and is the only poverty-stricken Yao[9] family in the whole village of Shun'an. They chose to live here because in the old days, when traditional agriculture was the mainstay, and each family had much more arable land per capita here than outside, so there was enough arable land to produce enough food, and there were many trees in the mountains, so there was no worry about finding firewood for cooking. In the 1990s and even the beginning of the twenty-first century, the hills of Shun'an Village were not so lush and full of trees as they are now, but trees were cut down by villagers to the extent that there were bare mountains, and some villagers even conflicted over a handful of hogweed, while scattered residents in the deep mountains did not have such a problem due to the lower population density. In addition, not only it does not worry about food and clothing living in the deep mountains, but also the diet structure is relatively rich. Aside from planting, they can also cut grass to raise pigs and goats, as well as gather, pick, and hunt for food. For these reasons, adult men living here had an advantage in getting married in the old days (before 2000), and matchmakers were willing to introduce girls for mountain men. However, nowadays, men living in the mountains are mostly bachelors, or there are many cases of wives running away after marriage. People living outside the mountains think that mountain people cannot find wives because the roads in the mountains are impassable and the transportation is not inadequate. In fact, the inconvenient traffic is only a superficial reason, because the traffic here is not convenient as always, but why the mountain people was still popular in the marriage market then? A more fundamental reason is that now the basic food and clothing problem has been solved, and modern rural women who have knowledge and seen the world are no longer simply satisfied with adequate or ample food and clothing, but also have a new understanding and pursuit of the quality of life and living requirements.

When we were still standing at the gap overlooking this family, the dogs kept by the people in the farm already started barking, and when we arrived at the back of the house, four or five dogs of this family already greeted us with barking. The sheep pen, chicken coop, vegetable garden and cultivated land in front of the house, the pond and water cellar behind the house, the wooden beehive under the eaves, and the pig pen and cowshed under the house, all indicate that this is a self-sufficient family. The head of the household let us go inside. Through inquiries, we knew that this old-style house was renovated in 1989. The head was born in 1971 and is still single whose mother died when he was in his 20 s. He currently has an elderly father, a 32-year-old younger brother, and a sister-in-law who is just in her early 20 s. The

[9] Yao is shorten form of Yao ethnic group. – Trans.

brother and sister-in-law already have three children: one is 4 years old, one is 2 years old, and the last one is just 50 days old. The two brothers, plus the sister-in-law, all have elementary school diplomas. The head of the household and his brother had previously worked in Liuzhou and Guilin, but they did not like the outside life and chose to return to the mountains. The head of the household and his brother now run home farming. They do farm work during the busy season, and usually also in the mountains to herd sheep and cattle. In addition, the head of the household also has an identity, Dao Gong, when the local marriage and funeral celebrations happen, he will be invited to chant and draw charms. His participation in such ceremonies can yield income of one or two hundred yuan each time. When we directly asked the head of the family why he didn't want to move out, he said the air outside was not fresh, while in the mountains the air was fresh, and the water he drank was spring water, and he held the leaves of a soybean in the ground and said: we don't use pesticides, we grow everything we want to eat, and we have to pay for everything outside. He was also afraid that the policy would change after he moved out and his life would not be guaranteed. When we were about to leave, the neighbor of the head of the family also happened to be talking in his house. The neighbor lives in a valley outside the mountain who also did not agree to move before, but afterward agreed to move for the sake of his children who were going to college outside. The neighbor said the house in the county was prepared for his own children, he himself will not go to live there, even if the government drove him to live.

We believe that the reasons the head of the household said for not moving are not fundamental as the root of the problem lies in the structural relationship of the family, especially the special position of the head of the household in the family. When we talked, the head of the household talked to us all the time, while his father, brother, and sister-in-law did not talk much. The poverty support cadres thought that the head of the household's brother and father were willing to relocate, but they did not have "a say" in the family, and the main resistance was the head of the household's own unwillingness to relocate. The economic factor is not the main factor for the head of the household to resist relocation, but once he had a house outside, his brother and sister-in-law would definitely go to live outside, so the big family will be disintegrated, and the authority of the head of the household will be dissolved, resulting in a de facto separation of the family. The head of the household does not have a child as a bachelor, so after such a separation happens, he will have no one to provide for him in his later years. The sister-in-law's mother's family is located less than 200 m away from the old house in the same valley, and she has an old-aged father, a mentally disabled brother, as well as a younger sister who is studying at the fourth grade in her elementary school. One of the reasons the sister-in-law's mother's family agreed to the marriage was that it was close to the head of the household, and that the daughter and son-in-law could provide some support to her family and also provide for them in their later years. The head of the household had been supporting the family on his own since he was in his 20 s, and he was worried that moving out would affect the integrity of the large family that he had worked so hard to build. Once there is such a house outside, the head of the household's brother and sister-in-law will have the possibility to live together outside independently, which is only a matter of time. It is this family structure and family relationship that makes the head of the household unwilling to move outside. Even if the support cadres said they could get a house for free and also continue to live in the mountains, the head of the household still expressed his firm refusal, because once such a house exists, it means that his brother and sister-in-law will leave him with their children at any time.

Although he knew we were here to mobilize him to move out, the head of the household still insisted on his reasons for not moving out, and the two sides' argument remained deadlocked around whether to move or not, but fortunately their attitudes and tone of their speech were still polite and amiable. When we were ready to leave, the head of the household insisted on keeping us for dinner, and asked his brother to catch a big rooster and kill it for us. We huddled on a big round table, eating the freshly killed chicken in an electric hot pot, sticky rice and rice wine with royal jelly. As we ate together, we realized that it was not easy for the head of the household to provide for such a large family, and everyone had to eat, so there must be his own intention. The head of the household and his brother do not drink, which is their habit, their father and neighbors proved that the two brothers do not drink, so the neighbors and the old father enthusiastically clinked glasses with us one by one, while the head of the household finished his meal early and laid down on a bamboo chair to watch the "CCTV News". He also pulled out a branch from the fire pit and used it to write a "bug" character on the wooden floor. The word "bug" means there are no biting bugs in the house. Being able to understand TV program, write, and read scriptures to people as a Dao Gong, it reflects that the head of the household is not uneducated, and we tend to think that he has his own concerns and plans. After we finished the meal, the head of the household insisted on sending us out of the mountain, and we repeatedly asked him not to bother to see us out, but he insisted on walking ahead with a lamp to show us the way, and kept walking for half an hour until he stopped at the last step into the village, which is also the first step to the mountain. The road lamp next to the road exactly shed light on the step, which made the junction between the concrete road in the village and the stone steps in the mountain, and formed a metaphor. The head of the household sitting on this last step, with bare sturdy dark upper arm, smoked a cigarette and had a rest. The next step was the flat concrete road and bright street lamp, where was not his responsibilities. After smoking his cigarette, he stepped into the darkness toward the mountains. He had become one with the mountain. Later, we learned through the first secretary in the village that this household was not relocated finally, and the poverty alleviation work team renovated this family's houses for two separated households in the same place, and built them new houses. The other family in the same mountain moved to the bottom of the mountain and lived in a house built by the government for poor families.

The majority of poor households are willing to move in the town, with only a few unwilling to relocate. For example, when we visited a household in the farthest tun[10] in the west of Shun'an Village, the head of the household was over 80 years

[10] Tun is also a type of name for village in China. It literally means a station or garrison. – Trans.

old and was preparing to drive his sheep up the hill in the sheep pen when we walked up to his doorstep. We thought he was like the household before, avoiding us by driving the sheep. It turns out that after a few minutes, he came back from the back of the house. He drove the sheep up the hill at first and then immediately returned to receive us. His wife, who had a stooped back, took stools from the inner room for us to sit on, and his son, who was in his 40 s or 50 s, brought out plantains, guavas, and pumpkin seeds to entertain us. The head of the household said to us that if we met the first secretary in the village headquarters later on, please help them ask the secretary when they were to move, as they wanted to move out early.

Just as the poor households in Shun'an Village gradually moved out of the village, the rich people in Shun'an Village came back to build new houses. In Shun'an village we found a number of more superior houses had been built or was being built, while some were even four- or five-story high villas. According to the local villagers, the people who own these "mansions" under construction are rich people who went out of the village of Shun'an. After they retire, they will return to the village of Shun'an, renovating their old houses or building new houses. These buildings are tiled with ceramic tiles on exterior surface, which looks very grand. We even saw a household building a luxurious villa in a place in the village where there was no hard-surfaced road and no electricity. After talking to the owner of the house, an old man in his 60s, we learned that the house was built by the old man's children, and the old man worked as a policeman outside. All of his three children were very successful as leaders outside. Their house was built on the basis of the old house where the old man's ancestors lived for generations. They intentionally left a few old houses around the new house as a kind of memorial. The cost of the house is more than 500,000 yuan. The children usually come here on weekends to stay for a few days, because there is no water or electricity on the mountain, so they prepare their meals that cooked at the bottom of the mountain and bring them up. Someone wrote a poem for the house, and the old man read for us: "the old house the old father left, a new palace the children has built; new idyllic countryside today has, the picturesque scene as poem depicts".

10.4 Conclusion

As the most important policy of "Five Measures for Poverty Elimination[11]" for targeted poverty alleviation and poverty eradication, the relocation to alleviate poverty is a basic livelihood project. With the implementation of the policy of the

---

[11] Regarding the question of "how to help," Xi Jinping has proposed five measures to be taken according to the specific conditions of poverty-stricken areas and impoverished populations:

1.Boosting the economy to create more jobs for the disadvantaged.
2.Relocating those living under adverse natural conditions.
3.Providing eco-jobs for the poor.
4.Improving education in poor areas.
5.Improving social security for poverty alleviation.

relocation project, centralized resettlement areas have come into being one after another, allowing the people to move from the mountain forests into new houses. How to strengthen the follow-up management of the centralized resettlement areas to ensure that the poor households can "move out, live stable and get rich" is an important problem that needs to be overall considered. The following conclusions can be drawn from the example of relocation in Shun'an Village.

Whether the relocated rural households can steadily increase their income or not is the key to stabilize their poverty alleviation, and it is also the biggest psychological concern of the poor households who are unwilling to relocate. The relocated population is still dominated by the "three left-behind groups". Some elderly people mainly rely on the meager pension, temporary relief, and a few of favorable subsidies, so we need to adjust the measures to local conditions and carry out targeted measures in the public health services and pension security system to meet the wishes of the sick having access to medical care and the elderly having care and provision. Adhering to the synchronous planning, synchronous promotion of relocation, resettlement and industrial support, making adjustments according to local conditions, making integrated planning, and vigorously developing specialty industries with immediate effects, yields, and sustainability are to ensure that poor households really move out to live a happy new life. They comprehensively implemented the transfer and connection of various agricultural policies and all kinds of protection policies, actively relocated people's households, registered properties, contracted and transferred land, sold and reserved properties, etc. They actively explored the management methods of the centralized resettlement sites for relocation, and innovated the household registration management mode of "separation of people and land" for the relocated population in terms of contracted land, woodland, collective economic benefit distribution among other benefits, as well as agricultural subsidies that could be handled in the original place of household registration, while other things related to social security, education, health care, welfare, aid and assistance, pension, disability subsidies, etc., could be handled in the village or community of residence. In a word, "relocation is the means, and getting rid of poverty is the purpose". During the conduct of relocation policy, it is necessary to help relocated people to get employed or start up their own business, so that the relocated people can broaden their income-increasing channels, and to ensure that the relocated poor population can "stabilize" and "get rid of poverty", and they will strive to help the needed, to achieve real poverty alleviation and to accomplish the real poverty eradication, which effectively enhances the sense of gain, happiness, and security of the relocated people.

References

Cheng, H. (2018). Easy Poverty Alleviation and Relocation: Striving to Achieve Real Poverty Alleviation, Real Poverty Alleviation and Real Poverty Removal. *China Economic Herald*, July 19, 2018.

Du'an County Poverty Alleviation Office. (2015). Implementation Plan for the Targeted Identification of Poor Households and Poor Villages in Du'an County. October 2015.

Du'anyao Autonomous County County Zhi Compilation Committee, Local Chronicles of Du'anyao Autonomous County, Guangxi People's Publishing House (2016).

Li, X. (2014). Building a New System to Improve the Achievement of Poverty Alleviation. China Old Area Construction, No. 9, 2014.

Li, Y. (2017). Relocating Poor Villagers Gives Them a Home and a Job. *China Economic Herald*, December 27, 2017.

Liu, Y. (2017). Achievements and Experiences in Poverty Alleviation since the 18th Party Congress. Qiushi Magazine, No. 6, 2017.

Lu, H. (2015). A Feasible Way to Implement Targeted Poverty Alleviation Strategy. National Governance, No. 38, 2015.

Tong, Z. (2019). The effectiveness and experience of poverty alleviation work since the founding of New China. China Reform News, August 6, 2019.

Wang, S., Guo, Z. (2015). On China's Targeted Poverty Alleviation. Guizhou Social Science, No. 5, 2015.

Yongsong Liao, Researcher, Institute of Rural Development, Chinese Academy of Social Sciences, with research interests in industrial economy and rural development.

Zongshuai Zhang, PhD student, Graduate School of Chinese Academy of Social Sciences, with research interests in rural society and regional culture.

Peng Wei, Senior Engineer, Guangxi Investment Group, with research interests in water conservancy engineering.

Chapter 11
Relocation to Alleviate Poverty Promotes Inclusive Village Development: Practice of Sanshanjing Village in Ningxia

Tongshan Liu

Abstract Relocation is an important way to protect the environment of ecologically fragile areas and solve deep poverty in rural areas. Ningxia is the main battlefield of relocation for poverty alleviation. A survey of Sanshanjing Village, a typical relocation site in Concentric County, Ningxia, found that initiatives such as improving infrastructure and public services in resettlement villages, strengthening compulsory education and labor skills training, and introducing industrial poverty alleviation projects are effective ways to enhance the willingness of poor people in ecologically fragile areas to relocate and support the inclusive economic and social development of resettlement villages. However, Sanshanjing Village faces problems such as fewer successful poverty alleviation projects and less targeted implementation of poverty alleviation work, resulting in low satisfaction of some people with poverty alleviation work. Therefore, it is necessary to improve the policy design of poverty alleviation (resettlers) relocation, to improve the inclusiveness, coordination, and comprehensiveness of relocation on the one hand, and to mobilize the people and social forces to improve the working methods and effectiveness at the grassroots level on the other.

Keywords Poverty alleviation and relocation · Targeted poverty alleviation · Inclusive development · Sanshanjing Village

At present, it is more difficult to get rid of poverty in deep poverty areas, especially in ecologically fragile areas, and a real problem in poverty alleviation is that the local land and water cannot feed the people living here. The implementation of the relocation project can effectively realize the poor people's "moving out of poverty-stricken place, changing the meager salary occupation and eradicating the poor root problems", which has been widely recognized by scholars at home and abroad. As one of the "Five Measures for Poverty Elimination" projects for targeted poverty alleviation, the relocation project for poverty alleviation has achieved outstanding results in recent years. By the end of 2018, China completed the relocation of about

T. Liu (✉)
Research Center for High-Quality Urban and Rural Development, Nanjing Forestry University, Nanjing, China

Case Studies of Targeted Poverty Reduction and Alleviation in 100 Villages, International Research on Poverty Reduction, https://doi.org/10.1007/978-981-95-0549-4_11

8.7 million poor population. As a form of relocation for poverty alleviation, ecological relocation is an important measure to build a well-off society in all aspects. Ningxia Hui Autonomous Region is the main battlefield of China's ecological relocation policy, and has initiated the relocation work for poverty alleviation since the 1980s. In order to solve the poverty problem, Ningxia has adopted the whole village relocation method to relocate the poor people who lived in the southern ecologically fragile areas such as Guyuan to the irrigation area along the Yellow River. By the end of the 12th Five-Year Plan in 2015, 1.16 million people had been relocated in an organized manner, accounting for more than 1/3 of the rural population. Through ecological relocation, Ningxia has been able to protect the ecological environment while effectively lifting poor rural households out of poverty. Therefore, studying the relocation of poverty alleviation in Ningxia not only helps to comprehensively understand the effectiveness of the practice of coping with regional poverty and ecological environmental protection in ethnic minority areas, but also can provide important references for targeted poverty alleviation and relocation in other places.

As the key county of returning farmland to forest and grass, Concentric County is the front-runner in the relocation of ecological resettlers to alleviate poverty in Ningxia. Since 2007, the concentric county has followed the idea of "people move with the water flows, water goes with people" by taking the lead in launching the county ecological relocation project in the Ningxia Hui Autonomous Region. Taking the "move out, live stable, and get rich" as the basic direction for ecological relocation and resettlement work, it has not only formulated and issued several policy documents, but also incorporated ecological relocation into the work assessment of departments at county-level and township governments. Its practice was written as a typical example in the "Twelfth Five-Year Plan" for ecological resettlers in the south-central region of Ningxia. In 2009, Sanshanjing Village in Xiaomaguan Township, Tongxin County, which is relatively rich in per capita arable land resources, was selected as one of the ecological relocation resettlement areas in the county as well as a typical model of ecological relocation. This paper selects Sanshanjing Village in Xiaomaguan Town, Concentric County, Ningxia Province, as the object of analysis, analyzes the measures and effectiveness of poverty alleviation relocation by "dissecting the sparrow", analyzes some challenges in existence, and then puts forward relevant thoughts and suggestions, with a view to providing experience and lessons for relocation in other places.

11.1 Major Measures and the Effectiveness

With the strong support of the local government, Sanshanjing Village makes ecological resettlers "willing to come" through infrastructure improvement and full coverage of public services; makes ecological resettlers "have stable lives" through compulsory education and labor skills training; makes ecological resettlers "getting rich" by promoting the economic development of the village through the introduction of poverty alleviation projects.

11.1.1 Improve the Infrastructure and Public Service System to Make Ecological Resettlers "Willing to Come"

A fully developed infrastructure and public service system is the basic precondition for ecological resettlers to be "willing to come". In recent years, the roads, water, satellite TV, and community cultural activities in Sanshanjing Village have been gradually improved.

In terms of infrastructure, hardened cement roads have been built in front of every household in Sanshanjing Village, the roads in the village are broad and unobstructed, and the bus line connected to Xiamaguan Township has also been opened smoothly. As Sanshanjing Village is a large village with ecological resettlers, with the opening of urban and rural buses and long-distance coaches, villagers can find a bus stop in a few minutes' walk and take public transportation to their destinations smoothly, whether they are going to Xiamaguan Township to go to the market, or going to school in Concentric County, or going to work or see a doctor in Yinchuan City, the provincial capital. When villagers want to sell agricultural products and buy daily necessities, thanks to the flat, broad, and hardened road which connects to the door of each household, large trucks can drive directly to the villagers' doorstep, which greatly facilitates the production and life of villagers. A 70-year-old villager told the author: "once upon a time, it may take a day to go from the old home to the market to buy things, when people generally drive donkey cart to go to the market, and with better conditions, some families may drive a walking tractor. At that time, the road was not good, apt to accident. But now I walk 10 min to the kiosk. If the village kiosk does not have what I want, I can take a bus in the village, and I can get to the town of Xiamaguan in half an hour for the traffic here is very convenient. What is more, because the road is wide and flat, heavier things such as purchased charcoal can be delivered to my doorstep, so I don't need my children to take care of me and I live very comfortably". By the end of 2016, Sanshanjing Village has all realized the tap water provision to the households. With the "double guarantee" of water, the residents of Sanshanjing Village, who suffered from a lack of water supply very long, no longer worry about drinking water problem. Communication signal for cellphone has covered Sanshanjing village, and satellite TV service has connected to every household.

The public services in Sanshanjing Village are also very well developed. In terms of cultural activities in the village, Sanshanjing Village has built a fully functional cultural activity center in the village, with cultural and sports facilities such as an activity center for the elderly, a village library, and a villager fitness field. A convenient financial service site of the Yellow River Rural Commercial Bank system has been installed in the village mini-supermarket, which can handle small withdrawals, money transfers, credit repayments, agent bill payments, and bank card balance inquiries for villagers, providing them with great convenience. For example, some elderly people do not need to go to Xiamaguan town, which is 7 km away, to pay medical insurance premiums and withdraw pensions, but can do so through the services from convenient financial service sites without "leaving home". The villagers' access to culture and entertainment activities as well as modern services is remarkably facilitated. In terms of village medical care security, Sanshanjing Village has established a clinic with two practitioners who hold certificates, providing medical care security for the whole village. The fact that there have been no deaths of children aged 0–5 in the village in recent years also indicates that the village's medical capacity and treatment level have been improved. In terms of housing security for village residents, new resettlers in Sanshanjing Village pay 16,000 RMB per family to receive a 1.2 mu[1] homestead and a brick house of 54 square meters. The elderly villagers can get a subsidy of 15,500 yuan to renovate their dilapidated houses, and can build their own houses on their homestead. Some of the villagers confessed in their interviews, "Compared to the dark house cave,[2] the new house is much brighter now".

11.1.2 Promote Compulsory Education and Labor Skills Training to Allow Ecological Resettlers to "Live Stable"

In order to allow ecological resettlers to "live stable", it is necessary to provide educational support and labor skills training. Education support can help "eradicate the root of poverty" and stop the intergenerational transmission of poverty. Labor skills training can help improve the employment support for ecological resettlers and enhance their human capital level to better achieve employment. With the increasing national investment in education in poverty-stricken areas in recent years, the teaching hardware, teacher level, and teaching quality of elementary school in Sanshanjing Village have been significantly improved. Those children in Sanshanjing Village who fail to enter high school after graduating from junior high school will attend technical secondary schools or technical schools with the financial support of the national "Dewdrop Project", while more and more children of ecological resettlers have entered high schools and further universities with the support of the national scholarship. At present, the ecological resettlers in Sanshanjing Village attach great importance to the education of their children, considering education as an important way to improve the economic status of their families and to raise their social status. Some villagers with better economic power even rent houses in Concentric County specifically for their children to receive better education and have their families accompanying them. Given that Sanshanjing Village is relatively large and many families live far away from the kindergarten, the Sanshanjing Village specially arranged funds for the village kindergarten to arrange a special school bus to pick up and drop off children. A resettled villager of relocated family said in an interview: "In the past, when I lived in previous hometown, my eldest daughter had to walk

[1] 1 mu equals 1/15 hectare. –Trans.

[2] "House cave" is a particular form of earth shelter dwelling common in the Loess Plateau in China's north. –Trans.

4 km to elementary school every day, and my children studying at junior high school had to go to Magaozhuang Township Middle School, which is 16 km away. Most of the mountain roads were not passable for bicycles, so they had to walk, which was very hard for them. At most 60 percent of the children in the village could go to junior high school, and the education quality was very poor. After moving to Sanshanjing Village, the government attached importance to education, and there are kindergartens and elementary schools in the village, and the teaching level of school teachers is much higher. My eldest daughter was able to develop her musical talent in Sanshanjing village elementary school and learned a musical instrument with outside funding, and now she comes to Yinchuan City to continue her music studies. It takes only 15 min for my second and third daughters to walk to elementary school from home, and my fourth and fifth daughters are in the village kindergarten, where they can have nutritious meals and grow up very robustly".

As a poor village, Sanshanjing Village has received more education support resources from all walks of life. The poverty alleviation work team in the village actively integrates social resources by expanding donation channels to donate money for schooling, and has carried out such activities as "helping students with love and letting their dreams fly", and organized some association members to carry out donation activities and distribute free study stationery and school bags for elementary school students. In addition, the poverty alleviation work team of Ningxia Department of Commerce stationed in Sanshanjing Village has also established a long-term tracking and support mechanism for the children from poor households who are studying in the village, and actively carried out projects such as hand-in-hand pairing support. In response to the problems of low employment skills of ecological resettlers and difficulties in matching the employment demand of the labor market, the village work team and villagers' committee often organize skills training for the villagers, such as welding skills, embroidery, cooking, and home car, which enhance the vocational skills of the villagers.

11.1.3 Introduce Poverty Alleviation Projects to Promote Village Economic Development, and Help Ecological Resettlers "Can Get Rich"

In order to make ecological resettlers "rich", it is necessary to take multiple measures to increase villagers' income and broaden employment channels by all means. Various poverty alleviation projects and the government's poverty alleviation policies have made important contributions to the cause of helping ecological resettlers of Sanshanjing Village "get rid of poverty and become rich". In order to promote industrial development, governments at all levels have actively introduced various industrial projects for Sanshanjing Village and given a lot of policy support. Sanshanjing Village gives full play to the spillover effect of the black donkey breeding industry poverty alleviation project to realize the employment of poor households and increase their income. The number of seasonal workers employed by the black donkey breeding base is more than 500, and the number of long-term employees is more than 40, of which 70% are officially registered poverty-stricken households with a monthly salary of more than 3,000 yuan. At the same time, according to the wishes of the poor households in Sanshanjing Village, the black donkey breeding base signed an agreement with the poor households to raise young donkeys, and the company provides young donkeys, forage and technical guidance after evaluating the price. After 3 ~ 4 months of breading, the company will purchase and sell the donkeys at market price, and each donkey can bring an income of 2000 ~ 3000 RMB. The introduction of industrial poverty alleviation projects has produced good economic benefits and provided a guarantee for ecological resettlers to "settle down". With various projects of ecological relocation and targeted poverty alleviation and subsidies introduced in Sanshanjing Village, the subsidy money has become an important source of income for villagers. For example, in 2017, villagers in Sanshanjing Village received an industrial development subsidy of 7,000 yuan per household to raise goats, and many villagers enjoy an annual minimum living guarantee of 1,920 yuan. Villagers who participate in the village's land transfer receive a rent of 100 to 200 yuan per mu. Villagers can also receive agricultural subsidies, old-age subsidies, and improved seeds subsidies from the state and the autonomous region. In 2016, the average monetizing income of poor households in Sanshanjing Village exceeded 40,000 yuan, a significant increase compared to the period before ecological relocation.

In addition, a variety of employment options have also achieved an increase in villagers' income levels. For example, He Yingli, a villager in Sanshanjing Village, opened a kiosk and installed the Yellow River Rural Commercial Bank system in the kiosk, which is mainly used to provide villagers with services such as small withdrawals, money transfers, credit repayments, and payment of medical insurance and pension insurance on behalf of the villagers. He Yingli will get 1 yuan service fee for helping villagers with phone bill payment online, and 0.5 yuan service fee for each payment of new agricultural cooperative medical insurance. Villagers can have cash from their improved seeds subsidy, agricultural subsidy, and even large amounts of cash from goat breeding in this kiosk. Some crippled older people can't even press the password, and the service provided by He Yingli's kiosk can effectively solve the daily needs of the elderly in the village. Because of the large population and the various needs of villagers in Sanshanjing Village, He Yingli can have a relatively substantial income only by running kiosk without doing agricultural work.

11.2 Challenges in the Face

Although Sanshanjing Village has improved the lives of ecological resettlers by improving infrastructure and public services, compulsory education and labor skill training, and increased the income of ecological resettlers by introducing various industrial poverty alleviation projects and striving for poverty alleviation policies, there are still problems such as a few number of successful industrial poverty alleviation projects, the degree of accuracy of poverty alleviation that needs to be improved, and discontentment of some people with the relocation for poverty alleviation.

11.2.1 A Few Number of Successful Industrial Poverty Alleviation Projects

Most of the industrial poverty alleviation projects implemented in Sanshanjing Village ended in failure. Some projects were aborted without returns to villagers. Some projects were interrupted due to enterprises' inability to operate. Some projects stagnated due to poor industrial benefits, and some projects under implementation yield no benefits yet. In-depth analysis of the reasons for the failure of industrial poverty alleviation projects discovers that there are mainly the following four aspects. First, the selection of industrial poverty alleviation projects has a strong subjective nature. The implementation process of industrial poverty alleviation projects is mainly promoted by government departments and village "two committees", and it does not mobilize the people, so villagers are not highly motivated to participate in poverty alleviation projects and even unwilling to cooperate. Industrial poverty alleviation projects are developed as a means to obtain government subsidies rather than as a way to get rid of poverty and get rich, which has intensified the poor households' thoughts of "passively longing for national assistance, expecting government grants and claiming for poverty reduction funds". Second, industrial development infrastructure construction is not perfect. Some industrial development itself can be successful, but some of the poverty alleviation industry projects focus too much on production support while ignore the integrity of infrastructure support and the development of product marketing channels, resulting in some projects aborted because villagers are not willing to develop. For example, in Sanshanjing Village, many greenhouses were abandoned before they were put into production due to the shortcoming of irrigation as well as the failure to achieve the initial goal. Third, the supporting method of industrial project is not science. Some poverty alleviation industries generated wrong market signals due to unscientific supporting methods, which led some enterprises to launch poverty alleviation projects mainly for the pursuit of financial subsidies. Some poverty alleviation projects are blindly introduced, which run with the herd, making it difficult for some projects to be promoted in depth according to local conditions and eventually fail. For example, the subsidies for land transfer of the 10,000 mu of Paeonia suffruticosa and Licorice planting projects were paid in three years. The enterprises did not conduct small area cultivation trials in the early stage, nor did they carry out cultivation technology demonstration and technology research and development of product processing, but directly promoted the projects by transferring large areas of land. Finally, due to the market depression and lack of efficient management, the project is abandoned halfway. Fourth, industrial development and the interests of villagers are not closely linked, which even emerges the phenomenon of severe decoupling from villagers and it is difficult to acquire the long-term support of them. For example, the benefits generated by the enterprise in developing the construction project of 10,000 mu of Paeonia suffruticosa and Licorice base have no other interest connection to the villagers in the village, instead of the payment of rent for the land transferred by the villagers.

11.2.2 The Degree of Precision in Poverty Alleviation Needs to Be Improved

Accurate identification and confirmation of poor households is the basic work of targeted poverty alleviation, which directly affects the poverty alleviation work. Due to the large number of villagers and the small number of cadres, some problems have emerged in the targeted poverty alleviation work of Sanshanjing Village. First of all, the "separate of households" confuses poverty alleviation with rural elderly care problem. The existing criteria for identifying poor households is that the per capita income of a household should be no higher than the local standard line for poverty alleviation. This has induced a large number of villagers to make some of their family members get poor by "Separating" their households. In Sanshanjing Village, many villagers, especially the elderly who have no source of income, became eligible officially registered poverty-stricken households by separating their household register from their sons' and other family members'. Among the 32 randomly selected officially registered poverty-stricken households, 15 of them became poor through "separating household register", and one of them even separated the husband's household register and then became officially registered poverty-stricken member due to the lack of labor. Among the 31 randomly selected non-status officially registered poverty-stricken households, 7 households also made their members officially registered poverty-stricken members by "separating their household registers". This practice of "separating household registers" confuses the elderly social security with poverty alleviation, wasting valuable resources for poverty alleviation and violating the spirit of targeted poverty alleviation of the central government. Secondly, there is a problem of "arbitrariness" in the identification of officially registered poverty-stricken households and households enjoying minimum living guarantee in Sanshanjing Village. In addition to the problem of "separating household registers", there is a lot of room for improvement in the "target" accuracy of poverty alleviation work. Among the 32 randomly selected poor households, as many as 20 should not be identified as poor households according to local standards, and the per capita net income of 6 households of the 20 even reached 10,000 yuan, far exceeding the standard for poor households. Several villagers told me that in 2011, the village used the "minimum living guarantee quota" to attract villagers cleaning the garbage in the village, but after a few months, these villagers just "enjoy minimum living guarantee" and no longer do the cleaning for the village. Finally, there are also many cases of "three haves" people who cannot be identified as poor households as they have public positions, cars, and shares, but become "households enjoying minimum living guarantee". Among the 31 non-poor households randomly selected, 6 of them were households enjoying minimum living guarantee. 1 of them had a per capita net income of 14,608 yuan in 2016 and a private car, but since 2017, two elderly people of this household started to receive 180 yuan of minimum living guarantee per month. As of August 2017, the number of people dependent on minimum living guarantee in Sanshanjing Village increased by 79 compared to 2016, reaching 463, accounting for 9.5% of the resident population. The "Minimum living guarantee", which was only available to low-income groups, has become a "big pot of porridge",[3] and the phenomenon of inaccurate poverty alleviation has emerged.

11.2.3 Some People Are Unsatisfied with Relocation for Poverty Alleviation

The relocation for poverty alleviation does not take into account the differentiated needs of some villagers as well. Coupled with the fact that there are not many successful poverty alleviation projects and the degree of precision of the village's poverty alleviation work needs to be improved, it has led to some villagers being less satisfied with the poverty alleviation relocation work.

On the one hand, the relocation for poverty alleviation fails to fully consider the change of living habits and lifestyles of the villagers concerned. Some resettlers are used to living in house caves[4] for a long time and do not adapt to the life in tile houses. Some interviewed villagers told me that the house cave life is warm in winter and cool in summer, so there is no need to burn charcoal in winter, no need to blow fan or turn on air conditioner in summer, and the cost of living obviously increases after relocating to Sanshanjing Village. Moreover, one resettler said that before moving to Sanshanjing Village, he could grow vegetables and food, but after arriving at Sanshanjing Village, the quality of the arable land allocated to him was too poor to cultivate, so he had to pay for all the vegetables and food, and his living expenses increased significantly. The change of living habits and the increase of living expenses lowered some people's satisfaction of relocation for poverty alleviation.

On the other hand, the effect of industrial poverty alleviation projects after resettlement is not satisfactory, since the poverty alleviation work does not fully mobilize the masses, which affects the satisfaction of the masses with the poverty alleviation work. A villager from Sanshanjing Village told the author, "The policies of the central government are good, but our place is 'high in the mountains and far away from the emperor'". In other words, he thought that some of the central government's

[3] Literally means that egalitarian treatment of individuals regardless of their performances, as everyone can have his/her own portion of porridge. – Trans.

[4] "House cave" is a particular form of earth shelter dwelling common in the Loess Plateau in China's north. –Trans.

poverty alleviation policies were good, but they were not effectively implemented at the grassroots level, so he was not very satisfied with the poverty alleviation work. The above two reasons lowered the villagers', especially the poor households', evaluation of poverty alleviation work in their villages. Among the 32 randomly selected poor households, a total of 62.50% of the poor households thought that the selection of poor households in their village was "very unreasonable", "not very reasonable", or "just so so"; 6.25% and 15.63% of the poor households thought that the arrangements of poverty alleviation projects in their village were "very unreasonable" or "not very reasonable", respectively. As many as 59.38% of the poor households were not satisfied with the effect of poverty alleviation in the whole village.

11.3 Reflections and Suggestions

The goal of relocation for alleviate poverty is to get rid of poverty, and the means is relocation. Compared with other means of poverty alleviation, the cost and risk of relocation for poverty alleviation is greater and higher. Therefore, unless in the prohibited development zones or restricted development zones in the National Main Functional Area Plan, or in areas with weakest resource bearing capacity, relocation for poverty alleviation should be the last option. To better implement ecological relocation, the starting point of policy design should be to improve the inclusiveness, coordination, and comprehensiveness of ecological relocation, by reasonably selecting the supporting industrial projects for the relocation area, and at the same time innovating the government's support mode for industrial development, mobilizing the masses and social forces, and improving the working methods and effectiveness of grassroots.

11.3.1 Improve the Policy Design to Improve the Inclusiveness, Coordination, and Comprehensiveness of Relocation

Firstly, truly respect the will and autonomy of the ecological resettlers to relocate. The relocation in many places does not fully take into account the subjective will of the resettlers, and there is a serious tendency of administration, which leads to greater grievances of the resettlers. It is necessary to differentiate the treatment of differentiated needs of different types of migrant relocation, respect the autonomy and spontaneity of villagers, and let them make their own decisions. The role of the government should be changed from referee to waiter, providing guidance and help as the main focus, supplemented by administrative orders. For ecological resettlers who can move to towns, they are allowed to dispose of their rural resource assets and are given certain subsidies to settle in towns; for ecological resettlers who are willing to move to the county or other areas, a differentiated subsidy policy should also be formulated to provide land, property and job; for those who still do not want to move in the face of various preferential and supportive policies, as long as the local resource carrying capacity allows it, and the location does not belong to a prohibited development zone or restricted development zone, they should be allowed to stay to live.

Secondly, in addition to strengthening community care, it tries to change the way of resettlement of ecological resettlers, from centralized resettlement to "flower arrangement". In recent years, a series of mass incidents in some areas of resettlement sites have sounded the alarm that concentrated poor households in the county have obvious negative effects. Therefore, in recent years, the Ningxia Hui Autonomous Region has begun to experiment with "flower arrangement" for ecological resettlers. The so-called flower arrangement is a method of resettlement in which ecological resettlers from a township or village are resettled in different villages or even different counties in a dispersed way, with only a few or a dozen households resettled in each village. From 2013 to 2016, Pingluo County of Ningxia once tried to resettle more than 1700 households of ecological resettlers from Xihaigu in a "flower arrangement" way. The main approach was that the government used ecological resettlement funds to acquire the contracted land and rural houses (together with homestead) of villagers who lived in the village, and ask them to give up their collective membership status, encourage them to move into the city so as to completely leave the countryside and quit their land. Then, the left land and houses, together with their collective membership status, will be transferred by contract to the ecological resettlers who moved to the village. Since Pingluo County is located in the Hetao Plain, also known as the "Saishangjiangnan",[5] and has a solid foundation for agricultural development, so the overall effect of "flower arrangement" for ecological resettlers is very good. The "flower arrangement" needs to give more community care to the resettlers and help them integrate into the community as much as possible.

Thirdly, comprehensive reform is used to protect the interests of the ecological resettlers. The ecological relocation involves all aspects of villagers' production and life. In order to avoid backtracking and reduce the hidden dangers of reform, comprehensive consideration and group efforts are needed during the formulation of policies for relocation. After compensation is done, the land and house property titles of resettlers need to be canceled and new titles will be obtained in the place where they move to. For ecological resettlers who give up their contracted land, homestead and other legal properties, they should be given financial compensation instead of transferring their properties to the state without compensation. In addition to land and housing, it is also necessary to take into account the grain subsidies, pension and medical insurance, ecological subsidies and poverty subsidies that will be given to villagers by the state, which should be transferred to them at the relocation site in a timely manner and allowed to be cashed in a lump sum to protect the rights and interests of ecological resettlers.

[5] Literally means the abundant place outside the Great Wall. – Trans.

11.3.2 Reasonable Selection of Industrial Projects, and Innovate Government Support Model for Industrial Development

First of all, there is a need for scientific selection of industrial poverty alleviation projects and reform of industrial support model. As far as household-based industrial support mode, it is difficult to make the industry bigger and stronger, and it is also difficult to achieve sustainable development. It is a must to completely change the result of industrial poverty alleviation. In other words, "year after year there are projects, year after year no development achieved". It is a must to adhere to local production factors and resource conditions as the basis in selecting the projects that meet product market demand, with high product quality, sales channels, development benefits, and robust driving capacity, suitable for villagers to develop their own planting, breeding, service, or secondary and tertiary industries. As for the introduction of new projects and new technologies, it is a must to adhere to the "three steps" principle of "one experiment, two demonstration, three promotion", and resolutely put an end to the industrial support model without experiment and demonstration, in a way of rushing headlong into mass action. Taking industrial park development as a focus point, it gives full play to the industrial clustering effect. Whether it is planting or breeding industry, it should be implemented in the park development. Planting projects should be clustered development, so as to unify farming, provide centralized technical services, and promote centralized product sales. Farmers carry out park-based farming management, so as to facilitate the construction of power and water supply facilities, provide farming technology services, make harmless treatment of manure, and implement farming environment management. Villages with good conditions can promote the integration of industries by introducing and cultivating leading enterprises.

Secondly, there is a need to strengthen the construction of industrial infrastructure and reform the phase of industrial support. After the scientific selection of industrial development projects, it should concentrate all industrial support funds, and must improve infrastructure construction in the various development phases of pre-production, mid-production, and post-production, so as to provide reliable infrastructure guarantee for industrial development. There is a need to increase the national subsidies so as to make centralized construction, and separate resources for each household use to improve the use of infrastructure construction efficiency. For example, to support the development of planting industry, it is necessary to concentrate material and financial resources to unify the construction of modern agricultural infrastructure such as water-saving irrigation facilities, protected land cultivation facilities, field roads, product storage, and cold chain transportation. To support the development of breeding industry, it must unify the planning and construction of breeding parks, water and electricity supply, forage processing, disease prevention and treatment, technical training, slaughtering, product storage and transportation, and other facilities. As the amount of arable land and yard area per household of ecological resettlers is small, it is not cost-effective for every household to purchase agricultural machinery, so part of the poverty alleviation funds should focus on supporting the development of socialized professional service organizations, such as the development of big agricultural machinery households, forage processing professional households, product distribution professional households, and other types of socialized service professional households, so as to provide socialized professional services for industrial development. The development of the industry should not only support the upstream production link of the industry chain, but also enhance the market capacity of the downstream sales link. It is a need to strengthen the brand building of regional agricultural products, actively organize "go out" and "invite in" activities for production and marketing, increase marketing promotion and publicity, support the development of rural e-commerce, so that it will effectively solve the problem of connecting production and marketing.

Thirdly, there is a need to increase financial support to extend the loan period of industrial poverty alleviation projects, to actively summarize and promote the financial poverty alleviation models such as "Fiscal + Finance + Industry + Poverty Alleviation" in Guyuan City, Ningxia, and "Village-Level Mutual Assistance Funds for Poverty Alleviation" in Yanchi County, to fully implement financial poverty alleviation projects, to expand the scale of loans for industrial development projects, to extend the coverage of loans for poor households, and to extend the industry support loan period. There is a need to support the development of local special advantage industries of agricultural business entities such as officially registered poverty-stricken households, big planting and breeding households, family farms, farmers' cooperatives, farm stays, and agriculture-related enterprises. On the basis of the current establishment of the poverty alleviation industry guarantee fund and the establishment of a financing guarantee company, it is needed to further expand the scale of the industrial poverty alleviation guarantee fund, to improve the loan guarantee capacity, and to increase the amount of loans for poverty alleviation industry.

Finally, it is needed to increase government guidance and strengthen the mechanism for integrating interests between industrial poverty alleviation projects and poor households. It is necessary to explore the construction of an industrial interest integration mechanism. As long as the agricultural business entities receive state financial subsidies, they must hire ordinary farmers, especially poor households, to help them get out of poverty and increase their income through a close interest integration mechanism. At present, in the industrial poverty alleviation, governments in all places are actively exploring development models like "guaranteed income + second dividends", and farmers' investment with land, capital, and other factors into the enterprise, and cooperative development relationship between enterprises and farmers, etc. The government should strengthen the guidance of agricultural enterprises, large-scale business entities and farmers, and encourage farmers to establish close interest linkage mechanisms with upstream and downstream agricultural enterprises or other large-scale business entities in the form of buying shares with agricultural products sales orders, land or capital, etc.

11.3.3 Mobilize the Masses and Social Forces to Improve the Way and Effectiveness of Grassroots Work

Firstly, it is needed to interchange the roles of third parties and grassroots cadres in poverty alleviation work, so as to change the mechanism of poverty alleviation at the grassroots level. At present, the government mainly assigns basic poverty alleviation work such as identifying poor households to village cadres, and then uses a third Party to evaluate the effectiveness of poverty alleviation. However, to speak subjectively or objectively, it is difficult for village cadres to wholeheartedly implement the central government's poverty alleviation policies, and the third-Party assessment is actually only an after-the-fact supervision, making it difficult to guarantee the effectiveness of poverty alleviation from the source. In order to do the poverty alleviation and elimination work solidly, carefully and well enough, a third Party without interests is needed to carry out this work specifically in the rural grassroots, especially in the villages. In the next step, it can be reversed to let the third-Party act as the main body of poverty alleviation work, and it will be responsible for the identification of poor households, the use and investment of poverty alleviation funds; let the grassroots government, village cadres and villagers jointly evaluate and accept the third Party's poverty alleviation work and its effectiveness. Let professionals do professional work, which is conducive to the implementation of poverty alleviation policies.

Secondly, it is needed to widely mobilize the masses, so that farmers really understand and participate in poverty alleviation work. At present, it mainly relies on the village "two committees"[6] cadres to push forward the poverty alleviation in many places, and it is reluctant to play the pioneering role of the village Party members, and even more unwilling and unable to mobilize ordinary villagers. Many villages have a large number of Party members, but the number of those involved in poverty alleviation work is small; yet even if the number of Party members involved in poverty alleviation work is large, the number of whom dawdle along their work is not small. To mobilize the masses extensively and let ordinary Party members and villagers participate in the identification of poor households and the use of poverty alleviation funds is an effective measure to fundamentally eliminate the problems of inaccurate identification of poor households and "leakage" of poverty alleviation funds.

Finally, the poverty alleviation funds from various departments and channels should be integrated and unified for use. It is needed to form synergy of various poverty alleviation funds to implement "combo blow" effect. The goal is to stimulate the endogenous motivation of poor households to get out of poverty on the basis of meeting their actual needs. Considering the uniformity of funds and goals, on the basis of improving the poverty alleviation mechanism at the grassroots level, we can try to integrate poverty alleviation funds from different departments and channels at the village level. For concentrated contiguous poverty areas or other areas with good conditions, under the precondition of fully ensuring the poor households to get out of poverty, the remaining poverty alleviation funds can be tried to use in the following

[6] Villagers' committee and the village's Party committee. – Trans.

two ways: first, they can be converted into rural pension insurance premiums to raise the level of pension protection for rural residents; second, they can be used to build village public facilities or purchase public services needed by villagers to improve the village's capacity for sustainable development.

References

Zou, Y., Liu, Z., Zheng, X., et al. (2019). Evaluating Poverty Alleviation by Relocation Under the Link Policy: A Case Study from Tongyu County, Jilin Province, China. *Sustainability, 11*(18), 5061.

Zeng, X., & Wang, S. (2019). Some Thoughts on Winning the Battle of Poverty Alleviation and Relocation. *Northwest Normal University Journal (Social Science Edition)*, No. 1, 2019.

Li, P. (2017). Implementing ecological relocation for targeted poverty alleviation. In Wang, X., et al. (Eds.), *Ecological Relocation and Targeted Poverty Alleviation—Ningxia's Practice and Experience*. Social Science Literature Press, 2017.

Liu, T., Zhao, H., & Yan, H. (2016). Rural Land Withdrawal: The Experience and Inspiration of Ningxia Pingluo Experimental Zone. *Ningxia Social Science*, No. 1, 2016.

Wang, X. (2017). Relocation and Targeted Poverty Alleviation: A Re-examination of Ecological Relocation in Ningxia. *New Horizons*, No. 2, 2017.

Wang, Z., Sun, H., & Zhang, G. (2020). Theoretical and Practical Innovation of Ecological Relocation: The Experience of Ningxia. *Journal of Shandong University (Philosophy and Social Science Edition)*, No. 4, 2020.

Tongshan Liu , Director of Research Center for High-Quality Urban and Rural Development, Nanjing Forestry University, professor and doctoral supervisor, mainly researching on rural land system and urban and rural green development.

Chapter 12
The Three First Secretaries Who Passed the Relay Baton of Poverty Alleviation: Poverty Alleviation Memoir of First Secretary of Shahao Village, Shanxi Province

Junxia Zeng

Abstract Located in the deeply impoverished mountainous area of Lvliang, Shahao Village has greeted three First Secretaries successively. The three First Secretaries completed the pass of the baton in poverty alleviation, which not only helped Shahao Village successfully complete the task of poverty alleviation, but also laid a solid foundation for rural revitalization. The first First Secretary, facing a poor and unmanaged village, took the lead and demonstrated the role of Communist Party members as a benchmarking flag; the second First Secretary built the village "two committee" team, established a standardized working system, improved the working ability of the team, and built the village's own development momentum; the third First Secretary set up a solid village "two committee" team. The third First Secretary built up the village "two committees" team, enhanced the development momentum of the village, improved the life of the villagers, sought the long-term development of the village, and strove to achieve the goal of "affluent Shahao, beautiful countryside". These three First Secretaries have not only completed the pass of poverty alleviation work, but also reflected the inheritance and evolution of poverty alleviation and supporting work.

Keywords Targeted poverty alleviation · First Secretary · Win the critical battle of poverty reduction · Shahao Village

---

J. Zeng (✉)
Institute of Rural Development, Chinese Academy of Social Sciences, Beijing, China

Case Studies of Targeted Poverty Reduction and Alleviation in 100 Villages, International Research on Poverty Reduction, https://doi.org/10.1007/978-981-95-0549-4_12

12.1 Thousand-Year History of Shahao, and Poverty-Stricken Shahao

Shahao Village is located in the mountainous area in the northwestern part of Xing County, Shanxi Province. It is part of the Caijiaya Township, which is 17 km from the township government. And the Caijiaya Township is the famous capital site of Jin-Sui border area[1] (liberated area). Shahao Village is located in a mountainous area with rolling hills and steep slopes. The total area of the village is 4.37 square kilometers, including 2979 mu[2] of arable land, mostly sloping land, and 400 mu of forest land. Shahao Village is an administrative village with 4 natural villages under its jurisdiction, including Shahao Natural Village, Three Eyes Spring Village, Nianta Village, and Wangjiaya Village.

Shahao Village has a long history, recorded as early as the Han Dynasty, and has been in existence for more than 1000 years. At the beginning of the liberation, there were more than 400 people in the village. At that time, the villagers of Shahao basically had no land, so they rented the land of the landlord from the nearby Yangjiapo Village, with a leased area of about 500 mu. During the land reform, every family was given a share of land. During the people's commune period, these lands were collected as collective land. In 1982, the village started to realize the land contracting system, and in 1994, the second round of land contracting started, when there were more than 600 villagers, and each person could get 3 ~ 4 mu of land. At that time, the village had a large population and was one of the vibrant villages in the eight villages in the countryside. In 2000, the villagers began to migrate on a large scale, and more than half of the villagers left, only 300 people were still in the village. Especially after the village elementary school was revoked in 2002, villagers took their children to the county or township to attend school, and there was hardly a school-age child left in the village. By 2017, the village had a household population of 755, with less than 150 permanent residents and about 70 households, and most of those left behind were old, sick, and disabled.

Within 1000 years in Shahao, poverty has also accompanied the ancestors living on this piece of land. Shahao Village is located in a deep poverty area, and in 2016, there were a total of 62 officially registered poverty-stricken households and 215 members among 245 households and 755 people in the village, with a poverty incidence rate of 28.5%. The economic income of villagers is very low, according to the survey, the per capita disposable income of Shahao Village villagers in 2016 was only 5072 yuan, accounting for only 41% of the national per capita disposable income of rural residents of 12,363 yuan, while the per capita disposable income of poor households

---

[1] *Zeng Junxia is an assistant researcher at the Institute of Rural Development, Chinese Academy of Social Sciences, whose main research interests are agricultural and rural talents and rural education.

During the War of Resistance Against Japanese Aggression and the War of Liberation, Jin-Sui border area is the main base of Communist Party of China (CPC) in the North China which is an important traffic position for Central China, North China, and South China and Shanxi-Gansu-Ningxia border region. – Trans.

[2] 1 mu equals 1/15 hectare. –Trans.

in Shahao Village was only 4,469 yuan, accounting for only 36% of the national per capita disposable income of rural residents.

Although there are a series of objective unfavorable factors such as geography, transportation, and history, the lack of subjective factor, "human", which is needed for development is also an important reason why Shahao Village has never been able to get rid of poverty, and these human factors are precisely what can be changed. These human factors are concentrated in the lack of a good "leader" and the lack of a good team of village "two committee" in Shahao village; they are also reflected in the villagers' own lack of development ability and willingness.

Shahao Village is not only a poor village, but also a village with a weak and slack Party organization. For a long time, the work of the "two committees" of the village was basically paralyzed, and it was impossible to lead the villagers out of poverty. The former secretary of the village Party branch had not only failed to serve the village collective and villagers for more than a decade, but also used his position to embezzle collective interest and personal interests of the villagers. According to the interviewed elderly people, as early as a dozen years ago, the former Party branch secretary contracted the government-ordered "providing drinking water access to household" project, yet in the result of jerry-building project, due to the pipes laid down in shallow earth, in the first winter, drinking water pipes were frozen to get cracked. Since then, all households can no longer have access to drinking water in their houses. During the term of office, the former secretary effortlessly developed his kins[3] as CPC members, which incurred conflicts among natural villages. In May 2016, the former secretary was dismissed by the villagers in a collective petition. There are 15 members in the Party branch of Shahao Village, 12 of them are over 50 years old, which is a serious aging of the organization; only 7 of them live in the village for a long time, and the activities of the Party organization cannot be carried out normally for a long time, which made the Party organization undisciplined and slack.

In Shahao Village, the villagers' weak ability to develop themselves is mainly reflected in their low skill level and education. 16 of the 62 officially registered poverty-stricken households lacked skills, which was the primary cause of their poverty; 60% of the officially registered poverty-stricken population accepted elementary school education, 30% had junior high school education, and only 10% have high school, technical school or higher education. Due to the low level of skills and knowledge, villagers can only engage in simple manual labor, which prevents them from earning a higher income to lift their family out of poverty. The villagers of Shahao Village are not willing to develop themselves, and this is reflected in the inactive development. For more than 30 years of poverty alleviation and development by government, the villagers in Shahao Village have been the recipients, and some of them have naturally been used to passively longing for national assistance, expecting

[3] A Chinese kin, lineage or sometimes rendered as clan, is a patrilineal and patrilocal group of related Chinese people with a common surname sharing a common ancestor and, in many cases, an ancestral home. – Trans.

government grants, and claiming for poverty reduction funds. Of course, it is undeniable that there are many poor households in Shahao Village who have to rely on the minimum living guarantee of government. Nonetheless, more poor households have the capability to achieve their own development through the government's help.

In order to help the Shahao of a 1000 year history to get out of poverty, it is necessary to have someone to lead, and then to cultivate the village's own team, and finally to build up the team for long-term development. The three First Secretaries from the Chinese People's Association for Friendship with Foreign Countries (CPAFFC in short) passed the baton of poverty alleviation on such a path to help Shahao to get out of poverty step by step.

12.2 The First First Secretary—Lead to Demonstrate and Guide

In December 2015, Shahao Village welcomed the First Secretary Cao Xiaowei. Secretary Cao, male, born in 1979, has a bachelor's degree and worked in the general office before he was stationed. When Secretary Cao arrived at Shahao Village, the village "two committees" conflicts were prominent, the "two committees" team was not united, basically in some state of work where no one was in charge and no one was doing anything. In addition, due to the previous secretary's behavior like deceiving superiors and subordinates and damaging the public interest to benefit himself over the years, the village cadres have long lost the trust and support from the villagers. The village Party branch has almost lost its appeal and cohesion among the masses. In face of such a poor village, the weak "two committees" team, and the alienated masses, Secretary Cao can do nothing but choose to take the lead. Only with his own achievements, he can let the village Party members and the masses in the village understand what is a real Communist Party member should be.

The first thing that Secretary Cao insisted on doing in the village is staying in and taking root in Shahao Village, so that the village cadres and the masses could see a "real officer doing real thing". Secretary Cao recalls, initially the village cadres thought that the upper administration just performed a show in the village, after a maximum of ten days and a half months he would go back. But they did not expect that he came and did not leave, as he had worked in the village for hundreds of days, and did not even return to Beijing on New Year's Day. It was only then that people slowly realized that this was not just a formality going through the motions, but a real officer. It is not an easy thing for a young man from a big modern city in Beijing to insist on working in the village where there was not drinking water to access, let alone anything else.

Difficulty in drinking water is the biggest difficulty faced by the villagers of Shahao, and for generations Shahao villagers had to fetch water to drink. People in the natural village of Shahao have to go to a small well a mile away to get water. People from Wangjiaya Village have to go to a centralized well source in the village to fetch water. The water quality of the well is contaminated and villagers say they can smell a foul odor. For the elderly left behind, getting water is the biggest difficulty. The distance to fetch water is far, and the road is rugged, especially on rainy days, making it even more impossible to walk. The difficulty of drinking water not only increases the burden of labor for villagers, but also restricts them from developing side businesses. Liu Xiying is a villager. When he was young, he made his own tofu and bricks and sold them in nearby villages. He carried all the water needed for production to his home on his shoulders, making more than 40 trips a day and walking dozens of miles to sell his products. After two decades, he is physically challenged with knee deformation, and he cannot keep on doing that.

Solving the drinking water problem is the primary goal of poverty alleviation after Secretary Cao stationed in the village. He spent three months alone looking for a quality and stable water source. He went through all the gullies and ravines in the village, and finally determined the final water source through repeated and detailed comparisons. He wrote a detailed research report and applied for 560,000 yuan of special funds from his institution, CPAFFC, and 200,000 yuan from the county water conservancy bureau, raising a total of 760,000 yuan for the drinking water project. The drinking water project lasted for 10 months, and Secretary Cao was on site almost every day, supervising the overall progress of the project and ensuring the quality of the work. In less than a year after Secretary Cao was stationed in the village, Shahao Village finally realized the tap water access to the village and in every household. The problem of drinking water for both humans and animals was fundamentally solved.

The introduction of tap water into households not only saved a lot of cost in fetching water for villagers, but also provided the basic conditions for villagers to develop their production. In addition, more than a dozen families who were always away from home returned to the village. They also had tap water access in their households, so that they will prepare for their life and production after they return to village in the future. The villages around Shahao Village, and the villages in the neighboring townships have not achieved drinking water access into the households, so the villagers of these villages are very envious of Shahao Village, and knew that First Secretary came with the tap water access. The villagers of Shahao Village are all grateful to Secretary Cao, who affectionately referred to the tap water as "Xiaowei[4] water". It is also because the villagers saw the Secretary Cao is a sincere, honest, and hard-working man, and he could bear responsibility without any grudge for the villagers to find water and draw the water, that the trust and sense of closeness those villagers gave the Secretary Cao steeply increased.

The road is also a serious problem that has been troubling the villagers of Shahao Village. Both sides of the public roads at the village level in the village are loess. When it rains and snows, the road is muddy and the vehicle skids; when it is windy, the sand is everywhere, which affects the safety of travel. Secretary Cao got 200,000 yuan of financial support from the county sanitation bureau and his institution, and purchased more than 4600 seedlings. He led forty to fifty villagers every day and spent half a month planting seedlings to complete the greening project on both sides of the village's public roads. In addition, with the help of the County Poverty Alleviation Office, Secretary Cao also repaired the dilapidated houses for 10 poor households in the village, built 91 new toilets, repaired more than 5600 m of farm machinery roads, and built 1 new communication tower, which greatly improved the infrastructure construction of Shahao Village.

[4] Cao Xiaowei is the full name of the first First Secretary. – Trans.

When our research group followed Secretary Cao to implement the household research, Secretary Cao would turn on the tap of every house to check the water quality and water output, and ask the farmers about the drinking water supply. When passing by the village road, he would also check the growth of saplings on both sides of the road, and when he found that some saplings lacked water, he would tell the village road guards to irrigate in time. It can be seen that the First Secretary has a strong sense of work responsibility, so that villagers can really benefit from poverty alleviation projects in the long term.

Secretary Cao not only does practical things for the people to change their material poverty, but also really cares about the people and relieves their emotional poverty. He has integrated himself into the village, becoming "half of the villager", and through Secretary Cao, the villagers can experience the care of the government and the Party, and build confidence in development. At the same time, in the interaction with the villagers, he knows the situation of each household well, which also lays the foundation for *targeted poverty alleviation work and helps to identify the real poor households and distribute poverty alleviation resources fairly.*

More than material poverty, what the elderly left behind in the village cannot tolerate is emotional poverty. The children of the elderly left behind in the village work outside all year round and seldom come home. Usually, when walking around the village, there is hardly a young person in sight. The old people lamented that it was difficult to find someone to talk to in the village. When Secretary Cao came to Shahao Village from Beijing, he liked to "visit villagers' homes and have nice chat with them". His daily communication with the villagers enhanced their emotions, and the villagers knew more of him and turned more supportive of his work. The villagers said, "Now that everyone in the village has left, it's hard to find someone to talk to. Secretary Cao came from Beijing. He came to our house to sit and talk with us, then we are very happy!"

After arriving at the village, Secretary Cao spent two months visiting the people, completing a research report on Shahao Village and familiarizing himself with the basic conditions of the households. He assisted the County Poverty Alleviation Office to investigate the actual situation of the officially registered poverty-stricken households in many dimensions, such as income, consumption, assets, education and health, and established the "Shahao Village Poverty-stricken Household Work Forms", which recorded in detail the family information, causes of poverty and measures to help the poor households. By holding a general meeting of all villagers and organizing discussions among villagers, 9 poor households were disqualified in strict accordance with the "eight no-entry" standard for poverty alleviation in Shanxi Province, and the final list of selected poor households was unanimously approved by the villagers.

During the 2 years Secretary Cao stationed in the village, he dine, sleep, work and live together with the villagers. In the forefront of everything, he will always take the lead, which moves Party members and the masses to follow, to fulfill the commitment of a Communist Party member to serving the people. The relationship between the villagers and Secretary Cao is changed from distant to close, and villagers also like to chat with Secretary Cao on their small household affairs; they also send their own home-made fermented rice, oil cake, and Wotou[5]; when it snows, he will go to sweep the snowy road to the toilets. Secretary Cao has laid a solid foundation for poverty

[5] Wotou, also called Chinese cornbread, is a type of steamed bread made from cornmeal in Northern China. – Trans.

alleviation in Shahao Village, and at the end of his two-year term, he officially handed over the baton of poverty alleviation to the second First Secretary.

12.3 The Second First Secretary—Set up a Team to Seek Their Own Development

In August 2017, Shahao Village welcomed the second First Secretary, Li Xin. Secretary Li, male, born in 1983, has a postgraduate degree and worked in the Party committee of the institution before. When Secretary Li came to work in the village, the face of Shahao Village had changed a lot under the leadership of Secretary Cao, realizing tap water access to households, strengthening the village roads, communications and other infrastructure, improving villagers' housing, toilets, and other environment; poor households received targeted identification and various targeted poverty alleviation policies, as well as materials and emotional sympathy; the institution of the First Secretary also invested nearly 2 million yuan in a new large farm for Shahao Village to develop industries. The relationship between the cadres and the people has also improved significantly, and the villagers have higher expectations and deeper feelings for the First Secretary.

The biggest problem facing Secretary Li when he took office was that Shahao Village did not have a sound and competent team. For a long time, the village's own development power and ability are not strong, simply relying on external help, so the village cannot achieve its own development. The development of the village cannot be achieved without a good team, but the "two committees" of Shahao Village are almost paralyzed. To build a good team and play the role of the grassroots Party branch as a militant bastion has become an important task of Secretary Li's poverty alleviation work.

Secretary Li carried out a series of Party organization learning activities and standardized daily Party activities to strengthen the Party's organization and discipline. By standardizing the learning activities of Party organizations, the consciousness and pioneering role of Party members have been significantly strengthened. At the end of 2017, during the second round of confirming land contracting authentic rights in Shahao Natural Village, Party members took the lead in the process of land allocation and took the initiative to give up the land, so that the matter involving historical disputes for more than 10 years could be solved in just one and a half months, ensuring the smooth implementation of the whole village's return to forestry. In daily life, Party members take the lead in resolving conflicts and disputes among cadres and masses, such as taking the initiative to persuade petitioning households to return and taking the lead in unloading fertilizer. The evaluation of Party members by the masses has improved significantly.

The number of Party members in Shahao Village is small, and the enthusiasm of Party members to attend the meetings is not high. Secretary Li criticized and educated the Party members who did not attend the Party meeting for three times, which improved the working style of the Party meeting significantly. Liu Guangxin, an old Party member who did not live in the village. There is only one shuttle bus running one round trip everyday from the township he lived to the village. He even attended the 2017 Party member meeting. He said, "I've been a member of the Party for so many years, so it would be a shame if I was criticized for not attending the meeting or expelled for not participating in the Party's activities". Whenever a large meeting is held, Secretary Li requires that no smoking is allowed at the meeting site. These requirements were initially difficult for the members of the village "two committees" to fulfil. When the research team came, the village branch members repeatedly took out cigarettes from their pockets to smoke, but they did not dare to break the rules, and as a result, they repeatedly put the cigarettes back into their pockets. The new Party branch's style of work has changed significantly, and its ability to work has improved significantly.

Secretary Li searched for the most suitable team candidates throughout the village to help form a new Party branch and cultivate endogenous poverty alleviation momentum for Shahao Village. Since the new Party branch was formed, the cohesion, centripetal force and driving power of the Party branch have been gradually enhanced, and two people took the initiative to submit applications to the Party branch and actively requested to join the Party organization.

The former village Party secretary of Shahao Village was removed from office due to personal integrity problems, and the Party organization team had been unsound for a long time and needs to be improved as soon as possible. Secretary Li reported the situation and exchanged opinions on the unsound Party branch team with the leaders at the township government on different occasions for many times, and actively sought for assistance. In November 2017, Secretary Li participated in the election of the village Party branch. The village has 14 Party members, of which 12 are over 50 years old, and the Party members are seriously aging. In view of that, Secretary Li insisted on promoting young person to serve as village Party branch secretary. On November 4, 2017, a new branch committee was elected in Shahao Village, with branch secretary Wang Jinwen, 44 years old, was a first-time village cadre; deputy Party branch secretary Ma Yingying (female), 61 years old, was a first-time village cadre; and branch member Wang Huayou, 65 years old, was a former village cadre. All the three Party branch members were recognized by the villagers for their character and ability. The interviewed village Party members said: Now this team is well chosen!

On the basis of the successful election of the Party branch, Secretary Li helped the villagers' committee achieve a fair and just election. Some villagers, seeing that the appearance of the village has greatly improved in recent years, especially the large pig farm project is about to generate revenue, vainly attempted to profit from the election of village cadres through illegal means. Secretary Li was determined to uphold the fair election of the villagers' committee and safeguard the fairness and justice of the village. The period of election lasts almost two months, when Secretary Li tempered the internal conflicts to ensure the smooth election process through his situation investigation, education, and persuasion, which foiled the election of bribery candidates. At the end of 2017, Shahao Village has finally achieved the sound and complete "two committees" of the village since May 2016, when the former village Party secretary was removed from office by the township Party committee due to personal integrity problems. The new team was elected with the main leaders both young and robust, and enjoyed high credibility, laying a solid organizational foundation for Shahao Village to achieve poverty eradication in 2018.

On December 5, 2017, a new villager's committee election was held in the village. A few months before the election, the former deposed secretary secretly recommended a villager surnamed Wang. The villager surnamed Wang saw that the village had the support from national-level institution, and the large pig farm would be put into operation soon, which he thought it was a profitable opportunity. With the help of the former secretary, the villagers surnamed Wang bought votes. After Secretary Li knew the situation, he went to report the situation to the township Party committee timely. Secretary Li warned the candidates for village director that he must adhere to the fair election; Secretary Li educated and persuaded the villagers, through the analysis of the candidates campaign intentions, work ability, service consciousness, etc. to help villagers to compare and identify candidates.

On the election day, a total of 298 villagers participated in the voting. The incumbent village director received 150 votes and the villager surnamed Wang received 136 votes. According to the principle of "double majority",[6] the village director-elect must receive more than half of the votes, that is, 149 votes, to be elected. The incumbent village director won by just over one vote, a very close victory. The villagers were very happy to say, "It's this one vote that shows that evil can never suppress good!"

On the basis of building up the village "two committees" team, Secretary Li improved the level of village governance by improving the working mechanism and ensuring democratic decision-making. At the same time, he attaches great importance to the publicity system of village affairs, standardized operation of village affairs, to make it sunlight operation. By promoting, implementing, and making public the policies, it increases the villagers' right to know and reduces their doubts.

Secretary Li insisted on the normalization of the villager's committee's deliberations, which made work informed and pooled the various ideas, so as to prevent the rule by the voice of one man alone and others do not know. After each meeting, he asked the participants to sign and fingerprint on the minutes book, to prevent them from eating words after they leave the door, or pretending that they did not know after the meeting. He helps members of the villagers' committee to develop a good habit of making work plans; helps to determine the priority of work and carry out work in an integrated manner to avoid repetitive work; helps the village director to distribute tasks in a reasonable way to improve overall work efficiency. In spring of 2018, the organization of confirmation of land rights is both a historical legacy and a core work that concerns the long term development of Shahao Village. In order to complete this work, the First Secretary concentrated human and material resources and energy, and assisted the villager's committee to hold several meetings, so as to reasonably formulate the work plan, arrange working staff, and take more than 40 days to fully complete this task smoothly and successfully.

In order to increase the transparency of village affairs and poverty alleviation policies, the publicity methods used by Secretary Li include: "Firstly, let the First Secretary speak, who will speak at meetings, at meals, and guide the talk with villagers. Secondly, let the branch secretary and village director speak. Mainly let them make scroll post in the WeChat groups of Party branch and villager's committee, for example, free screening of 'two cancers',[7]

---

[6] In the election of the "two committees" in villages, "double majority" refers to two specific majority requirements: 1. Validity. The number of villagers participating in the voting must be more than half of the total number of registered villagers, so that the election result is considered valid. 2. The conditions for election: candidates or alternative candidates must obtain more than half of the votes of the participating voters in order to be officially elected. – Trans.

[7] Government-offered medical services for female, i.e. screening for cervical cancer and breast cancer. – Trans.

poverty alleviation health policies, nurse training, social security medical insurance policies, etc., once a day in the morning and once in the evening to prevent being overwhelmed by invalid information. Thirdly, let the loudspeaker speak. Record the poverty alleviation policies related to Shahao Village, copy them to a USB disk, and play them regularly on the existing loudspeaker in the village". Matters of immediate interest to the villagers should be notified to the villagers in the form of holding village representative assemblies, villagers' committees and village assemblies, so that information will be transparent and open, and things must be done fairly and justly.

During the 2 years that Secretary Li stationed in the village, he not only set up a new village "two committees", but also established a brand new working system and mechanism, the enthusiasm of the village "two committees" in work was significantly increased, and the village governance and service capacity were also greatly enhanced. As for the village's poverty alleviation work, poverty alleviation difficulties, and future plans for poverty alleviation, Secretary Li organized the village "two committees" to fully discuss these issues. When encountering difficulties and problems, he first encouraged the village cadres to come up with their own solutions, instead of relying on the material assistance from the First Secretary's institution. As for the problems such as the historical dispute over land contracting, the future land acquisition for the village activity center, and the start-up funds for the village multi-grain processing project, the answers will be basically dependent on the village "two committees" to take the lead in solving these problems. During the research, I repeatedly heard the village director say: "We'll figure out how to do this". The enthusiasm and self-confidence of the village director in work were obviously enhanced. Secretary Li laid a solid organizational foundation for the poverty alleviation work in Shahao Village, and at the end of his two-year term, he officially handed over the baton of poverty alleviation to the third First Secretary.

12.4 The Third First Secretary: Strengthening Internal Strength for Long-Term Development

In August 2019, Shahao Village welcomed its third First Secretary, Meng Qingke. The Secretary Meng, male, born in 1977, with a bachelor's degree, worked in General Office before he stationed. When Mr. Meng came to work in the village, under the leadership of the previous two First Secretaries, the infrastructure of Shahao Village, such as water, electricity, and roads, was obviously strengthened. 1429 mu[8] of grain plots were returned to forestry, and 950 mu of barren hills were afforested. The head office of Economic Development Cooperative was established. On the basis of this, the pilot project of e-commerce was initiated through planting apple tree, pear tree, cherry tree, and introduction of new variety, "Matian No.1" walnut, and carrying out the agricultural "science and technology going to the countryside" activities. The position of Shahao Village Party branch and the upgrade and renovation of

[8] 1 mu equals 1/15 hectare. –Trans.

village health room were completed, and the village has full coverage of solar street lights, and cement road access to each household; the supporting institution invested 2 million yuan into the pig farm, which was put into use, and the 300 kW village photovoltaic power station invested by the county with 2 million yuan is completed and grid-connected. The village collective economic income reached 250,000 yuan per year; the "two committees" team is soundly developed, and the cohesion, appeal, and influence of the team are significantly enhanced, which puts the end to the predicament of "nobody do things, no money to do things". At the end of 2018, 85 households and 313 people were lifted out from poverty, and the poverty incidence was reduced to 0.53%, and the whole village was successfully lifted out of poverty.

The success of Shahao Village lifted out of poverty, to a large extent, depends on the First Secretary and the vigorous assistance from the institution of First Secretary. How to increase the soft power of the village, enhance the village "internal force", improve the quality of life of the villagers, and seek the long-term development of the village is a more difficult task and a more serious trial that the third First Secretary Meng faced.

Secretary Meng and the branch team fully exchanged their ideas, made in-depth study, and actively explored the current mission to achieve the smooth transition from poverty alleviation to rural revitalization. Firstly, to determine the goal of Shahao Village: set the "affluent Shahao, beautiful countryside" as the goal; secondly, to find the endogenous motivation of the village collective: to promote the spirit of Lvliang, "hard work, contribution to the overall situation, endless self-improvement, and dauntless innovation", so as to inherit the red gene, stimulate the innovation drive, and promote rural revitalization as the endogenous motivation; lastly, to establish the work idea of poverty alleviation and development: enhance the Party building, promote poverty eradication, develop rural characteristics industries, combine the increase of people's confidence and people's mastery of necessary knowledge and skills in poverty alleviation, and enhance the endogenous power, so as to build a beautiful and harmonious Shahao Village, and take the road of rural revitalization.

On the basis of the previous work of former two secretaries who took the lead and built the team, respectively, Secretary Meng continued to build up the team and enhance the endogenous power of the team and its development momentum. The First Secretary insisted on holding monthly "theme Party day" activities to strengthen the core leading role of Party building; insisted on strengthening the construction of grassroots organizations, improving the quality of Party members and enhancing the cohesion of the team as a key task, organizing the training for Party members and cadres, improving their theoretical level, ideological quality and ability to serve the people, focusing on the hot and difficult issues of concern to the villagers and doing good for them, leading Party members to win the battle against poverty and vigorously implement the rural revitalization strategy; insisted on the co-building of village Party branch with the Party branch of the General Office of CPAFFC so as to realize the goal of "educating Party members, promoting the Party branch, benefiting the people, and bearing fruits in poverty alleviation"; insisted on developing young Party members to expand the part organization with 2 comrades officially joining the Party.

To commemorate the 99th anniversary of the founding of the Communist Party of China, inherit and carry forward the glorious tradition and fine style of the Party, on the morning of July 1, 2020, the Party Branch of Shahao Village in Caijiaya Township of Xing County organized a "7·1" themed Party Day activity. Xu Ximing, Deputy Secretary of the county, Bai Yongbing, director of the poverty alleviation office of the county, the resident work team, the village "two committees", villagers' representatives and all Party members of the village participated together to celebrate the Party's birthday. Meng Qingke, the First Secretary of village chaired the activity under the theme "revisit the history of the Party, stick to the mission to take responsibility". The First Secretary lectured at the Party class, reviewed the glorious history of the Party, revisited the Party oath, preached the spirit of Lvliang, so as to further enhance the determination and willingness of all Party members to learn and implement the Xi Jinping Thought on Socialism with Chinese Characteristics for a New Era, and strengthened the determination and motive power of all party members and backbone cadres of the village "two committees" in staying true to the original aspiration, shouldering the mission, and striving for the most beautiful Shahao people.

Based on the building of the foundation of the village leadership, Secretary Meng improved the motivation and ability of the team to drive the development of the villagers, so as to improve the quality of life and culture of the villagers and the civilization of the village. The "two committees" of Shahao Village, with the assistance of Secretary Meng, carried out a series of activities to build the soft power of the village, such as the enhancement of Party building, promotion of culture walls at the villagers' committee compound and those in meeting room, focusing on "staying true to the original aspiration, shouldering the mission", and incorporating "People's aspiration for a better life is our goal" implicitly into the hearts of Party members, so that the idea of "carrying people in our hearts, relying on people for work, thinking of people in everything, and doing everything for people" takes root in the village "two committees". A flag stand was built and let the flag fly high over the village compound. The secretary made village rules and regulations with the "two committees" and villagers' representatives, established and run the "Impression of Shahao" WeChat Public Platform for Shahao Village, built the Shahao Village bookstore, improved the cultural and sports activities and fitness facilities, run a love laundry and a love supermarket, carried out the "Overwatching Family Tradition" activity, and developed a garden economy with the characteristics of the elderly in the village, which greatly promoted the knowledge level of villagers and sense of happiness in their lives, and the village civilization has become a common practice.

The "cultural and sports room" project in Shahao Village received a total investment of nearly 200,000 yuan, including a meeting room, a cultural and sports room, and a bookstore in Shahao Village, which meets the needs of daily meetings of village organizations and cultural entertainment of villagers. On the basis of the previous 360 books, the all staff of CPAFFC donated 1322 books and the associated enterprises of China Friendship Foundation for Peace and Development (CFFPD) donated 573 books, which meets the villagers' need for reading. The books cover topics such as agriculture, health, literature, history and Party building, and many are children's books, which attract many villagers to bring their children to read. In terms of caring for the lives of villagers, they implemented holiday visits and presented gifts, provided targeted assistance, and provided regular health examination for the elderly, distributed Essilor presbyopic glasses, applied for electric wheelchairs for the disabled with mobility difficulties, and actively contacted public welfare checkups and treatment for elderly patients with cataracts and other eye diseases; in the battle against the

COVID-19 epidemic, they were the first to contact villagers and donated epidemic prevention masks and "Dettol" antiseptic liquid to them. They strictly implemented the village epidemic prevention management system. The "Love Laundry" in Shahao Village was assigned to a dedicated person to manage who provided free laundry services for empty nesters, senior citizens and disabled elderly people over 60 years old in the village, relieving them of a great burden of household chores. The "Love Supermarket" gave full play to the role of combining poverty alleviation measures of "helping the poor's spirit first and then reducing the poverty itself". According to the environmental improvement work of village appearance and household appearance, the "two committees" of the village will regularly evaluate and score the villagers, and issue rewards, so as to stimulate the endogenous motivation of the villagers and improve their spiritual outlook, and effectively change the mindset of "passively longing for national assistance, expecting government grants and claiming for poverty reduction funds" of some poor households.

The foundation of Shahao Village's poverty alleviation and rural revitalization is always the prosperity of industry, and the cultivation and growth of local brands is the root of the prosperity of industry. Secretary Meng insisted on making achievements on the prosperity of local industries, developing the special multi-grains of Shahao Village, leading the village to build its own brand and culture, registering the trademark of "Shahao Village", establishing the sales platform of agricultural products of "Jinsui Special Products", and playing the role of the head office of Economic Development Cooperative of Shahao Village. In November 2019, the small multi-grains of Shahao Village entered the Changsha International Fair under the theme of "One Belt, One Road, and One World; One Township; One Product, and One Dream"; the "Jinsui Specialties" e-commerce platform was built to implement both online and offline sales, which continuously improved the economic benefits of the special industry in the village.

In the future Shahao, there will be tourist base for hiking, folklore experience base, art sketch base, etc., in the plans and blueprints of Secretary Meng and all the people of Shahao, which is the driving force and source of their efforts (Fig. 12.1).

Fig. 12.1 LOGO of "Shahao Village" trademark and "Jinsui Special Products" agricultural products sales platform

12.5 The Relay of the Three Secretaries' Poverty Alleviation Work

Three First Secretaries, the total of 5 years of successive assistance, Shahao Village successfully completed the task of poverty eradication. In December 2018, Shahao Village achieved the "removal of hat[9]" due to the poverty eradication in the whole village, and passed the national third-Party assessment of "removal of hat" in December 2019, passed the State Council Poverty Alleviation Assessment Team's random inspection in June 2020, and passed the State Council Poverty Alleviation Survey in July 2020. The support of the three First Secretaries is reflected in every bit of change of Shahao Village. The following is extracted from *the progress report on poverty alleviation in Shahao Village* by Secretary Meng in August 2020.

> *Through these years of vigorous support, Shahao Village has mainly achieved "twelve major changes". First, the "water" changed from the previous picking water to the mountain spring water access to every household. Second, the "road" changed from dirt roads, mud roads to cement hardened road to every household, so the villagers no longer trod mud road travel. Third, the "light" changed after the installation of 76 new energy street lights, lighting up the mountain village at night, to ensure that the villagers travel with convenience and safety. Fourth, the "house" changed from earth kilns and other dilapidated houses to safe and comfortable housing. Fifth, the "household" changed from 85 poor households lifted out of poverty to getting well-off. At the end of 2020, all poverty-stricken households reduced to zero. Sixth, the "collective income" changed from zero to 250,000 yuan, and it provided 45 public service jobs. Seventh, the "health insurance payment" changed, as the village collective paid for the villagers in entire village, at the price of 250 yuan per person, with a total of 109,000 yuan per year. Eighth, the "village collective agricultural machinery" changed. The new agricultural tricycle, small multi-grain processing equipment, micro-tiller, windmill, sprayer and other agricultural machinery worth nearly 170,000 yuan facilitated the villagers' production and life. Ninth, the "industrial model" changed with agriculture, transportation, photovoltaic power generation and other industries growing in full bloom and meteoric rise of mall multi-grain special industry. Tenth, the "environment" changed from the village appearance, household appearance, the villager's committee compound in a new look to various types of infrastructure gradually improved. Eleventh, the "two committees" team changed, as the team is becoming strong and vigorous. Twelfth, the "spiritual outlook" changed, as the villagers overcome the mentality of "passively longing for national assistance, expecting government grants and claiming for poverty reduction funds", and enhanced the endogenous motivation with a new spiritual outlook.*

The three First Secretaries completed the baton relay of poverty alleviation, in different stages of poverty alleviation, facing different poverty alleviation themes, highlighting different poverty alleviation work, achieving the continuity of the work of helping the village, and reflecting the long-term effectiveness of the First Secretary of the poverty alleviation system. The first First Secretary, facing an impoverished and unmanaged village, took the lead himself, demonstrating the role of Communist Party members as a benchmark and banner; the second First Secretary built the village "two committees" team, established a standardized work system, improved

[9] Hat metaphorically means poverty. When it is recognized a poverty-stricken one, the one will wear a hat; while one is lifted out of poverty, the one will be taken off the hat. – Trans.

the team's working ability, and cultivated the village's own development momentum; the third First Secretary built a solid village "two committees" team, enhanced the development of the village, improved the quality of life of the villagers, sought the long-term development of the village, and strove to achieve the goal of "affluent Shahao, beautiful countryside". The three First Secretaries not only completed the transition of poverty alleviation work, but also reflected the inheritance and evolution of poverty alleviation and support. In the past 5 years, the Shahao Village of a thousand years of history has been fundamentally changed, and the whole village has been lifted out of poverty, which has laid a solid foundation for rural revitalization.

References

Han, G., & Zhou, G. (2013). The Establishment of the System of Selecting and Assigning Cadres from Party and Government Organs to Poverty Alleviation in Rural Areas. *Journal of Theory*, No. 11.

Wang, Y., & Shu, Q. (2017). First Secretary Poverty Alleviation and Rural Leadership Supply. *Journal of the National School of Administration*, No. 1.

Yuan, L., & Wang, S. (2017). The logic of the "cadres in villages" system in practice: a case study of village C in southeast Fujian. *Journal of Huazhong University of Science and Technology (Social Science Edition)*, No. 3.

Yang, F. (2016). The First Secretary in the Village and the Change of Village Governance. *Learning Forum*, No. 2.

Chen, G., & Tang, J. (2015). A Trial on the Influence of Foreign "Helping Forces" on Villagers' Autonomy: An Investigation Based on the Work Practice of "First Secretary" in Village S of Shandong Province. *Journal of Tianjin Administrative College, Vol. 6, 2015. Journal of Tianjin Administrative College*, No. 6.

Xie, X. (2017). "Dual-track governance": an analytical framework for the poverty alleviation system of the "First Secretary"-a field survey based on Yuan village in Guangxi. *Journal of Nanjing Agricultural University (Social Science Edition)*, 3.

Junxia Zeng is an assistant researcher at the Institute of Rural Development, Chinese Academy of Social Sciences, whose main research interests are agricultural and rural talents and rural education.

Chapter 13
Rural Elites Drive Poverty Alleviation: Hunan Zhuigaolai Village Practice

Xiaomin Liu

Abstract This paper examines the practice and experience of village elite-driven poverty alleviation in Zhuigaolai Village, Phoenix County, Xiangxi Tujia and Miao Autonomous Prefecture, Hunan Province. Based on the investigation, we believe that the village elite-driven poverty alleviation is the most important cause for the remarkable effect of poverty reduction in Zhuigaolai Village. The important insight is that the driving demonstration of village elites is the key to poverty alleviation in poor villages in less developed areas, and also the key to rural revitalization in the post-poverty alleviation era. Therefore, active and effective support policies should be formulated to cultivate and develop more rural elites, and it is needed to build a linkage mechanism of rural elites driving for poverty alleviation in which rural elites will drive and help all villagers, including poor villagers.

Keywords Targeted poverty alleviation · Village elite · Zhuigaolai Village

13.1 Elite Participation: An Important Perspective for Analyzing Targeted Poverty Alleviation

Elite refers to those who have certain talents and are outstanding, shrewd and capable in some aspects. In this paper, rural elites refer to those who have the dual identity of farmers and elites, and also include elites among those who go out of village to do business and work. Therefore, drawing on the definition and classification of elites by many scholars at home and abroad, this paper classifies rural elites into political elites and economic elites. Rural political elites are "village Party branch secretaries, village directors and cadres of the 'two committees' and community leaders

X. Liu (✉)
Institute of Ethnology and Anthropology, Chinese Academy of Social Sciences, Beijing, China

Case Studies of Targeted Poverty Reduction and Alleviation in 100 Villages, International Research on Poverty Reduction, https://doi.org/10.1007/978-981-95-0549-4_13

who actively participate in community politics". Village economic elites are "the founders and managers of village economic organizations, such as the managers of village collective economic organizations, the managers of village economic cooperatives, the founders or managers of village private enterprises, as well as village economic experts such as large households of planting and breeding, marketing experts, agricultural technicians, etc.; and the outstanding people who go out to do business and work".

The Zhuigaolai Village is a village under the jurisdiction of Laershan Township, Phoenix County, Xiangxi Tujia and Miao Autonomous Prefecture, Hunan Province. It is located in the last mountain range extending eastward from Yunnan-Guizhou plateau, and a poverty-stricken village of ethnic minority in the core area of deeply impoverished county of national poverty alleviation Wuling Mountains region. The Zhuigaolai Village is a Miao ethnic group resided village, the total population of which is 286 households 1393 people, where more than 97% of the population is Miao people. In 2015, the per capita disposable income of rural residents in Zhuigaolai Village was 3503 yuan, ranking 15th among 19 villages in Laershan Town, equivalent to 48.1% of the average level in Phoenix County and 30.7% of the national average.[1] At the end of 2013, there were 120 poor households and 496 poor people in Zhuigaolai Village. The poverty incidence rate was 36.9%, which was 28.4 percentage points higher than the national average.[2] At the end of 2017, with the support of the village resident work team and driven by the village elites, the targeted poverty eradication work in Zhuigaolai Village was effective, achieving a per capita disposable income of 4873 yuan for rural residents and a poverty incidence rate of 1.5%, making it one of the first two villages lifted out of poverty among the 11 poor villages in Laershan Town.

The 286 households and 1393 people in the village of Zhuigaolai can be basically divided into three layers. The first layer is the affluent class. They are usually the elite groups in the village who are well connected, know how to socialize, and are good at seizing market opportunities with economic advantages, personal quality, influence, and other advantages. The number of such groups in the village is small, but they can mobilize other villagers and give demonstration in village production and life. The second layer is the middle class, most of which are those farmers who form a half-working and half-farming household livelihood pattern based on intergenerational division of labor, in which the relatively elderly parents of the family work in agriculture at home, while the young children with abundant labor

---

[1] According to the compilation and calculation of related data from *the China Statistical Yearbook 2016, Hunan Statistical Yearbook 2016, Phoenix County Statistical Yearbook 2015,* as well as *"the Laershan Township Information"* (provided by the Laershan Township Government), and *"the Reports on Targeted Poverty Alleviation Work from 2015 to 2018 in Zhuigaolai Village"*.

[2] The information was obtained from a questionnaire survey of Zhuigaolai village conducted by the research team in February 2017.

force work outside the home, and the family has both farming and working income, which largely improves the income of farmers' families and becomes the middle layer of the village. Of course, there are also a small number of middle-class farmers who mainly rely on moderate scale planting of cash crops (such as tobacco farming) or "high-quality rice + paddy fish", and engage in a certain scale of farming to obtain a stable income from agricultural operations. The third layer is the low-income class, with 119 officially registered poverty-stricken households and 522 officially registered poverty-stricken people in the village. The main reasons for poverty are lack of effective labor force, lack of cash, illness, and large expenditure on education. According to incomplete statistics from the research group, there are more than 30 households at the affluent layer of the village, accounting for about 12% of the total number of farming households in the village; at the low-income layer, there are about 120 households, accounting for about 42% of the total number of farming households in the village[3]; the middle layer accounts for about 46% of the village.

It has been argued that rural elites, as one of the important mainstay of rural public governance, play a bridging role between the government, the market and ordinary villagers, and have an obvious driving effect on poverty alleviation. Based on our three research visits to Zhuigaolai Village from 2017 to 2018, this paper will examine the practice and experience of poverty alleviation driven by rural elites in Zhuigaolai Village, in hope of providing some inspiration and reference for poverty alleviation and rural revitalization in other poor villages.

13.2 Political and Economic Integration: The Participation Model of Rural Elites in the Poverty Alleviation

The main cadres of the village "two committees" are the political elites of the village, as they belong to the affluent layer of the village, and they are also the economic elites. The following are a few cases to illustrate the development of village elites in Zhuigaolai Village and the practices and characteristics of poverty alleviation through industry.

[3] At the beginning of 2017, there were 119 officially registered poverty-stricken households in Zhuigaolai Village, including 106 average poor households with 498 people, 12 poor households enjoying minimum living guarantee with 22 people (including 7 households with 14 people enjoying minimum living guarantee, while the other 5 households with 8 people supported by both the minimum living guarantee and poverty alleviation), and 1 orphan household with 2 people. Through the acceptance assessment, it was realized that 106 poor households with 498 people were lifted out of poverty at the end of 2017, and they became the officially registered poverty-free households, but basically they were still at the low-income layer in the village.

Case 1

The village Party secretary dared to try the "high-quality rice" dry field seedling method, driving villagers, including poor households, to develop the "high-quality rice + paddy fish" industrial project for poverty alleviation.[4]

I was born in 1970, attended the Phoenix County Health School in 1991, and became an intern at the Laershan Town Hospital after 1994. Then I worked as a school nurse at No.1 Middle School of nationalities from 1995 to 2001, and got repaid during the discharge of temporary staff and substitute teachers. When I was a school nurse, my salary was 240 yuan per month, and during the time I was a school nurse, I often paid home visits and earned 300 ~ 400 yuan per month. After I stopped working as a school nurse, I rented a store in Laershan Township from 2002 to 2007, by selling medicine and visiting patients, I could earn more than 1800 yuan a month. Meanwhile, my wife and I also farmed, raised pigs, and ran a small business.

My family has raised pigs since 2001 and one sow all the time, which gives birth to two litters of piglets a year, with usually more than ten piglets per litter. My family sold piglets for more than 10,000 yuan last year (year of 2017). The piglet price is 15 yuan per catty, so one pig can be sold for almost 800 yuan. My family's first bucket of gold came from raising pigs. My wife is a teacher of private school in the village. Besides teaching classes, she is a handy person when she returns home, and she is mainly responsible for raising pigs. My wife was a hardworking, thrifty woman, and she cleaned the pig pens very well and raised pigs for more than ten years and no pig fever ever happened, so pig raising was always a stable source of income for my family. Several pig farmers in the village (including poor households) often came to my house to consult about the experience of raising pigs, so there was rarely any pig fever in the village. At that time, my family was the first family in the village to buy a motorcycle and color TV, and villagers came to my house to watch TV, and I was also one of the first families to buy a car.

Since 2008, I have started to work as a village cadre. At first, I was the director of stability maintenance, and at that time my subsidy was 2400 yuan a year. At the same time, I served as the village doctor, and my compensation was 1000 yuan a year, and it has increased to more than 9000 yuan a year in the past few years, as the amount of compensation was offered according to the village population scale. In 2014, I was elected as the village Party secretary, and now the subsidy for the village Party secretary is about 15,000 yuan a year.

In addition to working as a village cadre, village doctor and raising pigs, I also contracted other people's land to grow rice. My family has 4.8 mu[5] *of paddy fields and 2 mu of dry land under contract. Since 2001, we have contracted 10 mu of land without paying rent but a little rice. In 2018, my family planted a total of 8 mu of paddy fields and 7–8 mu of dry land for corn, which is mainly used for feeding pigs.*

[4] Interview code: 20180923WULX.

[5] 1 mu equals 1/15 hectare. – Trans.

In 2016, the County Agricultural Bureau implemented the "high-quality rice" project in Laershan Township and arranged for technicians to be stationed in the village to carry out dry field seedling cultivation of new varieties. The test field selected at the beginning was a 120 mu of contiguous dry fields of No. 1 and 2 village group. However, people in the village had never heard of raising rice seedlings in dry field and were afraid to try it. Then the technicians came to me, and I thought I could try it, so I convinced the villagers in the group to join me in experimenting with rice seedlings raised in dry field. The success of dry field rice seedling raising not only reduced the labor burden as it does not need to go to the paddy fields when sowing seeds, but also increased and stabilized the grain yield, and furthermore, it laid the foundation for the development of the "high-quality rice + paddy fish" industry in Zhuigaolai Village. In this process, I learned the knowledge and farm management methods under the guidance of technicians, recorded the growth of seedlings and gave feedback to them, and hereby I not only obtained new agricultural technology, but also established a good relationship with the county agricultural bureau.

In 2017, the Ministry of Agriculture issued a notice on "the pilot implementation plan of the Special Appointment Program for Agricultural Technology Promotion Service in poor areas", and Phoenix County was appointed as a pilot county for the grassroots work of the special appointment program for agricultural technology promotion service, and the county agricultural technology promotion center recruited five specially appointed agricultural technicians. It is because of the good cooperation with the Agricultural Bureau in 2016 and before, I was hired as a specially appointed agricultural technician for the rice industry in Phoenix County, and could get more learning opportunities and also earned 24,000 RMB per year for my work.

As a pilot county of Special Appointment Program for the Grassroots Agricultural Technology Promotion Service, the county provided seeds, fertilizers and pesticides at a discounted price of 100 yuan per mu for all villagers participating in the "high-quality rice" project. The seeds are of high-yielding good variety that has been tried and tested in the local area for the first two years, and the fertilizers and pesticides meet all ecological standards and have low toxicity. In the process of planting and promoting "high-quality rice", I followed the "high-quality rice" production management process provided by the county agricultural bureau and encouraged everyone to adopt a standardized model for field management, such as following a unified, standardized fertilization and same amount of pesticide application at the same time. When I encounter problems, I will deal with them in a timely manner, and if I can't deal with them myself, I will contact the county agricultural technicians to come and deal with them on site. For example, during the time when I promoted "high-quality rice" planting in my village, one day a villager surnamed Long approached me and asked why his rice was still infested with insects even though it met the requirements. At first, I had no experience and could not explain, so I immediately contacted the relevant experts of the county agricultural bureau who came to the farmer's field for consultation, and the experts concluded that the ratio of farmer's pesticide to water did not meet the standard, and found that it had signs of insects spreading to the adjacent rice fields. After the experts' diagnosis and explanation, the villager surnamed Long understood the serious consequences of his momentary negligence and non-compliance with the standard operation. In the first year, some of the villagers were only tentative to follow me to plant "quality rice" who also encountered some small problems, so I gave back these problems to the county agricultural bureau, and since 2017, the county agricultural bureau has began to implement the "unified system of pesticide treatment and problem prevention" in Zhuigaolai Village, that is, to organize "pesticide team"[6] *to make unified use of pesticide according to the unified standard, or unified spraying of pesticides with drones. This solves the problem that it is difficult for every household to apply fertilizer and pesticide in a regular and consistent way to reach uniform standard, so the effect is very good. Not only did rice pests or diseases disappear, but the ecological and efficient production of paddy fields was also achieved—due to the unified use of low-toxicity pesticides, the fish raised in the rice fields could continue to survive and grow after the pesticides were applied. The project of "high-quality rice + paddy fish" implemented in Zhuigaolai Village had smooth success and got the approval of most villagers.*

I plan to transfer 100 mu or 200 mu of land from Songtao County, Guizhou Province next year (year of 2019) to grow "high-quality rice". I have already contacted the village director over there, from whom I am waiting for a reply, so I think there is no problem.

Case 2

The village director took the lead in demonstrating large-scale cultivation of "high-quality rice", registered the trademark of "Laershan Zhuigaolai" for high-quality rice, and made efforts to open up various sales channels.[7]

I am 44 years old (year of 2018) and graduated from junior high school. When I was young, I went to Taizhou, Zhejiang Province to work for 3 years as a wire puller, and did other jobs such as syringe. Then my eldest uncle got sick (who was my adoptive father), so I came back to take care of him, and haven't worked outside anymore since then. Nonetheless, since 25 years old, I have been killing pigs and selling pork in town, and doing some small businesses furthermore. My family's financial situation is considered wealthy in the village, and we bought a pickup truck two years ago, so we are one of the families in the village to own a private car earlier.

In 2015, the old village director of Zhuigaolai Village passed away and I was elected as the acting village director, and in 2017 I was officially elected as the village director. The subsidy for the village director is 1000 yuan per month. In the past few years, we have been engaged in targeted poverty alleviation, and as the main village officials of the "two committees" of village Party branch, we are busy every day, so we can no longer do business such as killing pigs, and our family income has been affected. Fortunately, from 2017 onwards, the various village affairs have gone smoothly, and I have been engaged in running some other industries, so my income has increased, and it is not less than the previous income from doing my business.

[6] The village organized the "pesticide team", which specially recruited slightly younger villagers by the county agricultural bureau, including slightly younger members from the poor households.

[7] Interview code: 20180922WUQF.

Since 2016, the county agricultural bureau has been promoting the "high-quality rice" project in the village, and the momentum of "high-quality rice" development is very good, and there are great prospects for development mainly owning to relatively good soil and climate, which is more suitable for large-scale cultivation of "high-quality rice". Through the technology promotion and training of "quality rice" by the county agricultural bureau, villagers have basically mastered the advanced planting techniques, as the planted rice sent to the provincial test, and get the experts' approval. The quality of the rice from the Zhuigaolai Village is very good and the rice is rich in selenium, so it is possible to apply for the trademark of the product and increase the selling price of the rice. It is also based on this situation, the resident work team in Zhuigaolai Village from Phoenix County Poverty Alleviation Office invested 160,000 yuan to build a rice processing plant, which was completed and put into operation in October 2017 and is owned by the village collective, and I contracted the plant in my personal name with an annual contract fee of 12,000 yuan. In 2017, I had a plentiful harvest of 20,000 catties[8] *of high-quality rice, and I purchased more than 10,000 catties of grains in the whole village. The purchase price of the grain was 1.8 ~ 2 Yuan/catty, which was higher than the purchase price in previous years or in other places. Subsequently, I rented a storefront in Jishou City, the capital of Xiangxi Prefecture, and my son was responsible for the sales. According to the quality of the rice and the total amount that supporting departments and organizations purchased, the prices of rice were set at three levels, which were 3 yuan/catty, 4 yuan/catty and 5 yuan/catty. I also use my personal relationships to sell high-quality rice in the hospitals, schools, the county administration for industry and commerce, and other departments of government, which won a good reputation of the rice from Zhuigaolai in Phoenix county and Jishou City. I think the future trend of the development of Zhuigaolai high-quality rice is to take the route of e-commerce and supermarket sales. Therefore, in 2017, I started to apply for the registration of the agricultural product for "Laershan Zhuigaolai" brand of high-quality rice, and in October 2018, the registration was approved. I plan to expand the rice processing plant, buy a dryer and a sifter.*

I want to expand the cultivation scale of "high-quality rice" next year (year of 2019), and I have already discussed with the Party branch secretary to transfer 200 mu of land from each of the two households for "rice" cultivation, so that it will be easier to mobilize other villagers to further expand the scale of production. In addition, there is more land in other villages that can be transferred, so it will not be a problem to transfer land. I think that to develop industry at home may not be as good as being a boss or running business outside, but it is not necessarily worse than outside employment. I have an ideal, which is to expand the scale of the village's "high-quality rice", expand the rice processing plant to make "high-quality rice" industry bigger and stronger, in addition to open a flour processing plant to make rice flour, sweet potato flour, etc., *so as to promote the development of the village industry, which will not only benefit my development but also drive the development of the village, including poor households.*

Based on the above two cases, combined with field research, some simple conclusions can be drawn.

[8] A Chinese measure equal to 500 g. – Trans.

Firstly, village Party branch secretaries and the village directors are currently both political and economic elites. Both of them went out and grew up to be economic elites through their own efforts at first, and then were elected as the main village cadres and returned to the village to become village political elites. Our research in Zhuigaolai Village also found that the main cadres of the village "two committees" (village political elites) are economic elites who have received relatively high levels of education and have experience in non-agricultural work such as running business or outside employment. In other words, compared with ordinary villagers, economic elites who have human capital, economic capital, and social capital at the same time can more easily obtain political capital in the village and become political elites. Moreover, some economic elites do not take their own initiative in becoming political elites, but the local government takes the initiative to embrace them in order to improve the quality of the members of the village "two committees". Of course, being a political elite does not affect their statuses as economic elites, and to some extent, it may consolidate their capital as economic elites.

Secondly, the elites' drive has enabled the smooth implementation and rapid development of the "high-quality rice" industrial poverty alleviation project in Zhuigaolai Village. As some studies have argued, rural elites have the modern mindset of being the first to perceive changes in factors and agricultural prices, and are often the "primary action group" for institutional change, leading innovation in agricultural operation practices as potential profit finders.[9] Compared with ordinary farmers and poor households, elites often have obvious resource advantages and higher ability to cope with social risks, and they often play the leading role in the poverty alleviation action system, showing certain "charismatic authority" characteristics, which makes villagers regard them not only as wealth leaders, but also as model figures in village governance. The villagers see him not only as a wealthy leader, but also as a model figure in village governance, and voluntarily accept his leadership.[10] The industry poverty alleviation project of "high-quality rice" encountered predicament at first in the Zhuigaolai Village, because villagers did not dare to try the dry field rice planting method, which made the project uncompleted. This is because before that, the villagers' rice production was basically direct for their own consumption, that is, self-sufficient, so they followed the traditional rice planting, fertilization, pesticide application, and other farm management as always, which basically guaranteed their own family's food provision. As for the new agricultural technology such as "dry field rice planting method", they worry about the result and risk, and they dare not take any action without reassurance. This requires political elites with a certain degree of risk resistance to be the "charismatic authority" and the "first ones" as the main village cadres. Once the village political elites themselves act first, ordinary farmers, including poor households, are likely to follow suit and

[9] He Jun et al. "The community logic of the evolution of agricultural business practices in China—a case study based on two rural communities in Fenyang City, Shanxi Province," China Rural Insights, No. 2, 2017.

[10] Zhu Tianyi, "A Study on the Interface between State and Society by Rural Governance Elites in Targeted Poverty Alleviation—A Practical Analysis of XS County, Jiangxi Province", Socialism Studies, No. 5, 2016.

regard the village elites as wealth leaders, so that the project can be implemented and furthermore, the purpose of industrial poverty alleviation can be realized.

13.3 Participation Effectiveness: Industry Cooperation, Resource Linkage, and Perception Change

According to our three studies in Zhuigaolai Village, in 2016, more than 100 households in Zhuigaolai Village participated in the "high-quality rice" project, which covered more than 80% of the poor households. Both ordinary villagers and poor households can participate in the "high-quality rice" poverty alleviation project, while the treatments they enjoy are both same and different. The same thing is that all participating households can enjoy the infrastructure construction of the project in the beginning phase of implementation, such as the construction of country roads and water channels, the technical training of high-quality rice cultivation, as well as the unified management of fertilizers and pesticides provided by the county agricultural bureau and the village. The difference is that in order to support the poor households' industrial poverty alleviation, the resident work team of the county poverty alleviation office provides subsidies of 300 yuan per mu for the poor households. The village director, village Party branch secretary, and other village cadres also persuade and mobilize poor households to participate in the high-quality rice industry, promising them that the rice will be purchased at the agreed price after harvesting. In this way, the production cost is borne by the county poverty alleviation office's resident work team in the village, and the sales channels and risks are borne by the village's political and economic elites, so that the officially registered poverty-stricken households will actively participate in the development of the "high-quality rice" industry. The price of high-quality rice is much higher than the previous ordinary rice, and the income of poor households' agricultural operations is greatly improved, which has contributed to the poverty alleviation of poor households.

Since 2017, the yield of "high-quality rice" in Zhuigaolai Village has been 1000–1200 kg per mu. Not only has the yield increased, but farmers' production costs have also been reduced. The county agricultural technology promotion service special appointment program provides farmers with seeds, fertilizers, and pesticides at a preferential price of 100 yuan per mu, and WULX, the Party branch secretary, as the specially appointed agricultural technician, organizes a team to apply fertilizers and pesticides in the village, which greatly reduces the cost of purchasing seeds, fertilizers, and pesticides by farmers themselves, and further reduces the labor-hired and management costs of farmers. Under the current situation of increasingly convenient agricultural socialization services,[11] rice and other agricultural production becomes not too difficult, and the disadvantaged groups with lower labor capacity and poor

---

[11] Field research found that during the rice harvesting season, some people from Jiangsu brought harvesters here to help farmers harvest at a price of 200 yuan per mu, and the result is very good, faster and cheaper than hiring labor.

labor skills can also operate a certain scale of rice cultivation. Poor and disadvantaged groups operating rice cultivation are not only of economic significance, but also increase agricultural operation income, plus important social benefits. Focusing on rice production, the poor and disadvantaged groups can orderly organize their production and make living in the countryside, thus improving their self-confidence with production and life, which in turn improves their social interaction and social status in the countryside, allowing them to get out of poverty not only economically, but also spiritually. Therefore, at present, the industrial poverty alleviation project mainly focusing on "high-quality rice" is widely recognized by almost all villagers, including poor households, in Zhuigaolai Village. Under the guidance and drive of the village "two committee" cadres led by WULX, a number of officially registered poverty-stricken households have developed industrial poverty alleviation projects based on "high-quality rice", and their income from agricultural operations has steadily increased and they have getting out of poverty. Some ordinary farmers, including some officially registered poverty-stricken households, have the developing trend of becoming large agricultural households among other "economic elites" through the development of "high-quality rice" and other agricultural industries. The following typical cases can vividly illustrate.

Case 3

WUTG, an out-of-poverty household.[12]

I was born in 1963 and studied in the 5th grade of elementary school. In 2014, I was rated as an officially registered poverty-stricken household, and I got out of poverty at the end of 2016. The cause of my poverty was "poverty due to education cost", since my son studied in the university in other places with high costs, and I have relatively smaller amount of arable land.

I got married in 1983 and have two daughters and one son. Both daughters have been married off. My son is 25 years old and graduated from Yiyang Academy of Fine Arts in Hunan in 2016. When my son was studying in Yiyang, his tuition fees were quite expensive, with the state subsidies and an education loan of more than 20,000 yuan, and I covered my son's living expenses. It is because of the high cost of my son's education, my family was rated as the officially registered poverty-stricken household in 2014, and in 2016 my son graduated from college and now works in Beijing, and my family is lifted out of poverty.

[12] Interview code: 20180922WUTG.

The total number of my brothers and sisters is 7. After I got married and separated my household registration from my family's, I have relatively small amount of arable land, with only 1 mu of paddy land as well as 1.2 mu of dry land. In 2017, I planted 9 mu of rice, all of which was "high-quality rice", and spent 800 yuan to rent 8 mu of paddy land from other people, which yielded more than 8000 catties of rice. I sold more than 5000 catties at the price of 2.5–2.6 yuan per catty. I hired more than 10 workers and spent more than 700 yuan on labor. The rest work was all done by my wife and me. We also has a sow that gives birth to two litters a year, each with about 10 piglets. The piglets will be raised just more than 30 catties and sold at 15 yuan per catty, and sometimes pigs will be raised up and sold, so we can have an annual income of tens of thousands of yuan. The dry land is planted with corn, which is enough for the sows to eat. Because I am of the officially registered poverty-stricken household, the government offered me pigs, chickens, ducks and baby fish etc. *for my production in 2015 and 2016. Last year, the government gave me 3 pigs, 20 chickens and 20 ducks, all of which my family raised up and sold the fat pigs, and we will sell some of the chickens and ducks when they grow up, with some left for our meals, and had an income of 5000 yuan. This year, no more pigs were given to me, because I got out of poverty. I also have a female cow at home, which I breed myself and sell the calves.*

I had never gone out of the province to work, only helped others paint houses and other things in the vicinity. Now that I'm older, I don't paint houses anymore, and in the past two years I've been working as a pharmacist for pharmacies and herbal companies in Phoenix County. My father understands Miao medicine, and I read the Miao medicine books left by my father, so I also understand Miao medicine somewhat. I worked 8 months in 2017, with food and housing covered by companies, and earned about 2000 yuan per month with 4 days off per month. In 2018, because the wife's poor health, I worked only 7 months.

I think my family's life is getting better and better. In the village, except for those few households with minimum living guarantee, most of the officially registered poverty-stricken households are similar to my own family and get out of poverty. If the industry can develop steadily, as long as we are willing to work, we can also do odd jobs in the vicinity, and there are many opportunities. Our lives will be better and better and we will not return to poverty.

Case 4

WANGFS, a household out of poverty.[13]

I was born in 1973, was rated as an officially registered poverty-stricken household in 2014, and passed the inspection and got the approval for poverty elimination in May 2018. The cause of poverty is "poverty due to education", since my family has too many children, i.e. 5 children, with insufficient workforce and a heavy burden, and my two daughters were studying outside, which cost more.

[13] Interview code: 20180922WANGFS.

I didn't graduate from junior high school. At that time, I was studying in the prefecture traffic school, majoring in auto mechanics, and studies for 3 years (from 1997 to 1999), and the annual tuition cost was more than 1000 yuan, and I had to pay for living expenses. My family had no money, so I didn't complete the education. After that, I went to work in Guangdong for less than a year and came back, following masters as apprentice. Then, I went to Jiangsu for a job, and worked in a steel pipe factory. I married at the age of 25 and had five children, the first four children are girls, and the fifth is a son finally. The oldest daughter is 20 years old and is studying at Xiangtan Vocational College, with an annual tuition fee of 12,000 yuan and monthly living expenses of more than 1000 yuan. The second daughter, born in 2004, is a grade-3 junior student at Huaxin School, where she got enrolled in the 6th grade at the elementary school as she was selected for good performance in a competitive exam. Now the tuition fee is 4600 yuan per semester and the living expenses are 800 yuan per month. The second daughter is a good student and is studying in the top class, so she will be directly promoted to the high school of Huaxin School. The third daughter was born in 2010 and is studying in the third grade at the town elementary school, free of tuition and fees, and enjoying a subsidy of about 1000 yuan per semester. The fourth daughter, born in 2012, is studying in the first grade at the town elementary school, free of tuition and fees, with a subsidy (about 1000 yuan) per semester. The youngest son, the fifth child, was born in 2017 and is just over one year old. I was fined a lot of money for this unplanned birth.

My family has contracted more than 1 mu of paddy land and 4 mu of dry land. In the past, we mainly grew tobacco, and the main source of income for our family also depended on growing tobacco. Over these years, I have basically contracted other people's fields every year. I pay a rent for some fields, usually 100 to 200 yuan per mu, which depends on the quality of the field. The rent for tobacco fields is higher, 500 yuan per mu. As for some fields, I do not pay rent, and I will give 100 pounds of grain per mu. All are negotiated and confirmed by mouth, and every year I will negotiate about the price. In 2017, my family's farming situation was like this: 12 mu of rice, all were "high-quality rice"; 50 mu of tobacco; 10 mu of corn; and 30 pigs. The rent for the land cost more than 10,000 yuan and more than 2000 catties of grains. The cost of hiring labor for tobacco planting is about 20,000 yuan. I seldom hire labor for rice planting as fertilization and pesticides application are all covered by the village, and my main work is sowing, transplanting and harvesting. When it comes to harvesting, I hire laborers, which costs about 1000 yuan. Last year, the rice harvest was late by more than a month because of the rain, but the quality of the rice was not affected and the yield was more than 800 catties per mu. In this year, the rice yield is higher, with more than 1000 catties. Tobacco is sold at the contracted price with the tobacco station. Growing tobacco is much harder than growing rice as it requires careful management, and the costs and risks are relatively high. In 2017, there were 7 to 8 households in the village who grew tobacco for many years and they had some experience. Last year, 24 pigs were slaughtered, 10 small ones (about 100 catties), and the earning was more than 40,000 yuan, and 6 will be slaughtered this year. After getting married, my family started to raise pigs, only one or two at the beginning, but more in recent years. Now it is not easy to hire workers, the young and strong laborers have gone out to work, and most of those left behind are old people and women aged 50 and above.

They generally tended to hire female workers because the wages of female workers are relatively cheaper, and female workers are more patient and careful.

Since I am an officially registered poverty-stricken household, besides the various agricultural subsidies that we all have, it seems that there is an annual subsidy for industrial poverty alleviation (about 2000 yuan). The government also offers pigs, chickens, ducks, seedlings, etc. *and the seeds of "high-quality rice", fertilizers, pesticides are also subsidized. The children go to school in the town, whose tuition is free of charge and they are subsidized. My family also received a small government interest-bearing loan of 50,000 yuan for three years.*

Finally, I think that the national policy is so good, as long as I am willing to work, there is no problem to get out of poverty and live stably. Now there are more children, and as long as they can study, I will do my best to support them to study more.

Case 5

LONGAC, a large rice grower.[14]

I am 64 years old this year (year of 2018), married, graduated from elementary school, and I am the leader of the second village group. I was a soldier in Guangxi for 5 years, after completing the military service, I have been farming, and no experience of working outside. My wife is 56 years old and we have 4 children, including 1 son (second in line) and 3 daughters, all of whom have grown up and have their families.

My family had 22 mu of arable land to farm in 2018, including 4.5 mu of my own contracted land, 4 mu of rented land without rent, and the other 13.5 mu of rented land with rent (about 400 yuan/mu). Of the 22 mu of land,15 mu were planted with rice, 1.5 mu of paddy fields were used to farm fish. The rest of the fields are planted with kiwifruit and pepper.

In 2015, I started to rent land from farmers in my village group who were working outside and I responded to the county's call by growing commercial vegetables, but I never made any money due to poor sales. I like and am good at growing rice, so I planted 12 mu in 2017 and sold more than 10,000 yuan. 15 mu was planted in 2018. This year, I have hired laborers at the price of 120–150 yuan/day for men and 100 yuan/day for women. This year, I mainly use a harvesting machine to harvest the rice, which comes from Jiangsu and costs 200 yuan per mu, while I still hire laborers to harvest the 1.5 mu of paddy fish. The harvesting machine is very good, fast and cheaper than hiring labor. In 2018, rice harvest was very good, and I think my rice harvest is the best in the whole village, as I follow the Party branch secretary's guidance, manage my land quite well and the weather is good. The yield can reach 1000–1200 catties/mu. I think the advantage of growing rice is that I can sell as much as I want in the current year, and if I can't sell it, I can pack it up and save it for the next year's sale, so I am going to continue to expand the area of rice cultivation in the future. I will still rent others' land annually with verbal agreement. Last year, we sold 3000 catties of rice to the village director at the price of 2.8 to 3 yuan per catty, and the village director packed it and sold it for 4 to 5 yuan per catty. The rest rice was sold by myself

[14] Interview code: 20180921LONGAC.

at the market, and the unsold rice of 5000 catties was saved. In 2018, more than one catty of paddy baby fish was invested, and only 1.5 mus of paddy field was used due to the water source and management problems.

There are 26 officially registered poverty-stricken households in the second village group. I think the government's support for officially registered poverty-stricken households is good, but the government does not support people like myself who work hard, such as preferential loans, so I still have some problems with that in my mind. Of course, this does not affect my enthusiasm for growing rice. I just love to grow and want to grow, so I am especially willing to participate in the village's "high-quality rice" project.

From Case 3 to Case 5, we can draw the conclusions about elite-driven industrial poverty alleviation, i.e. some of the officially registered poverty-stricken households have been driven by the political and economic elites led by WULX to develop industrial poverty alleviation projects, which are mainly centered on "high-quality rice", and their agricultural income has steadily increased and they have been lifted out of poverty. Some ordinary farmers, including some of the officially registered poverty-stricken households, have the trend to develop into economic elites through the development of agricultural industries such as "high-quality rice". We can also draw the following conclusions based on the other cases we made in Zhuigaolai Village.

Firstly, in a typical poor village like Zhuigaolai Village, the main causes of poverty for poor households are lack of labor, lack of capital, illness, and schooling. For families with many children and high costs of children schooling that leads to high household expenses, most of them are temporarily poor and relatively easy to get out of poverty, like the Case 3 and Case 4. On the one hand, as the children complete their education and get employed, the family expenses will be reduced and the income will be increased, so they can get out of poverty soon; on the other hand, under the comprehensive promotion of the policy of targeted poverty alleviation, the education policies of poverty alleviation are put in place everywhere, so the risk and phenomenon of "poverty due to schooling" will be reduced. The research also found that the villagers of Zhuigaolai Village attach more importance to their children's education, as long as their children can study, they are willing to pay for their children's schooling, and try to provide their children with quality educational resources. The Huaxin School of Phoenix County is a school run by the local people but subsidized by the state with relatively high teaching quality. The school tuition and living expenses are relatively expensive, but the villagers, including poor households of Zhuigaolai Village, as long as their children are admitted to Huaxin School, basically will send their children to the school, which invariably increases the education expenses of villagers' families.

Secondly, except for those households enjoying the five guarantees or minimum living guarantee without working ability, and those special poor families with disabilities or serious diseases, who need the government's social security to get out of poverty, all other officially registered poverty-stricken households can rely on the development of moderate scale of special agricultural industries and other "odd jobs" to get out of poverty. In short, hard work can help people get rid of poverty. Our research in Zhuigaolai Village found that Case 4 is not rare.

Although there is not much arable land per person in the village according to household registration, about 80% of the young and strong laborers work outside for a long time, so their land can be transferred to those who stay in the village to farm. In this way, the constraint of land resources is relatively small, and it is possible to develop moderate scale agriculture as long as one is willing to do it, and thus it is feasible to develop scale agriculture to improve labor productivity and thus increase income steadily.

In the implementation of the "one industry with three-zation"[15] strategy, the development of tourism industry, Phoenix County has been constantly promoting the industrialization of agriculture, which has also brought opportunities and policy support for the Zhuigaolai Village. Because of its special geographical environment, rice cultivation and vegetable cultivation have become the key industries supported by the county. In addition, the development of tourism industry in Phoenix County over the years has led to the prosperity of the related catering industry, and the demand for rice and vegetables is constantly increasing. Such development opportunities not only attract some people to engage in large-scale agriculture in the countryside and become "big farmers", but also provide those who stay at home to work in agriculture or take care of their families with more opportunities for "employment in farming" and other "odd jobs". It can be said that the income from farming is not the only income of the laborers who do not go out to work at home. Most of them are engaged in non-farm activities in the village or town, or become hired laborers engaged in farming work for other economic organizations or farming households in the village or town, while manage their own agricultural production. Thus, in addition to income from agricultural operations, most of them have a certain share of income from wages and labor services.

Thirdly, the endogenous poverty alleviation driven by village elites is the most important cause for the remarkable effect of poverty reduction in Zhuigaolai Village. According to our research, village elites not only play a significant role in driving industrial poverty alleviation, but also play the role of resource linkers, and play a very important role in driving poor households to go out to do business, work, and local "odd jobs". For example, in her interview with us, the director for women affairs of Zhuigaolai Village told us that she often receives all kinds of work opportunities from the government, from "big farmers", and from bosses of other places, and usually they will approach her first, and then she will mobilize the people. Sometimes she will also use her political resources. For example, when going out to attend meetings, she will contact some people outside to seek employment opportunities for the village. It can be said that in Zhuigaolai Village, the "matrix effect" of "one woman driving a group of women to work" has been formed. The village director for women affairs

[15] The "one industry with three-zation" refers to: giving full play of the advantages of ecological and cultural resources with Phoenix characteristics, on the basis of making bigger and stronger ecological and cultural tourism industry, the county vigorously implements the "tourism + " strategy. Through developing the tourism industry, it will drive the industrialization of agriculture, new industrialization, and new urbanization and further drive the development of the tertiary industry.

told us that as long as people are willing to work, they will be busy working every day and they have work almost every day.[16] In the above-mentioned cases, the "big farmers" also reflected the same problem. Since most of the young and strong laborers are working outside the village, there are now sufficient opportunities for "odd jobs" in the village, and sometimes it is difficult to hire workers during the busy season. Almost all the farmers we interviewed in the village said that they had work almost every day as long as they were willing to work. In addition, in the process of targeted poverty alleviation, the village elites in Zhuigaolai Village pay special attention to reflecting on the current local development reality and development prospect, and attach importance to the spread of new ideas and concepts, which further enhance the poor people's awareness of self-reliance, independent struggle and initiative to get out of poverty, and have a potential influence on the poor people's ideology and lifestyle.

In summary, because village elites are familiar with local resources and have a strong sense of community with village households, they can easily lead to a change in the mindset of poor groups and form an endogenous poverty alleviation model with strong sustainability. We believe that the village elites in Zhuigaolai Village have a greater role in driving the livelihood and development of households, and the endogenous poverty alleviation driven by the village elites is the most important cause for the remarkable poverty reduction effect in Zhuigaolai Village. The important insight is that the driving demonstration of rural elites is the key to poverty eradication in deeply impoverished villages and the key to rural revitalization in the post-poverty eradication era. Therefore, it should actively and effectively formulate the supporting policies to cultivate and develop more rural elites, and build a linkage mechanism of rural elites driving and helping all villagers, including poor farmers, to alleviate poverty.

References

Chen, G. (2004). Capital Accumulation Strategies of Rural Community Elites in the Late 20th Century. *Journal of Jiangsu Administrative College*, No. 6.

He, J., et al. (2017). The Community Logic of the Evolution of Agricultural Business Practices in China—A Case Study Based on Two Rural Communities in Fenyang City, Shanxi Province. *China Rural Observer*, No. 2.

He, X. (2000). Village Elites and Community Memory: A Two-Dimensional Framework for Understanding the Nature of Villages. *Social Science Series*, No. 4.

Lv, S. (2006). *Rural Sociology*. Social Science Literature Press.

Xia, Z., & He, X. (2017). Half Work and Half Farming and China's Progressive Urbanization Model. *China Social Science, 12*.

Zeng, M., Zeng, W. (2017). Rural Elite Participation in Endogenous Poverty Alleviation: An Example of Relevant Practices in W city, Guangxi Autonomous Region. *Theoretical Guide*, No. 1.

[16] Interview code: 20180922FUNVZR.

Zhong, R., & Li, F. (2017). Analysis of Different Subjects' States in the Center for Targeted Poverty Alleviation in Villages of the Plugged-in Poverty Areas. *Journal of Northwest Agriculture and Forestry University of Science and Technology (Social Science Edition)*, No. 2.

Zhu, T. (2016). A Study of the Interface between State and Society by Rural Governance Elites in Targeted Poverty Alleviation—A Practical Analysis of XS County, Jiangxi Province. *Socialist Studies*, No. 5.

Liu Xiaomin, a researcher at the Institute of Ethnology and Anthropology, Chinese Academy of Social Sciences, whose main research interests are ethnic economy and anti-poverty in ethnic areas.

Chapter 14
Lighting the Way for the Villagers in the Corner of the Deep Mountains: An Example of Helping Poor Households in the Village of Bingga, Guizhou Province

Lidan Song

Abstract Guizhou is located in the poverty-stricken contiguous mountainous areas in the hinterland of Yunnan-Guizhou-Guangxi stony desertification, where it is difficult for the farmers to get out of poverty through individual production by themselves, let alone getting rich, due to the harsh natural conditions. One household after another household suffered a lot from long-term poverty and diseases. Before organizing them to form a collective economic accumulation and eventually to "make blood" by themselves, the state and society need to input a large amount of resources to help them get rid of their individual hardships at first and then seek collective common prosperity. This process is destined to be difficult, but it is a necessary path for the Republic to forge ahead and "leave no one behind".

Keywords Targeted poverty alleviation · Stony desertification · Bingga village

Guizhou is the home town of "Keichousaurus". 300 million years ago, there was a turbulent sea above the Yunnan and Guizhou. With the uplifting of the earth's plate, the sedimentary rocks under the sea rose upward and were scoured by the rain and shined by the sun, gradually forming a beautiful scenery consisting of peak forests, caves, underground rivers, canyons, lakes, and so on. But this "bonsai" like beautiful place is one of the poorest areas in China. It takes thousands of years to form a thin layer of soil on the surface of the rocks, but human development and the scour of wind and rain can quickly make the soil layer loss, so "stony desertification" has become the most terrible natural phenomenon here, where people can only grow some corn, potatoes, peppers, and other crops that do not need much nutrients in the barren soil of the rock nest, and survive on them.

Special Note: The real names of the family cited in these cases in the text have been anonymized.

L. Song (✉)
Institute of Marxism, Chinese Academy of Social Sciences, Beijing, China

Case Studies of Targeted Poverty Reduction and Alleviation in 100 Villages, International Research on Poverty Reduction, https://doi.org/10.1007/978-981-95-0549-4_14

In Guizhou, where the sky never clears for three days, the rainfall is not small, but due to the lack of vegetation on the ground, with underground caves and rivers crisscrossed, surface water often seeps into the ground without knowing where it goes, and people on the ground suffer a lot from water shortage. The poor soil and the limitation of water use have made this province, which is surrounded by mountains and no plains to support it, underdeveloped for a long time. The Qianxinan Buyi and Miao Autonomous Prefecture, which is located in the southwest corner of Guizhou, is one of the poorest regions in Guizhou. 71.5% of the total area of the prefecture belongs to the "most fragile environment for human survival", karst terrain, and is in the hinterland of "the poverty-stricken contiguous mountainous areas of Yunnan-Guizhou-Guangxi stony desertification": 7 out of 8 counties and cities in the prefecture are the state-level poverty-stricken counties (cities). There remain 432,000 people to be lifted out of poverty during the 13th Five-Year Plan period, which is the main battlefield of the whole province and national poverty reduction. In 2014, the average poverty incidence rate of townships in Qianxinan prefecture was 56.91%, 17.52 percentage points higher than that of the province.[1] There are 35 ethnic groups, including the Buyi, Miao, Yi, Hui, and Han, living in Qianxinan, and the population of ethnic minorities accounts for 42.47% of the total population of the prefecture.[2] There was a high poverty rate. In the 1990s, it took a day to travel from Xingyi city, the capital of Qianxinan prefecture, to Guiyang, the provincial capital. Before the start of targeted poverty alleviation, time also seemed to come to a standstill in the mountainous villages of Qianxinan, where slash-and-burn farming, thatched huts, and mud roads were still common sights.

The terrain of Bingga Village, Yuzhang township, Yilong New District, Qianxinan Prefecture, slopes gently, and the soil is relatively fertile. However, the tension between population and land is increasing. Nowadays, the arable land per capita is only 0.91 mu[3] and the villagers are very poor. In October 2009, Comrade Li Keqiang, then Vice Premier of the State Council, walked into a drafty thatched hut in the village of Bingga, and he was shocked by the poverty here, pointing out that "we should effectively solve key livelihood issues in accelerating development".[4]

Nowadays, a series of supporting measures such as the renovation of dilapidated houses and targeted poverty alleviation have transformed the old appearance of the village of Bingga into a new one. The villagers, who have lived with silence and poverty for many years, finally see the roads repaired to their homes, the streetlights lighting up the darkness, and their lives getting better and better. The villagers of Bingga expressed great appreciation for the policy of targeted poverty alleviation,

[1] Deng Boxiang, "Targeted Poverty Alleviation: 400,000 People Get Out of Poverty in Qianxinan in 3 Years," Guizhou Ethnic Newspaper, August 21, 2014, p. B1.

[2] Chen Zuyu: "New chapter of national unity and progress in Jinzhou", Guizhou Daily, January 5, 2019, p. 1.

[3] 1 mu equals 1/15 hectare. – Trans.

[4] Xie Dengke, "Li Keqiang's Inspection in Guizhou: Effectively Addressing Key Livelihood Issues in Accelerating Development," October 20, 2009, People's Daily - People's Daily, http://politics.people.com.cn/GB/1024/10218952.html, December 3, 2017.

saying that thanks to the Communist Party, the roads were repaired to their doorsteps, which is so convenient! Everyone has the hope that life will be better.

Although the lives of households lifted out of poverty in the Bingga Village are still far from well-off, for them, "Targeted Poverty Alleviation" provides a strong impetus to break away from the old life track and gives them more possibilities for the future.

14.1 Hospital Services Will Come When Get Sick

Yang Xiaohua, a villager lived in the Mianzhe second village group of Bingga Village, was born in 1954. He and his wife have 2 girls and 2 boys as villagers who live in the rural areas believe in "more sons and more blessings", and they have a family of 6. But in the village of Bingga, apart from planting a few mus[5] of corn and barley, they have no other way to get more income, and their lives are stretched to the limit. Due to the heavy burden of the family, he and his wife are always in overload. The long years of labor work caused him a strange disease in his 40 s: the soles of both feet were full of corns, except for the center of his feet. This makes him walk like stepping on a thorn, with stinging pain, so he had to use a sharpened knife to remove the thick layer of callus skin before going to bed every night to feel a little better. Worse than that, he also suffered from serious lumbar disc herniation, which made him barely walk without a walking stick or touching the wall. In 2016, Yang Xiaohua's annual family income per capita was only 1206 yuan. Yang Xiaohua also wanted to go to the hospital for treatment, but thought that the treatment was so expensive that he had to suffer in silence for many years. When it really hurts too much, he goes to the village pharmacy to buy some painkillers, which is considered as treatment.

The lumbar disc herniation is a consequence of years of overwork, and how come the Yang Xiaohua's feet full of corns? In the busy season, farmers will start to work before dawn (the sun rises, it will be too sunshiny). They generally do not eat breakfast. When the fieldwork finished, it will be almost at noon. After going back home, they will hastily have some food and rest, and then go to work in the afternoon. When the stars appear in the sky, they will rush home. Why do I say rush home? As after the fields were distributed to the family, good and bad fields are located in different places. The distance from home to different fields is quite far. After returning home, have a light meal then, it will be another day. People should eat breakfast at 7 to 9 am, otherwise they are very prone to gastrointestinal diseases, and dinner should be eaten before 7 pm, but they usually eat at 8 pm. In the long run, the stomach and intestines are naturally weak.

In terms of food, their food is very coarse, mostly coarse grains and vegetables. This seems "healthy" to the city people, because the city people eat too much fine grains and meat, eggs and milk, so they should eat more simply. But rural people need more fine and nutritious food after physical work, and the lack of meat and fat in the

[5] 1 mu equals 1/15 hectare. – Trans.

diet does not allow the skin to get the normal moisturizing. Long-term irregular diet, eating too coarse, all make their intestines and stomach meridians[6] damaged, and stomach gas could not descend. Plus, farmers work in the fields for years. Moisture often penetrate into the body through the feet, as weeds, rocks and other objects frequently hurt their feet, and the natural skin of the feet is severely damaged. Due to blockage of the stomach meridian, the stomach gas does not descend, which will make the skin of the feet do not moisten, and the feet veins cannot work, so it is difficult to metabolize the dead skin on the feet. With dead skin piled up in a piece, a foot full of corns is formed.

In 2016, Yang Xiaohua's weak gastrointestinal system was completely collapsed after a wedding drink, and he vomited blood out of his mouth, even "vomited up a big bowl" (in the words of his eldest son). The family took him to the county hospital, where several bags of blood were transfused, with each bag costing more than 800 yuan, the total cost was more than 3000 yuan, which they had to borrow money from others. At that time, he and his family did not know about the new rural cooperative medical care (referred to as "new rural cooperative"), so the cost was not reimbursed.

In 2017, the supporting cadres learned that Yang Xiaohua's lumbar disc herniation had seriously affected his quality of life, so they suggested that he go for surgery and told him that he could leave the cost documents for reimbursement. So, Yang Xiaohua went to the county hospital for the first time in his life and had the corresponding surgery, which cost about 110,000 yuan in total, and his family helped him get reimbursed about 100,000 yuan of medical expenses with the "new rural cooperative" this time, leaving more than 8000 yuan unpaid, and the town reimbursed him more than 5000 yuan according to the relevant policies, and his family only spent about 3000 yuan. Yang Xiaohua and his family had never thought about this welfare before. After the surgery, Yang Xiaohua finally lived a normal life, and he told everyone that the national policy is good; otherwise he could have lost his life.

Unfortunately, the good times did not last long. In 2019, Yang Xiaohua suddenly fainted and was sent to the hospital, as he was diagnosed with a brain hemorrhage caused by "something growing" in his brain. With the experience of the last reimbursement, his family decisively sent him to the hospital. After seven consecutive surgeries, he was in a coma in the ICU for 81 days before waking up. In the past, Yang's family would have given up on saving his life, but it was the "new rural cooperative" medical insurance for major illnesses that Yang Xiaohua was able to be saved for such a long time, and after his condition improved he was transferred to a general ward for treatment. Yang Xiaohua's medical expenses for this treatment alone amounted to 290,000 yuan, and according to the highest standard of reimbursement in Guizhou Province, he was reimbursed about 200,000 yuan by the "new rural cooperative", and the rest of the expenses were borne by his two sons. Although Yang Xiaohua finished his poor and unhealthy life in July 2019 (at the age of 65), he and his family were very grateful for the support he received from the state in his later years.

[6] This is a term in traditional Chinese medicine meridian system. – Trans.

After Yang Xiaohua's death, we interviewed his youngest son, Yang Yilong. According to his report, except him, his sister and brother have already had their families, and his brother still lives with his parents after marriage, but "money is counted separately", and "the family is not divided with separated household registration". Yang Yilong was born in 1989, and this year (hereinafter referred to as the year of 2020) he was 31 years old but he was still not married. So he missed the appropriate age for marriage. Now his peers are married, and he became the left ones. At present, the ratio of men to women in rural areas is reversed compared to that in urban areas, that is, there are more men than women, and once men miss the marriage age, and their economic conditions are not superior, there is basically no hope of getting marriage.

When Yang Xiaohua was hospitalized in 2019, his four children took turns caring for him. As Yang Yilong said,

> *Although most of the money spent for my father's treatment was reimbursed, we still had to pay tens of thousands yuan by ourselves. For example, the patient next to his hospital bed, who also had a brain hemorrhage, was cured by taking a medicine that cost more than 300 yuan per pill (i.e. An Gong Niu Huang Wan), and recommended us to buy. We bought some for more than 3000 yuan, but it turned out to be useless. In addition, my father's hospitalization cost 40 yuan per day for liquid food and 200 yuan per day for VIP fee, all these expenses and those expenses that exceeded the limit of reimbursement could not be reimbursed. The 15,000 yuan that I earned through work were spent, and my brother also spent 15,000 yuan, but it was not enough, so my brother and I borrowed 20,000 yuan each ...... my sisters were only responsible for buying some food, so they spent some money, and their own families also had no money. I have not gone out to work, as during the year when my father died, I had to stay at home with Mom. 5 mu of my family's land was returned to the forest, where we planted fir trees, and the trees have not grown up. There are still about 5 mu of land left, where we planted some dark grains (barley), I do not know how much it can be sold this year. Last year, it can be sold a few yuan a catty; this year, the price may be more than 1 yuan, then it can be sold for 8,000 ~ 10,000 yuan. My family raised two sows and sold nine piglets for 1,500 yuan each. Sometimes the village asks us to work at the "base" (the industrial base run by the enterprise in the village), and they may work for about one month a year for 100 yuan a day. The money we borrowed is likely to be repaid this year (the year of 2020).*

Generally speaking, Yang Xiaohua's two sons paid more than 70,000 yuan for his treatment, including a debt of more than 40,000 yuan, which was obviously extremely low debt for 81 days of ICU treatment.

Yang Xiaohua's life was tormented by illness and poverty, but fortunately, in the last days of his life, he caught up with the good policy of targeted poverty alleviation, so he was able to stay in the hospital again and again, and his family did not have to bear a debt too heavy for his treatment. It is not uncommon for villagers like Yang Xiaohua who suffered from serious illnesses and disabilities due to the unreasonable lifestyle caused by backwardness and poverty. In the planning of rural revitalization strategy, it is very important to pay attention to the improvement of farmers' lifestyles and provide the necessary knowledge of self-care to reduce the possibilities of poverty and returning to poverty due to illness.

14.2 Children Want to Study so Support Her

He Yunxing, a Han Chinese villager of Bingga Village, was born in 1980. He was rated as an ordinary poor household before he was lifted out of poverty in 2015, and the cause for poverty was lack of capital and technology. After assistance, the annual income per capita of He's family reached 3324.8 yuan by 2015. He Yunxing had three children, the eldest daughter is 21 years old and is studying in the No.2 secondary school in Xingren City, and will take the entrance examination of Gaokao[7] in 2020. The second is a son, 18 years old and has graduated from the Qianxinan Excellence Vocational and Technical School in Xingren City and is currently doing an internship. The youngest daughter died of an illness in 2016, at the age of 13. According to He Yunxing, the family's poverty is mainly caused by the large number of children and the heavy burden.

When asked He Yunxing how he got out of poverty, he said that he mainly received education subsidies.

> *The oldest girl is studying in high school in Xingren County, and the poor family will only be charged more than 1,100 for half a semester, and other expenses, such as accommodation and water fees, are exempted by the state. I pay more than 600 yuan per month for her living expenses. After graduating from junior high school, my son studied computer at a vocational school in Xinren for three years. The tuition fee for half a semester was also more than 1100 yuan, and the state also exempts him from other fees. But the monthly living expenses are more than 1,000 yuan that will be given to the school. The two kids can receive a total of 3,000 yuan of education subsidy for half a semester, i.e. 6,000 yuan a year.*

When asked how much He Yunxing spends on education each year, he said it was a few thousand yuan. I asked, "That's not right, is it? After all, tuition fees and living expenses for two children cost at least 12,800 yuan a year". He said, "I can't do the math, as I stopped studying in the third grade of elementary school". During the research, I was always confused by the villagers' calculations. They always said they couldn't remember how much they earned or spent, and the figures of the same item often fluctuated. Maybe it is the less education they receive that made their poor calculation. No matter how, in He Yunxing's mind, the education subsidy given by the state is very helpful.

In order to help him settle his poverty alleviation account, after repeated inquiries, He Yunxing recalled the things one after another.

> *Our family has more than two mu of land to transfer. The rent of transferring 1 mu is 400 yuan and the other is 600 yuan, so I can get more than 1,000 yuan a year. I rented five or six mu to other people to grow flue-cured tobacco, and I can get more than 2,000 yuan a year. Food needs to be bought, and we don't live at home, so we usually buy our meals in the city. My wife and I help people make bricks in the nearby town called Wantun, and we can earn 230-240 yuan a day. In this way, we work more than 20 days a month, earning more than 4,000 yuan.*

"It's only 4000 yuan for two people. Why don't you change to a higher salary job?" He Yunxing said, "We are uneducated, so we have to do hard work". He

[7] China's annual College Entrance Examination. – Trans.

Yunxing and his wife earn more than 40,000 yuan a year, plus land dividends of more than 3000 yuan and minus education expenses, there does not seem to be much money. So He Yunxing continued to "confess": "We still have that 100,000 yuan of Huinong agricultural loans, borrowed from 2017, and it is a three-year loan, and then the village let us buy some shares, the annual dividends of 5000 yuan". It turns out that like the other villages as well. As the Bingga Village cannot find good investment channels, they mobilize poor households to invest 100,000 yuan of agricultural loans per household into the village company, and then there will be 5000 yuan of "dividends" per year for every poor household. According to the current benchmark interest rate of one-year deposit in the central bank, which is 1.5%, one-year interest for 100,000 yuan deposit is about 1500 yuan. In the absence of better development, it is still good for the poor households who can have such an income, but unfortunately this loan can only be borrowed for three years. Frankly speaking, if poor households can find a good way to make a group investment in industry, then the Huinong agricultural loan is really a hen that can lay golden eggs.

He Yunxing said at the beginning that he had two children. Only when asked if he had been reimbursed for medical insurance, did he mention that he had a younger daughter who, in 2016, became ill with a "distended stomach and she was not saved". The medical expenses were reimbursed by the state for more than 20,000 yuan. When it comes to this past, although he voiced a bit of sadness, he seemed to talk about someone else's family affairs, and asked his wife if the child was 11 or 13 years old at the time and how many years has it been since she died? Rural people are usually not as emotional and sensational about these unpredictable tragedies as city people. It is not that they are not sad, but they don't have the energy to express broken-heartedly. Like an old woman we met in the mountains, she mentioned that she had given birth to 11 children, nine of them girls, and that they all died not long after birth. Her expression was also very light.

I asked He Yunxing: "Rural people generally do not like to let girls study, so why is your girl still in high school at the age of 21?" He Yunxing said, "She failed to go up to the next grade at elementary school for two years, so she is now in her senior year of high school. We are not educated, so we have been working hard. The girl likes to study, so we support her study, in that hope that she will be educated well in the future". They are really good parents, because there are many girls here who graduate from junior high school, get married and have children, and live in the countryside for the rest of their lives. But this is not only because the couple of He Yunxing is open-minded, but also it is more realistic that He Yunxing family caught up with the good policy of targeted poverty alleviation, and enjoyed the state poverty alleviation measures from loans, education and other aspects, so he has the courage to let his daughter to pursue their dreams. Although the score of his eldest daughter's college entrance exam is not ideal, plus ethnicity identity of 20 points, the total score is only 321 points (daughter's ethnicity is inherited from her mother's Miao), so she has decided to go to work. With a high school degree, she will certainly not repeat her parents' days of moving bricks on construction sites, but can find a more decent job in the city.

He Yunxing is very grateful for the state's poverty alleviation measures and said that after the targeted poverty alleviation, the days are gradually getting better. These days may still seem too poor for us, but for them who could only survive in the past, it is a very great thing that their children can receive vocational education, take the college entrance examination, and have a better future than them.

14.3 The State Back Me up in Husband's Family

Yang Dani, Han nationality, from Bingga Village's cedar group, was born in 1971, 49 years old this year, but her face is gaunt, and her fingers are rough, with a lot of white hair, so she looks not much different from the 60-year-old. When she was 22 years old, Yang Dani's own uncle convinced her "honest" father to marry the nephew of her uncle's wife, Mr. Yang Zhongyi. At that time, Yang Dani did not know anything about love, and she also did not like Yang Zhongyi, a "non-speaking" dummy. But her parents were persuaded by her uncle's rhetoric, and she had no choice but to marry him. I asked, "why you agreed?". She said, "I didn't know why, but my parents decided to do it".

Yang Dani is illiterate, as she never went to school, her parents are also illiterate, and the idea of "intermarriage brings family closer" led to the marriage. After the marriage, Yang Dani found out that her husband not only could not speak, but his brain was also confused and had mental illness. But there it was, she had to "marry a chicken, then follow the chicken; marry a dog, then follow the dog". What goes beyond her expectation is, the whole family-in-law treated her badly. Originally, she treated her parents-in-law as her parents, but her mother-in-law was always picky on her and abused her, and her brother-in-law and two sisters-in-law also targeted her, making her feel way miserable and disappointed. During the whole process of dialogue with her, Yang Dani would constantly mention the harm her mother-in-law had done to her, and the relationship between her mother-in-law and daughter-in-law is still very tense today. Since Yang Zhongyi is a "disabled person", Yang Dani is responsible for all the family affairs, and she has to put up with the difficulties her mother-in-law made for her day and night, and her body and mind are getting weaker. In this way, she also gave birth to three children one after another and raised them to adulthood.

The eldest daughter was born in 1995 and is 25 years old this year (hereinafter referred to as the year of 2020). She feels sorry for her eldest daughter.

> *My eldest girl was a good student. She passed the high school entrance examination, and was admitted to No.1 middle school (refers to the Xingyi No.1 middle school, the local top middle school), but she told me, "Mom, grandmother quarrels with you every day, so you should not live with her. Let's repair the old house, and you move out to live by yourself, then I go to work to earn money ......" and then she went to work. In that year, she was only 15 years old, and got married 17 years old. She met my son-in-law during the days she worked outside, and he was a farmer from Sichuan. She has 2 children, one is 8 years old, and the other is 3 years old. What I regret is, I didn't support her with her education, and she married too far away to me, so no one accompanies me around.*

It is obvious that Yang Dani and her eldest daughter have a very good relationship, and her eldest daughter saw her pain in her eyes and could think for her, but the person who understands her best is married in a distant province, and it is difficult to meet her. By now, she hasn't met the youngest child (3 years old) of her eldest daughter, which is the thing she regrets most.

The second girl is 23 years old. She did not do well in school, who did not study in the third year of junior high school, because she did not want to study and then went to work. Now she is married in Ceheng, a poor county in Qianxinan Prefecture. It takes just two hours away to travel by car. Her family (referring to the son-in-law's family) is also poor and has two children, a boy and a girl. The son-in-law treated her badly, often beating and scolding her, and when she came back with the children, I persuaded her to go back. I told her "do not divorce, only divorce adults, not divorce with children (referring to the situation for divorce. It does not matter if adults divorce without children; if adults have children, adults should not leave - the author's note), as the children are in the need of parents to raise them together; family needs both father and mother. You see I also did not divorce, bringing up three of you". Then she did not divorce.

Yang Dani's youngest son, 21 years old, is living more comfortably than his sisters. He first went to vocational school for three years in Anlong (a county in Qianxinan Prefecture), then went to work for two years and felt it was too hard for life, and asked to go to vocational school in Tongren (the capital of the Tongren region in Guizhou Province). This year is the third year of education and he is about to graduate. "Tuition is 9000 yuan per year, living expenses is, as he said, 30 yuan a day, and the two girls[8] help me send money to him, otherwise I can not afford it". It is not uncommon in rural areas for daughters to help their parents raise their sons. Anyway, he stays in Guizhou where the price is relatively low. The two vocational schools he attended were not included in the national compulsory education system, so the six years of tuition and living expenses will be paid by his mother and sisters. It is also deplorable that rural boys now generally do not know how to farm, and some still require their parents to provide for their own living expenses at city standards.

When it comes to her husband, Yang Dani has a lot of grievances, "he does not know anything, he does not know the pigs I fed at home, cattle are also fed on my own, he can not do anything. He doesn't even know that some people bully me". In rural areas, men are the main labor force, Yang Dani not only used to farm, but also raise pigs and feed cattle, take care of three children and parents-in-law, so her work is so intense that she suffers from sickness.

Two years ago I helped the village cooperative to make bacon, then there was no place for the old house, so I could not make the smoked bacon. I also fried chili noodles to sell, but after a year I could not fry because when I fried chili I would cough and could not breathe, even wearing a mask is useless, so I did not make that.

My body hurts everywhere. The teeth are almost lost, so dentures cost me two to three thousand yuan, and now I can not eat hard things, and have to drink conjee every day. The cervical spine is also bad, and I have asthma so serious that I can not eat when it got worse. I just pick some herbs and eat them myself.

---

[8] I.e. the two daughters. – Trans.

In this year, Yang Dani is only 49 years old, but her teeth are lost, so it is obvious that her long-term overwork resulted in kidney deficiency that loosened her teeth. She also suffers from the asthma because of the disharmonious relations between the mother-in-law and daughter-in-law that leads to her mentally unhappy, her feeling of depression, and weakened pulmonary function. Many diseases do find their roots in life!

Yang Dani, struggling with poverty and hard work, finally saw the light of day in targeted poverty alleviation. Yang's family now has 5.9 mu of land transferred to the village's "kiwifruit base" and receives an annual transfer fee of 3000 yuan. The village also gave her family a Huinong agricultural loan that is specially provided for poor households, which she invested in a company that the village invested, and could receive 3000 yuan of interest per year for three years. I did some calculations for her, but the money was not enough to pay for her son's schooling, so where did the rest of her income come from? Yang Dani said,

> *My family's old house had so many leaks, and the village Party branch secretary Zheng saw it and said my house was so dilapidated that the state (dilapidated house renovation) gave 18,500 yuan to fix it, and then someone wanted to buy it, so I sold it to him who developed it into farm stay, and I got 48,000 yuan. The money was not given to my mother-in-law because secretary Zheng and they thought it belonged to me, and my mother-in-law's family hated me even more and scolded me everywhere. The new house I built was next to my old house, so they (the farm stay operators) said they would like to rent it for farm stay too. The contract was signed yesterday for 7 years, and the rent for the first three and a half years is 18,000 yuan, and the rent for the next three and a half years will be dividend that depends on the earnings. Thanks to the government, otherwise my family's money would be in the hands of my mother-in-law and her sons and daughters!*

In Yang Dani's mind, the government has become her "mother's family", helping her to do justice and solving her housing problem after renting out her house.

> *The village found a place for me to live. I lived in the village office at first, paying 50 yuan a year for three rooms, but there were small rooms and not connected to each other, so I couldn't make it a parlor (it is a local custom to place the family' sacred memorial tablets in a place equivalent to a parlor - note from the author). Later, the village found a house in town for me for the rent of 420 yuan per year, with two rooms and a parlor. Yet my son said he wanted to get married, so I wanted to rent an extra house, and it was almost done.*

"And what other income does your family have? Your husband has mental problems, and the cause of poverty is written as 'due to disability'. Have you received any help from the state?" I asked. Yang Dani said, "He has applied for a disability identity and receives a monthly allowance of more than 300 yuan". It's not a lot of money, but it's enough to cover the basic needs of a family for rice, flour, and oil in the local countryside.

For this rural woman, her family was not a place to accommodate her and support her, but a burden that she had to support with all her efforts. She also raised up her children desperately in the belief that "this family cannot be broken up". She is constrained by traditional ideas, just like poverty. Even though her husband was mentally handicapped, even though her in-laws were critical of her, and even though she bore the burden of raising the family, she still struggled to support them, and taught her daughter not to divorce, because children need to grow up in an intact family. This is certainly a great aspect of rural women, but it is also a source of their misfortune. Her poverty and lack of education prevented her from leaving her penniless home, because this home was the only place she could settle. The only thing she can rely on is her sensible daughter. Her good fortune is that she has finally waited for the "targeted poverty alleviation", and the burden of life is finally lifted by the state.

We are now living better than before. Thanks to the Communist Party, thanks to secretary Zheng and you, cadres, everyone who saw me would help me and care for me. Without them, I wouldn't have the money for my house.

Yang Dani's eyes glittered with tears and she kept saying thanks. Let's hope this bitter woman can live a better life!

14.4 The State Raised My Disabled Son

Yang Anrong, who lived in Bingga Village, born in 1953, has long years of outdoor work, and his skin is brownish yellow like dried bacon, and his head lines and figure-of-eight pattern are deeply embedded on his face like knife carving. Silence is his tag and what praiseworthy thing is he was much clearer than others on the numbers and calculations.

He has two sons and a daughter. The oldest son, Yang Dalei, was born in 1977 and had meningitis when he was a child. Due to the limited conditions the local medical treatment have, adults thought the child had fever, got through difficult situations, and then he would be fine, yet it turned out to be "burned his brain" and became a "disabled". When he was more than 20 years old, his parents found another woman for Yang Dalei, who also "burned her brain" because of meningitis, and they formed a family. Fortunately, they gave birth to a boy and a girl who are normal children. Yang Dalei's eldest daughter was born in 2002, and in this year she is 18 years old, attended a year of vocational school in the provincial capital of Guiyang. She said she could not study anymore, so recently she returned home and did odd jobs in the city of Xingyi, and washed dishes in restaurants, etc., with food and accommodation included, the current job offered a month's salary of 1600 yuan. Yang Dalei's son studied in the private junior high school in the city of Xingyi, and half a year of his tuition cost 7260 yuan, and a month of living expenses was two or three hundred yuan, so a year of total expenses was nearly 20,000 yuan. The boy also did not get admitted to the high school, so he went to Xingren City to attend vocational school. It is said that he made electronics-related studies, and the school tuition was cheap, costing 1020 yuan half a year, and living expenses for half a year were 1300 yuan. Due to a series of reforms in recent years, there is a serious shortage of enrollment quota in public junior high school in Guizhou province, so many rural children have to go to private middle schools due to their poor educational foundation, as they cannot get admitted to good public junior high schools, which brings a heavy burden to their families. The tuition of vocational schools is very cheap, which is somewhat surprising.

I asked Yang Anrong who would pay for the tuition and living expenses of Yang Dalei's two children? He replied,

> *Yang Dalei and his wife had bad brains, but their family have 3 acres of land, planting barley and baogu (i.e. corn), and my wife and I will take them to plant. If you do not care about them, they will sit by the field for a day and will not do anything. They can't make much money by growing that stuff, so it's us - old couple that helped them. We rented 10 mu of land to grow flue-cured tobacco, with the rent is 500-700 yuan per mu, plus our own land which is 16 mu, so we can collect about 1300 catties of tobacco each year. Minus the cost of 10,000 yuan (including the cost of renting land and baking tobacco leaves), we have an income of more than 20,000 yuan.*

I asked, "During the education of your two grandchildren, their tuition and living expenses will cost at least 30,000 yuan, and your income is not enough". Yang Anrong nodded his head and, with my prompting, went on to do the math: "Yes, there was an education subsidy. The two children could get about 625 yuan every six months". I asked, "You and Yang Dalei are both poor households, so what kind of help do you get from the government respectively?" Yang Anrong said,

> *Yang Dalei and his wife have a monthly minimum living guarantee, but I do not know how much money will be given to his bank account. The money is still very useful (the village cadres pointed out that there are more than 500 yuan, which guarantees the living of the three people). I got a renovation of my dilapidated house, and they sent someone to fix the house, and gave me 1500 yuan for buying colorful tiles (i.e. buy colorful tiles for the roof decoration). The government gave Yang Dalei's family 35,000 yuan to help him build a new house with three rooms (a parlor and two bedrooms). Yang Dalei could not get an education loan for his children's education because he is disabled. But he and I got the 'Huinong agricultural loan' for poor households, and we both get 5,000 yuan of dividends every year (only for 3 years).*

In this way, he and his son have reached the standard of "the two assurances and three guarantees"[9] to get lifted out of poverty.

I then asked, "You have a son and a daughter. Do they help Yang Dalei's family?" "The younger son's family gives his brother more than 2000 yuan a year, but the daughter's family itself is poor, and she herself has been sick for the past two years, so she didn't give any money". When it comes to the youngest son, the old man seems to feel a bit relieved.

> *Both of them are working in Guangdong, and each has a monthly salary more than 4,000 yuan, so we take care of the two children here. One is studying in preschool and the other in fourth grade. Both live on campus, five days a week, and the school manages them well. The elementary school is free of charge, but the preschool charges 1,750 yuan for six months. Every year, our youngest son's family gives us 5,000 to 6,000 yuan as subsidies.*

Yang Anrong is 67 years old, and his partner 65 years old. They have to do farm work every day, but also cook for Yang Dalei' couple. At the weekends, they also

[9] The Two Assurances and Three Guarantees refer to assurances of adequate food and clothing, and guarantees of access to compulsory education, basic medical services and safe housing for impoverished rural residents. – Trans.

have to look after the grandchildren, so the days are busier than the city workers. Even so, they did not complain, as in their words, they lived a very quiet and uneventful life. Fortunately, the country's targeted poverty alleviation policy has given them a lot of help, which is also considered a blessing in misfortune!

14.5 I'm Fine as Long as My Son is Fine

Yang Anxing, living in the cedar forest group of Bingga Village, a Miao person, was born in 1968 and is 52 years old. At this age, Yang Anxing is already the grandfather of his eight children. While his peers give birth to children later in life in Beijing and other large cities, whose children may still study in elementary school. He has three sons, the oldest of whom was born in 1986, meaning that Yang became a father at the age of 18. His sons have also started their families early and have a large number of children and grandchildren. The only regret is that Yang's wife passed away six years ago (2014). Currently, Yang's three sons are all working in Guangdong, and he lives at home alone, widowed, with his second son's four children, two of whom are studying in elementary school and two in kindergarten. When the children go to school, he gets up early in the morning to make breakfast for the children, sends the younger ones to kindergarten, and then goes to the fields to work; in the afternoon, he picks up the children from kindergarten and then makes dinner, and he cleans up the house and does housework before the busy day is over.

When Yang Anxing's family was identified as a poor household in 2014, their annual income per capita was only 2792.73 yuan. The family has a total of 4 mu of arable land, 2.5 mu of paddy land, and 1.5 mu of forest land. Now the forest land is planted with cedar trees, 1 mu of arable land is transferred to the village cooperative, and the rest of the land is planted with corn and barley for a small amount of money, and the family's main income still comes from their sons working outside.

> *I planted corn to feed livestock, pigs, chicken. Now there are only five large chickens, as most die from chicken's plague. The price of pigs this year is too high. I can not afford to buy piglets, so did not raise pigs.*

Yang Anxing pointed to the empty pigpen with his finger, and his tone was full of helplessness.

Like other poor households in the village, Yang Anxing has also benefited from the "targeted poverty alleviation" program. He also used 100,000 yuan of "Huinong agricultural loans" to buy shares in the cooperative, so he could receive 5000 yuan of dividends per year for three consecutive years, which expired last year (2019). Yang Anxing said.

> *I used the 50,000 yuan of special loans to buy three cows, each 7,000 yuan, and bought feed. There were two calves bred during the two-year period, but then the cattle suffered from "No. 5 disease" (referring to foot-and-mouth disease), so I had to sell all five cows, although I did not make much money, but at least the loan was paid off.*

The "targeted poverty alleviation" policy also provided the family with 18,500 yuan for renovating their dilapidated house, and they built a 120-square-meter bungalow with a large parlor and two bedrooms for 27,000 yuan. "My second son and I live in this house, and my eldest son built his own two-story building on the slope behind us". Yang Anxing said, "The state takes good care of our poor households, so this is beyond doubt".

After the death of his wife, as his sons went out to work one after another, in 2016, Yang Anxing's family got lifted out of poverty, and he said,

All three sons are working in Guangdong, two of whom work in construction sites and one in a factory. I don't know how much they earn every month, but it depends on whether they can find a job or not. This year (the epidemic year) it is not good, so there are few jobs. My second son sends me 1,000 yuan a month because I help him take care of his children. You ask me where I buy meat. I go to the street by bus, and pay 5 yuan to stop at Jiaoluo (village) street, 10 yuan to Tunjiao (town), and 16 yuan to Xingren (county). I go to the street once a month. As I don't have a refrigerator, so I buy meat for one or two meals. Every morning the four kids get up, and I cook breakfast for them, I make noodles with some oil, sometimes with eggs, and they go to school after eating, which is a 20-minute walk away. The school has a meal prepared for them at noon, and they come back at night for another meal, just good enough to get by. The state is so good to us, the poor families that we don't even pay for our children's education in elementary school. Kindergarten is a private school, and it costs 800 yuan per kid for half a year, which is 3,200 yuan per year for two children. My son will send the money when he pays the tuition.

"My partner has been dead for 6 years. It was chronic tuberculosis. At that time, there was no such thing as reimbursement, so I spent tens of thousands yuan but she was not cured". "Isn't tuberculosis treatment free of charge by the state? Why did you spend tens of thousands yuan?" I asked. "I don't know, but it cost tens of thousands yuan anyway! If only it were now, there would be reimbursement". Yang Anxing said with regret.

She died in June, and her body rested in the parlor for more than ten days. At that time, we could still do the burial, according to our Miao rules. We are 'wooden comb Miao', so we needed to play Lusheng,[10] *drums. During those days, the acquaintances in the village and relatives came over, and we prepared meals for them. When guests from afar arrived, they would also have meals. Tables, benches, bowls, all of these were taken by the people in the village from home. We bought food, did cooking with more than ten people who were helpers, and no need to pay them. This is like doing work, as you help my family, and I will also help your family. We do not distinguish between Miao, Han and Buyi people here, as we are all similar and have a good relationship.*

"So how much did it cost?" Yang Anxing thought for a moment and said.

I spent 38,000 yuan. I bought two pigs. As one cost for 4,000 yuan, two for 8,000 yuan. She was buried in my own land, and her coffin cost 7,000 to 8,000 yuan! I didn't make a tombstone, as one cost more than 10,000 yuan and that was too expensive, so I didn't get one. Just take the bricks to cover up the grave. I accepted condolences from relatives, who gave me 1000 yuan or 800 yuan, and acquaintances gave me 100 yuan, 50 yuan. I don't

[10] It is a musical instrument with multiple bamboo pipes, each fitted with a free reed, which are fitted into a long blowing tube made of hardwood. It most often has five or six pipes of different pitches, and is thus a polyphonic instrument. – Trans.

remember how much I received, but I gave it all to my sons anyway, because my eldest and second sons paid for these arrangements, each paying 18,000 yuan. In the future, if someone else's family prepare for such an occasion, they will have to pay back at least 150 yuan for a 100 yuan of condolence and 300 yuan for a 200 yuan.

Through calculation, if the funeral is held 12 days, with the total expenses of 38,000 yuan, it is necessary to spend about 3160 yuan per day. For a family with annual income per capita of only 2000 yuan, this is undoubtedly a huge expense. The culture of holding big events in the countryside has not yet changed substantially, said a farmer's wife during our research.

If there are (red and white[11]) events and we do not attend, then when we hold event, others will not come, so we have to even borrow money to attend. So far, I have borrowed more than 10,000 yuan, and I need to get back the money I sent out, as we also have to hold events.

With so much money being spent on such unproductive expenses, it is even more difficult to develop production in rural areas where funds are in shortage. In the village of Tangyue, Pingba District, Anshun City, Guizhou Province, it stipulates that no gifts are accepted in red and white ceremonies, and the village collective provides the venue and personnel to hold red and white ceremonies, which in a short time puts a stop to the bad practice of gift-giving that has been spreading for decades. And it is worthwhile for the villager's committee of Bingga Village to learn and practice.

Yang Anxing's family was very poor, but as his three sons became adults and worked outside the province, the family economy was much better. In rural areas, working is the quickest way to get lifted out of poverty. At present, it seems that collective economy is the key for farmers to get out of poverty and get rich in the future, and it is also the key to organize farmers to realize the third leap in agriculture. The rural revitalization strategy should put more attention on the development and growth of collective economic organizations in the future. In this way, we can make our agricultural security more secure, our agricultural economy more profitable, and farmers' life with more dignity.

References

Cheng, E., Lu, X., & Xu, H. (2006). Diversification of Collective and Cooperative Economy Models Should be Advocated for Building a New Socialist Countryside. *Economic Journal*, No. 12.

[German] Engels. (2012). The French-German Peasant Question. In Marx Engels, *Selected Works* (Vol. 4), People's Publishing House.

Jiang, G. (2019). What Does It Really Take to Ensure Food Security. *China Rural Discovery*, No. 1.

Lenin [USSR]. (1995). Petty-Bourgeois Socialism and Proletarian Socialism. In *Lenin's Selected Works* (vol. 1), People's Publishing House.

Li, S. (2019). Relevant Reflections on the Strategic Opportunity Period in the New Era. *Marxist Studies*, No. 10.

[11] In Chinese tradition, red event means wedding; white event means funeral. – Trans.

Mao, Z. (2009). On the People's Democratic Dictatorship. In *Selected Works of Mao Zedong* (Vol. 4), People's Publishing House.
Wang, H. (2016). *The Road to Tangjiao*. People's Publishing House.
Yan, H., & Chen, Y. (2015). Characteristics and Directions of Agricultural Capitalization in China: Bottom-Up and Top-Down Capitalization Dynamics. *Open Times*, No. 5.
Zhang, W. (2006). New Socialist Countryside Construction Requires Reform and Development of Rural Collective Economy. *Socialism with Chinese Characteristics Research*, No. 5.

Lidan Song is an associate researcher at the Institute of Marxism, Chinese Academy of Social Sciences, with research interests in Marxist class theory.

Chapter 15
Increase the Spirit and Confidence in Targeted Poverty Alleviation and Targeted Poverty Eradication: Based on a Study of the Village of Ori in Qinghai Province

Cunying Long, Jun Nie, and Yi Chen

Abstract With the in-depth promotion of poverty eradication, spiritual poverty alleviation has become an important measure to get rid of poverty and prevent returning to poverty in poverty-stricken areas. Poor people are the main beneficiaries of our poverty reduction battle, and the main body and main force of poverty eradication and achieving prosperity. Stimulating poor people's awareness of poverty eradication is to support poverty eradication with endogenous motivation. The author examines the work of targeted poverty alleviation and targeted poverty eradication in the village of Ori in Qinghai Province through a field survey of the village. Through questionnaires and interview materials, we can understand the development and production and living conditions of the village, explore the problem of the poor people with the spiritual poverty alleviation during the work of poverty eradication in Ori village, and think about what cultural ideas affect the development of the endogenous power of the people. While helping increases their spirit and confidence has become an important part of poverty alleviation work, some poor people have the idea of "passively longing for national assistance, expecting government grants and claiming for poverty reduction funds" and do not take the initiative to solve the problem of family poverty. At the same time, some poor people have reached the standard of poverty eradication, but they are reluctant to get lifted out of poverty. Based on this, increasing the spirit and confidence has become an important way out of poverty for the poor people.

Foundation Project: Results of Targeted Poverty Alleviation and Elimination in 100 Villages-Case Studies; Base Project for Social Development Research of Ethnic Minorities in Northwest China (XBS10).

C. Long · Y. Chen (✉)
Ningxia University, Yinchuan, China

J. Nie
North Minzu University, Yinchuan, China

Case Studies of Targeted Poverty Reduction and Alleviation in 100 Villages, International Research on Poverty Reduction, https://doi.org/10.1007/978-981-95-0549-4_15

Keywords Targeted poverty alleviation · Increasing the spirit and confidence · Endogenous motivation · Ori Village

15.1 Overview of the Ori Village and the Production and Life of the Villagers

15.1.1 Overview of the Ori Village

The hills meet the flat land and after a few turns we reached our field point where the houses came into view and the tiredness from the driving car went far away. The quiet village added vitality to the land. A few pedestrians walked along the road, expressing curiosity about our arrival. We observed each other and began to explain our intentions of visit. The villagers were so simple, and after knowing our intentions, they gradually became familiar and enthusiastic. The Ori Village is situated on a plateau with an average altitude of over 3000 m and is surrounded by hills not far away. The village consists of 6 village groups, 1 of which is Han group and 5 of which are Tibetan groups. The majority of the villagers are Tibetans, and there are 274 households and 1001 people in the village, 231 households and 864 people from ethnic minorities, and more than 60 people with disabilities, and the number of laborers accounts for more than 50% of the total population of the village. The villagers mainly grow crops such as highland barley and rape.

Ori Village is located in the northeast of Qinghai Lake, only 15 km away from Qinghai Lake in the west, less than 2 km away from the government site of Ganzihe Township in the south, and 50 km away from Haiyan County in the north. At the same time, it is a national poverty-stricken village with deep poverty. Through the mapping survey and targeted identification at the end of 2015, 77 poor households, accounting for 28.10% of the total number of households and 220 poor people, accounting for 21.98% of the total village population, were identified to be included in the targeted poverty alleviation plan, among whom 70 households with 203 people are ordinary poor households; 7 households with 17 people are households enjoying minimum living guarantee. In 2017, the number of poor households was increased to 76 households with 253 people after the "retrospective re-examination" of the officially registered poverty-stricken households.

In 2016, Ori Village still faced major difficulties and challenges in infrastructure construction, public services, economic development, village governance, and targeted poverty alleviation. In terms of road traffic, the roads between villages are basically cement roads, but there are only 12 km; in terms of TV communication, the village has wired radio and TV, but there are still 13 households without TV sets at home, and the villager's committee has not yet been equipped with networked computers; in terms of maternity and childcare and healthcare, the village has one clinic and one pharmacy.

15.1.2 Villagers' Production and Living Conditions

Housing Conditions. In recent years, through the implementation of the policy of renovating dilapidated houses and relocation of poverty-stricken households, the housing conditions of some farmers and herdsmen have been greatly improved. As for villagers' houses, most of the houses are made of bricks and cemented, decorated in modern style, but of course there are some Tibetan cultural elements, and the houses are comprised of three rooms side by side. Clean floor tiles are laid, the walls are painted white and hung with various pictures, various tea sets are placed on the dining table, a large sofa is placed in the middle, and some of the appliances are equipped to meet the needs of the owner's family. The house is structurally safe and cleanly decorated, giving it a spacious and thriving feeling. For example, the house of uncle A is comprised of three rooms side by side, next to two bedrooms, and the house is paved with a little brown floor tiles. It looks neatly decorated and tidied up.

Now we live very well in a brick house, basically have everything at home, unlike our older generation who lived in a clay house, when the conditions were poor, so nothing was special. Now that we are old, the house can be cleaned up as long as you love it. Look at this floor, paved with floor tiles, and we usually have to use a mop to clean up. Sometimes when there is water, it is inconvenient to clean. The home is usually bright and clean, and we also place some flowers and plants (for decoration)[1] .

Of course, in addition to the immobilized safe house, they also have summer pasture tent houses, which are much simpler, as the tents can be moved, the living supplies inside are very few, and they are mainly to provide herdsmen with the usual living quarters.

Living Conditions. Compared with the past, the living conditions of villagers have changed a lot. In terms of income and expenditure, regarding the "net household income in 2016", a large proportion of households have a net income of more than 10,000 yuan. There are only a few of households who have fixed income sources. Most of them have income from agricultural business, for example, some families sell their cattle and sheep to increase their income. Other people mainly work and grow crops as their source of income. As for expenses, a large part is mainly for paying living expenses, and also for building houses. For example, the main source of income for Z's family is working, while the main expense of the family is the treatment of her mother's illness, which requires long-term treatment.

My family's income is mainly from what we, two young people, work outside, and the old people sometimes grow something on land at home, and there is no income from farming. We go out to work in the county, so I can get almost 3,000 yuan a month, my wife worked in the restaurant with a salary of more than 2,000 yuan a month. My mother is sometimes in poor health, who has a chronic disease, so we often buy her medicine. We also buy household items, something for children education, and usually buy some clothes, and there is no money left.[2]

---

[1] Interviewee: A, male, 72 years old, Tibetan, interviewed in his home in August 2017. All names have been processed according to professional requirements.

[2] Interview subject: Z, male, 46 years old, Han people, interviewed at the roadside in July 2017.

Household Property Status. Through the questionnaire, we can see that the ownership of household durable consumer goods such as TV sets, washing machines, refrigerators, cell phones, and motorcycles is relatively high among the farming and herding households in Ori Village, and the material capital is relatively abundant. Among them, TV sets have the highest ownership rate of 96.67%, followed by refrigerators or freezers with 80.00% in respondents' homes, while the ownership rate of various agricultural machines/ agricultural facilities is lower, only 1.5% ~ 8.5% because it is a pastoral area. Many young people have smartphones. As in interview with G, the family has a son who drives a big truck outside and has a good economic income. The family has built a particularly large house with luxurious decoration, which is paved with marble floor tiles, etc. The family has a refrigerator, TV, water heater, car, etc. Judged from his family's house and home living materials, it is a prosperous family with rich family properties in the countryside.

The capital resources of farming and herding families in the Ori Village are rare, as the family income is relatively limited, and the production and living expenses are relatively high, so most families have no savings. Family has less turnover of funds. When there is an urgent need for money, they mainly turn to borrowing money from friends and relatives, or the bank loans, etc. Especially like the expenditure of building a house, the capital in need is large, so many villagers will choose to borrow money from their relatives, at the same time this is also the performance of their mutual help.

In terms of health and medical care, the Ori Village is located in the plateau, with high and cold and wet climate, so many elderly people have chronic diseases, but herders are not clear about the medical reimbursement. Only a small number of villagers can be reimbursed. On the one hand, people do not know how to apply reimbursement; on the other hand, some diseases are not in the scope of reimbursement, or only when people must be hospitalized, they can get reimbursement. For example, a grandmother L, who has heart problems, often needs to take medicine, and also has pain in her hands and feet often, so she takes a mixture of various medicines, and also uses local herbs to wipe her hands and feet, but these medicines are not reimbursed.

Labor and Employment. Except for those disabled, seriously ill, and those studying in school, the labor force of the average herder's family is still relatively abundant. The elderly can work in the field and herd animals, the young people mainly herd animals, and the children help the family herd animals after the holidays. Only the limit of their labor is relatively long and their labor burden is heavier. Through developing agricultural and herding production, doing business and working outside, the farmers and herders also obtain corresponding labor income. There are three family laborers in F's family, mainly herding and farming, and everyone undertakes labor work.

> *Our family has five people. The children's grandfather stays at home to do some farm work, while two children are still studying in school, the children's mother and I often go out to herd, so the family affairs are taken care by the elderly, and the children are older enough and we do not need to manage them. We just usually pay some living expenses for them. In*

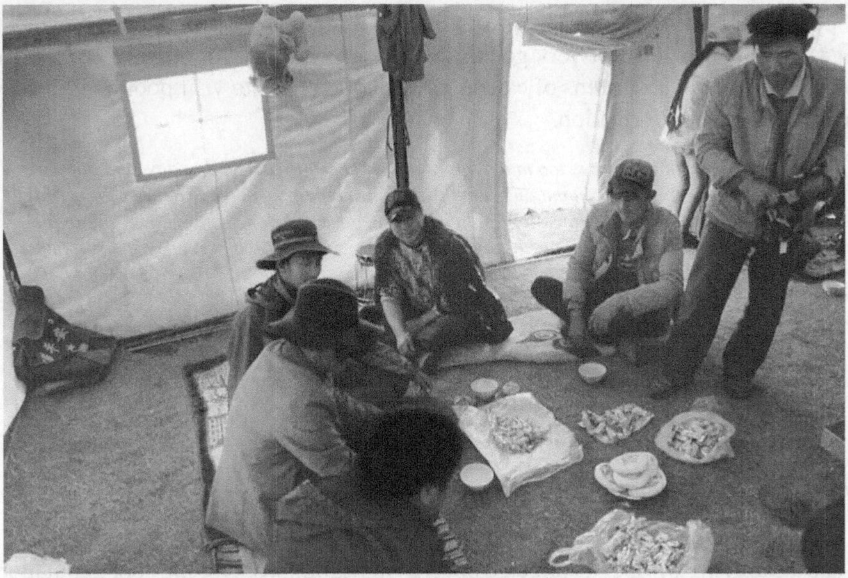

Fig. 15.1 Villagers gather in tents at the summer ranch

our rural areas, as long as you can move, you can't stay idle, as you have to do something, so that the family can live ever after. When we are not busy, we will also stay at home.[3]

Social Ties. Social relationship networks can be divided into formal social relationship networks and informal social relationship networks. Formal social relationship network mainly refers to the relationship network between farmers and herdsmen and some formal social organizations, such as families of farmers and herdsmen need to contact with cooperatives, which provide services such as agricultural products sales, processing, transportation, storage, and technology and information related to agricultural production and operation. There is the strong economic mutual assistance among them. Informal social relationship network refers to the relationship between farmers and herdsmen and their neighbors, villages, and relatives and friends, which is an inevitable way of behavior in people's daily activities and hence makes our life more colorful because of informal relationships. Neighbors visit and help each other, increasing the emotional communication between people in the village. This is also the main social network of people in the Ori Village (Fig. 15.1).

Poverty Alleviation and Poverty Eradication. The villagers have their own different views on poverty alleviation and poverty eradication. Some villagers think that it is not fair in rating poor households. This situation occurs mainly because they do not understand the policy and people only observe the superficial things. There is also a part of non-officially registered poverty-stricken households that have an unbalanced mentality because they do not enjoy the poverty alleviation policy. Regarding

[3] Interviewee: F, male, 41 years old, Tibetan, interviewed at the roadside in July 2017.

the effect of poverty alleviation, most villagers think it is good, and a small number of villagers think it is not very good. Resident cadres often fill out a large number of forms, as many as dozens of categories, and often have to visit poor households' homes to collect information.

> *Villager R thinks that there is too much information needed to collect in a day, and often we don't have time to stay at home and have to wait at home once we are needed to provide something. Some poverty alleviation policies are good, but I don't know about the implementation. But well, we still have to rely on ourselves, and we feel that it takes much time to fill in all these forms in a day.*[4]

15.2 Main Measures of Targeted Poverty Alleviation and the Effect

15.2.1 Main Measures of Targeted Poverty Alleviation

Take the lead in carrying out targeted poverty alleviation work for the poor population according to the "two lines in one" standard. Qinghai Province proposes to carry out the targeted identification of the poor population according to the "two lines in one" standard, i.e. combining the line of minimum living guarantee and the line of poverty alleviation, in which the line of poverty alleviation is based on the per capita annual net income at the end of 2015, that was 2970 yuan. Strictly carry out the "four red lines" for identifying poor households. Disqualifying resolutely those who own cars worth more than 30,000 yuan, those financially supported, and those owning commercial houses and stores, from enjoying the targeted poverty alleviation. After understanding the causes of poverty through visits and research, detailed records are kept such as illness, disability, economic income, whether they are included in minimum living guarantee, housing problems, number of cattle and sheep, and grass area, and promptly sorted out and summarized.

Excellent cadres are selected to be stationed in the village to help poor families. Poor families will be assigned a cadre to help them. Families with any problems or difficulties can discuss with their own cadres on solution. For example, some families have difficulties in supporting their children in schooling due to economic problems, and in such cases, they can consult with their cadres to see if there are any education policies to help them. Farmers and herdsmen who do not have a thorough understanding of various industrial and economic development projects and investments can also consult with family supporting cadres. The cadres stationed in the village to carry out poverty alleviation work is an effective means of targeted poverty alleviation under the new situation, and is a pragmatic move to adapt to the change of poverty alleviation and effective integration of project funds. In order to complete the task, the supporting cadres have to work "day and night", and sometimes

[4] Interviewee: R, male, 38 years old, Tibetan, interviewed at the roadside in July 2017.

they are too busy to have meals in the village all day. As C said, the supporting cadres are too busy.

> *The cadres work very hard and often come down to help us register various information. Sometimes there is no food to eat at noon on a hot day, so I occasionally ask them to eat a little at my house, yet they are afraid of bothering us. Sometimes they will call us in advance to inform us what information is needed from higher authorities. (We) cooperate with each other. Sometimes, if there is anything you don't understand, just call and ask the cadres, as they know more and serve us really well.*[5]

The "double help" mechanism helps poor people to get rid of poverty. The point-to-point supporting departments and organizations of Ori Village include Medical Administration Bureau of Haibei Prefecture, Herd Institution of Heibei Prefecture, Public Security Bureau of Haiyan County, and Veterinary Station of Haiyan County. After investigation of the actual problems of the Ori Village, these supporting departments and organizations play various advantages to introduce projects and apply funds to help farmers and herdsmen develop their economy. The support from the supporting departments and organizations plus the supporting counties in Shandong make contribution to the poverty eradication for the poor people of Haiyan County.

The "retrospective re-examination" of officially registered poverty-stricken households is to realize the dynamic adjustment of the poor population. The number of poor population and the number of officially registered poverty-stricken households are dynamically adjusted. In 2017, in order to ensure the accuracy of poverty alleviation, the village organized a comprehensive "retrospective re-examination" of the officially registered poverty-stricken households, mainly to check whether the selection of poverty alleviation objects in the village is accurate, whether the support mechanism is reasonable, whether the use of poverty alleviation funds is put in place, and whether the problems of poverty alleviation are real, etc. Poverty alleviation is a dynamic management process, and it is the foundation for winning the battle against poverty. Supporting cadres will check which families are suitable for poverty eradication, as in the process of economic development, some families should be removed from the "hat"[6] due to their income increase; while there are also some families affected by illness, sudden circumstances, and family calamities, they can also be included in the poverty-stricken households.

15.2.2 Poverty Alleviation Policy Innovation and Implementation Effect

Medical Aid Policy. In 2015, the Qinghai Provincial Department of Human Resources and Social Security formulated the "Qinghai Provincial Action Plan for Medical Security and Aid for Poverty Alleviation" to implement medical security and aid to

---

[5] Interviewee: C, male, 54 years old, Tibetan, interviewed in his home in July 2017.

[6] Hat metaphorically means poverty. When it is recognized a poverty-stricken one, the one will wear a hat; while one is lifted out of poverty, the one will be taken off the hat. – Trans.

fight poverty for the officially registered poverty-stricken population. The villagers live in the plateau area for a long time, and some of them suffer from heart disease, hypertension, arthritis, etc. The health assistance has helped many officially registered poverty-stricken families to overcome the difficulties in access to medical treatment, and in this way to improve the health index of the villagers. At the same time, each officially registered poverty-stricken household will have a supporting doctor to take care of them. The research of D's family shows that they can consult the family doctor for any health problems.

> *We, poor households, have family doctors. Those doctors from hospital and village clinic will come to help us register information, help us measure blood pressure, diagnose illness, etc. We can ask them what medicine to take if we have any (physical) problems, and they need to know about our family's health, saying that it is to register everyone's (physical condition). If we have problems, they can help us figure out what to do.*[7]

Ecological Protection and Services Policies. In 2016, the Qinghai Provincial Government formulated the "Qinghai Province Ecological Protection and Services Action Plan for Poverty Alleviation" and set up 43,100 ecological public welfare posts in the province, distributing these public welfare posts to officially registered poverty-stricken households, one poor person for one post with a monthly salary of 1800 yuan per person. At present, there are 11 poor households in the Ori Village working on the ecological public welfare posts. In addition, each village group has a public welfare cleaner post, which is mainly responsible for cleaning up the garbage in the village and earns a few hundred yuan a month.

Industrial Poverty Alleviation Policies. In 2015, the Qinghai Provincial Poverty Alleviation and Development Bureau formulated the "Notice on the Key Work of Industrial Poverty Alleviation Projects in 2015", which stipulates industrial support for officially registered poverty-stricken households. Differentiated support standards for agricultural and pastoral areas are adopted to support the poor. For example, in 2016, the Ori Village distributed industrial funds to the officially registered poverty-stricken households in accordance with 6400 yuan per capita in pastoral areas, and the total amount of funds was 1.28 million yuan. The officially registered poverty-stricken households make full use of the funds for industrial development to households to purchase ewes and other livestock to develop animal husbandry.

Financial Poverty Alleviation Policies. In 2015, the Xining Central Branch Bank of the People's Bank of China, together with the Provincial Poverty Alleviation Bureau and the Department of Finance, issued the "Financial Support Action Plan for Targeted Poverty Alleviation in Qinghai" and launched the "530 Credit Loan" project. The officially registered poverty-stricken households with development projects, labor capacity, capital needs, and good credit could apply for "530" small loans for poverty alleviation from local host banks, i.e. credit loans of less than 50,000 yuan, within 3 years, at benchmark interest rates, with local finance and poverty alleviation departments subsidizing interest rates for such loans at benchmark interest rates, so that poor households could enjoy zero interest rate loans. There are 27 officially registered poverty-stricken households in the village who applied for the loans,

[7] Interviewee: D, male, 62 years old, Tibetan, interviewed in his home in August 2017.

and they used the money to develop industries and so on. At the same time, there are also policies on relocation, education assistance, living subsidy, and mutual funds for poverty alleviation.

The main manifestations and reasons for the lack of endogenous motivation of the poor are:

15.3 The Main Syndromes of Insufficient Endogenous Motivation Among Poor People and Its Cause

15.3.1 Traditional Ideas of Resting on the Existing State

For some of the herders in the Ori Village, their diet structure is mainly beef and mutton, dairy products, etc. The basic living conditions can provide the families self-sufficiently. They are not accustomed to expanding the scale of cattle and sheep into industries, or allowing their families to have capital economic accumulation, and are relatively traditional in their thinking. For example, herder X's family has six members, two children are studying in school and live on the campus, while the husband and wife herd their livestock together with their parents in the pasture. The family has 14 mu of pasture, 34 cows, and more than 100 sheep, and their home (tent) in pasture is very simple, with only a carpet and some pots in the tent. X told us that what they usually eat is mutton and milk, and they didn't need to spend money at home, as children's meals and boarding were all taken care by the school, so there is no need to sell cattle and sheep to make money. Unless someone in the family is sick, they will sell some cattle and sheep for money and go to the doctor, only then will they consider turning cattle and sheep into money. Even if the family has free money, they will not let it be capital costs, as they will only use the money to buy more cattle and sheep to raise, and increase the number of cattle and sheep.

From the above examples, most poor households have insufficient endogenous motivation, and a large part of the cause is the traditional cultural practices, the cultural concept that the local land and water can feed the people living there well, and the traditional life has formed an entrenched thought. They do not dare to try a new way of life, due to anxiety about all kinds of uncertainties in the future and fear of difficulty in adapting to the new production and living environment. Accustomed to the original hard life, some poor people prefer to keep the obsolete living conditions. There are also some people who have the idea of getting out of poverty in their minds, but are not willing to do hard work. At the same time, the Ori Village is located in a remote area, and the economic development is relatively lagging behind. As people live far away from the town, and the land is vast and the population is sparse, it is not easy to go to the town. For these reasons, some villagers are not open-minded and continue to be satisfied with their original living environment.

As anthropologist Oscar Lewis's theory of the "culture of poverty" enlightened, we need to analyze the phenomenon of poverty from a sociocultural perspective. People who live in poverty for a long time unconsciously form a whole set of culture that influences the behavior and values of their children and their offspring or those around them. This makes their original poverty situation continue to spread and form poverty groups. It also shows that the culture of poverty itself can be self-perpetuating and self-sustaining. Just as a certain cultural pattern, as opposed to individual behavior, its choice of behavior includes the way of treating people, cultural practices, plus various rules and customs in the field of politics, economy, social interaction, etc., which evolve into customs through formalized ways and eventually form a cultural pattern of a nation. Such a living custom has formed a cultural pattern, and people's ideology is not easily changed by other new ideas.

15.3.2 The Culture of Poverty "Prides Oneself on Being Poor" Breeds

Targeted poverty alleviation not only pays attention to the material level, but more importantly, to helping the poor people establish the concept of "poverty as shame" in the spiritual level. Only by establishing this concept can villagers abandon the idea of "passively longing for national assistance, expecting government grants and claiming for poverty reduction funds". When the government implements some industrial projects to help the poor, it provides the poor people with material and technical support for development. However, some herders simply put their hopes on the government, as they neither participate in the development at all nor do anything themselves, just want to sit back and enjoy the benefits, hoping to get subsidies. Through the survey, it was found that some poor households in the village had the ideology of "proud of being poor". For example, during the research, in family K, the child said to his father, "when is our family going to be a poor family?" This idea has two conspicuous syndromes. One is that some farmers and herdsmen competed to be poor households, and some non-officially registered poverty-stricken households claimed that they were poorer than the officially registered poverty-stricken households. This is not that they really wanted to be poor households, but they complained that there were some unfair phenomena in the process of targeted poverty alleviation. The second syndrome is that poor households are unwilling to get out of poverty. Some of the officially registered poverty-stricken households refused to get out of poverty even though they have reached the standard of poverty eradication.

Such as Bai Guangfu. Bai Guangfu suffered from pulmonary heart disease, hypertension, heart disease, and other diseases, and has been taking medication for years, and has basically lost his ability to work. Only his wife could do labor work, which caused his family life full of difficulties. In 2015, the family was rated as the officially registered poverty-stricken household through the targeted identification work. In 2016, his family received various poverty alleviation measures, and achieved an income of 30,000 yuan (Bai Guangfu served as doorman at the people's bank of

Haibei prefecture with a monthly salary of 1700 yuan; his wife, Meng Zhanhua, did cleaning work there too, with a monthly salary of 800 yuan. There was an annual income of 30,000 yuan in total), plus net property income of 600 yuan (the family enjoyed the dividend from Xingsheng yaks breeding industry developed by Xiang Qibu, a villager of Dezhou Village of the home town), the policy income from ecological protection was 4290.64 yuan (100 mu of summer pasture per person, his family has 2 persons, so it was 200 mu in subtotal. And the annual subsidy for non-grazing pasture was 12.28 yuan/ mu, so it was 2456 yuan in subtotal; 8 mu of land was returned to forest, and the annual subsidy for returned land was 160 yuan/ mu, so it was 1280 yuan in subtotal; the annual direct subsidy to grain producers was 69.33 yuan/ mu, and there were 8 mu in subsidy, so it was 554.64 yuan in subtotal), the income from minimum living guarantee was 3540 yuan, the income from pension subsidy was 1714.8 yuan (Bai Guangfu enjoyed the monthly pension of 142.9 yuan), and social aid and subsidy of 200 yuan (the supporter, Zhang Shaoxing, donated cash to him in November, 2016). The whole family realized a total income of 40,345.44 yuan in 2016, with a per capita disposable income of 20,172.72 yuan. According to the standard for poverty eradication of per capita disposable income of 3316 yuan in 2016, Bai Guangfu's family should be lifted out of poverty. The work team of poverty alleviation and the cadres of the village "two committees" went to his home several times to verify his income and persuade him to actively remove his identity from poor households, but he kept on excusing himself, maintaining that he should continue to enjoy the treatment of poor households.

The poor households in targeted poverty alleviation enjoy "high welfare" given by the state. High welfare is prone to a moral scourge that causes waste of social resources and national laziness. High welfare provided by the state is a kind of public goods, just like eating from the same big pot[8] under the planned economy system, inducing everyone to make the most of it, and thus will lay the moral scourge. The specific manifestations are: the underutilization of social security resources under high welfare, such as the waste of medicines and other medical resources in publicly funded medical care; some people are not actively to look for jobs when they could be employed, and excessively enjoy the leisure brought by social security and unemployment insurance, as well as choose to retire early; over-reliance on the state, weakening the enthusiasm and ability of self-accumulation and self-sustainment; etc. Once these phenomena become widespread, social resources will be seriously wasted, and the national spirit is no longer positive, and economic development will be affected.

It is a common belief among the poverty alleviation cadres in the Ori Village that the poverty alleviation policies given by the government are too favorable, covering almost every aspect of the production and life of poor households, and that various preferential resources are applied on the poor households, which has cultivated their habit of "sit back and enjoy" and "resting on the laurels". In the process of targeted poverty alleviation, the government has absolute dominance over the allocation of

[8] I.e. "everybody eating from the same big pot", which is an equalitarian treatment of enterprises and individuals regardless of their performances. – Trans.

anti-poverty resources, while poor households receive these resources for free. For more than 3 decades, the state has attached great importance to anti-poverty work and invested a lot of human, material, and financial resources. This means that once farmers and herdsmen become officially registered poverty-stricken households, they have access to large sums of money for production and living and other policy support. In addition, some poor households worried that after getting out of poverty, compared with other poor households, they will not continue to enjoy the treatment of "poor households", but also lost the care and help of supporting cadres, so psychologically they will inevitably have a sense of loss and deprivation. In the long run, the majority of farmers and herdsmen will compete to become poor households, and poor households are not willing to get out of poverty, so the number of poor households can only be increasing, and the situation of poverty can only be more and more serious, which turns out to be such an ending as "poverty alleviation year after year, but poverty remains year after year" and "poverty is never-ending". More seriously, the state invested a large amount of funds for poverty alleviation will put a certain pressure on the government's finances, which will inevitably lead to a fiscal deficit in the long run, thus affecting the economic and social development of the whole country.

How can we eliminate the poverty culture of "taking pride in poverty"? First of all, poverty elimination needs to increase people's confidence. It is needed to strengthen the sense of responsibility of poor households. As the saying goes, "Poverty elimination needs to increase people's confidence at first, then people will be diligent to make hundred industries thrive". Poverty alleviation cadres should pay more attention to spiritual help when provide material help. "To solve the problem of spiritual poverty and lack of endogenous motivation of some poor people, grassroots cadres need to effectively change their concepts. In the specific work, strengthen the education and guidance of the poor masses; vigorously develop rural culture, promote the core values of socialism; innovative industrial poverty alleviation mechanism, enhance the participation of the poor masses, to produce a sense of participation in poverty alleviation so as to drive the sense of gain in getting out of poverty, to prevent the poor masses from waiting and seeing in the process of poverty alleviation". In the daily work of poverty alleviation, poverty alleviation cadres should pay attention to the guidance of public opinion, through building beautiful villages, simplifying folk customs, choosing the right development path among other strong measures, to help poor farmers and herdsmen establish confidence and courage, promote self-reliance among the poor masses, awaken the awareness of the poor masses to take the initiative to get out of poverty, fully mobilize the subjective initiative and creativity of everyone to get out of poverty and get rich, so that the poor masses know shame of poverty and take courage, everyone refuses to be poor households, and they will actively get out of poverty after reaching the standard.

Secondly, the temporary policy subsidies should be appropriately reduced to optimize the income structure of the poor. The excessive temporary policy subsidies given by the government to poor households are an important reason why it is difficult for poor households to get out of poverty. For this reason, the government should use more poverty alleviation funds for various poverty alleviation projects related to the increase of poor households' business income and wage income, instead of directly subsidizing poor households. For example, increase labor skill training funds and hold regular labor skill training courses to improve the labor and employment skills of poor farmers and herdsmen, promote employment of poor farmers and herdsmen, and increase wage income; provide poor farmers and herdsmen with more funds for industrial development or a large sum of funds for industrial project to help them expand the scale of animal husbandry and develop ecological tourism. By appropriately reducing temporary policy subsidies and increasing financial support for industrial development, we can stimulate the endogenous motivation of poor farmers and herdsmen, increase the proportion of stable income, and optimize the income structure of poor farmers and herdsmen, etc.

Finally, accountability system is established to guarantee the accurate identification. At the present stage, poverty alleviation cadres are to a certain extent in control of poverty indicators and deliberations; therefore, it is necessary to insist on "retrospective re-examination" and "re-identification" of targeted poverty alleviation for a long time, and establish a severe accountability system. When there is off-target thing discovered, the most severe accountability will be launched on the relevant departments, organization, and personnel. Through the implementation of a strict accountability system, it can prevent the poverty alleviation cadres from including relatives and friends into the identification of poverty, and safeguarding the fairness of targeted poverty alleviation.

15.3.3 Lack of Awareness of Learning Skills

In the Ori Village, due to its location in a remote and deeply impoverished area, the transportation is inconvenient, the information to the outside world is blocked, and the poor people lack awareness of making a living with modern skills. The herders do not know advanced breeding techniques except traditional herding techniques, and their awareness of industrial development is weak. In view of this, training can be used to learn breeding techniques, making meat products of higher quality. Also, Ori Village lacks the capability for the deep processing of livestock products, so the added value of livestock products is low. By accepting new ideas, herdsmen can take advantage of the village's beef and sheep meat resources to carry out primary processing of livestock products, and make air-dried meat and cold meat with ethnic characteristics through the way of "cooperative + poor households". At the same time, we can also realize the deep processing of livestock products with external force. For example, yak meat can be made into spicy sauce, which is more economical than the original primary processing.

For the new generation of young people or herders with less pasture at home, working in economically developed areas is undoubtedly a good way out, and this is also one of the paths for the poor to get out of poverty, such as short-term skills training under the "Dewdrop Project" and support for entrepreneurship and employment. However, some poor people think that these training programs are not useful, and even if I learn them, I can't find a job, and since the Ori Village is remote, people don't want to go so far to work. Also, they don't have any skills, so they don't know what kind of work they can do in the city, and they can't adapt to the new modern way of life, and they fear everything outside, so they are not willing to go out to work.

15.3.4 Limited Education Level

Compared with developed areas, education in deeply impoverished areas is in a disadvantaged position, which somehow makes it more difficult for them to go into society and more likely to fall into poverty. In terms of children's education, there was an elementary school in the village, but it was abolished in 2012, and now all school-age children are collectively sent to the boarding school in Haiyan County. In our research, compared to the past, children's education is relatively better now. Many local herdsmen do not understand Chinese and only communicate in Tibetan. The educational results of local children are not ideal, as many of them go out to work after junior high school, and some will go home to get married and have children early, or follow their parents to herd animals at home. For example, M, a young man, got married not long after graduating from junior high school and gave birth to a daughter the next year. When he got married, he was 16 years old, and his wife was almost the same age. In the young man's perception, they can get married as long as they do not study, and there are many early marriages around them, so naturally this way will not affect him. In their view, it is enough for them to study in junior high school, and there is no point in going to technical school. The lower the level of education, the higher the incidence of poverty. Due to the low level of education, poor people have limited knowledge of many social resources, which is unfavorable to their use, and therefore they have fewer opportunities for personal development in society.

15.4 Conclusion

The strategic idea of targeted poverty alleviation and poverty eradication represents a multi-dimensional and sustainable poverty alleviation idea, which does not imply the construction of a region with only capital investment, but more importantly, a systematic study of the special poverty-causing factors, the degree of poverty, the feasibility of poverty eradication, and the comprehensive development of the poor themselves. The report to the 19th National Congress of the CPC also clearly points out that "it is our Party's solemn commitment to resolutely win the battle against poverty and let the poor and poor regions join the people of the whole country to enter a comprehensive well-off society". The fight against poverty is a complex work, and multiple subjects are needed to participate in it for the efficiency and precision of its work.

In the fight against poverty in the Ori Village, there are various factors that have restricted the economic development of the area for a long time. At the later stage of poverty eradication, there existed a phenomenon that some of the poor people who had already got out of poverty returned to poverty, with the idea of "passively longing for national assistance, expecting government grants and claiming for poverty reduction funds", as well as the poverty culture of "being proud of poverty" spread, which resulted in the poor subjects lacking endogenous motivation for development. In view of this, the only way to motivate the poor people to get out of poverty and get rich is to increase people's confidence and help them acquire necessary knowledge and skills. Only by helping the poor people with ideas and concepts can we stimulate the motivation of the poor subjects, thus forming the function of blood-making by themselves, which can make the village's economy develop sustainably and finally win the battle against poverty.

References

Excessive welfare is a trap for economic development. People's Daily, August 11, 2015.

Fang, Q. (2012). The Revelation of Poverty Culture Theory on Cultural Poverty Alleviation and Suggestions for Countermeasures. *Guangxi Ethnic Studies*, No. 4.

Kong, X., & Zhou, X. (2019). Fostering Will and Wisdom: The Essence of Poverty Eradication—Learning from Xi Jinping's Important Discourse on Poverty Eradication. *Guangxi Social Science*, No. 10.

Li, Y. [U.S.]. (1988). Ruth Benedict, Cultural Patterns, translated by Wang Wei and others. Sanlian Bookstore.

Nie, J., & Shuang, X. (2019). An Empirical Study on the Performance Evaluation and Influencing Factors of Targeted Poverty alleviation in Tibetan Areas of Qinghai. *Journal of Northern University for Nationalities (Philosophy and Social Science Edition)*, No. 1.

[U.S.] Ruth, B. (1988). Cultural Patterns, translated by Wang Wei and others, Sanlian Bookstore.

Xi, J. (2017). The Tutorial Reading Book of the Report of the 19th Party Congress. People's Publishing House.

Yu, Z., & Yan, G. (2017). Poverty Alleviation First Helps the Will of the People to be Diligent and Prosperous. *Xinhua Times Review*, June 22.

Wang, C., & Zhang, H. (2019). The Theoretical Value of the Strategic Thought of Targeted Poverty Alleviation and Poverty Eradication. *Theory and Reform*, No. 1.

Zhang, J., & Li, W. (2019). Practical Exploration of Stimulating the Endogenous Motivation of Poor People to Get Out of Poverty with Great National Spirit. *Journal of Lanzhou University (Social Science Edition)*, No. 6.

Zhang, Y., & Xu, K. (2019). Poverty Characteristics of Deeply Impoverished Ethnic Areas and the Construction of Coupling Mechanism of "Helping Will" and "Helping Wisdom": Reflections on the Research of Ganzi and Liangshan States in Sichuan. *Journal of Central South University of Nationalities (Journal of Humanities and Social Sciences)*, No. 5.

Cunying Long , a doctoral student at Ningxia University, whose research interests are social research and social change.

Jun Nie , a lecturer at North Minzu University, whose main research interests are ethnic sociology.

Yi Chen , a doctoral student at Ningxia University, whose research interests are public administration.

Chapter 16
Industrial Poverty Alleviation in a Li Village: Poverty Alleviation Practice of Da'an Village, Baisha County, Hainan

Jin Pan

Abstract This paper mainly introduces the process of poverty alleviation in Da'an Village, Baisha County, Hainan Province, through developing the leading industry of natural rubber and other special planting and breeding industries, and also expounds on how to play the leading role of cooperatives in poverty alleviation and the problems in the process of poverty alleviation: shortage of arable land may hinder the development of special industries; poverty alleviation may create new problem of "imbalance"; the problem of development and leading ability of cooperatives; the lack of endogenous motivation of some villagers for development.

Keywords Targeted poverty alleviation · Cooperatives · Hainan · Li people · Da'an Village

The Li people live mainly on Hainan Island and are the earliest inhabitants of the island. The Li people have their own special living environment and ethnic culture. The research object of this paper, Da'an Village, is part of Da'an Town, Baisha Li Autonomous County, Hainan Province, which is a typical Li Village. Through the analysis of the case of targeted poverty alleviation in Da'an Village, a Li Village, it can provide insights into poverty alleviation in Li inhabited region and even in the whole minority region.

16.1 Basic Information of Da'an Village and Its Area

At the national level, Hainan Province, despite its small area and population, is characterized by a small number but large proportion of poor people in its population. In 2015, there were 477,000 rural poor people in 116,000 households living in poverty in the province, with a poverty incidence rate of 8.9%, higher than the national average

---

J. Pan (✉)
Institute of Rural Development, Chinese Academy of Social Sciences, Beijing, China

Case Studies of Targeted Poverty Reduction and Alleviation in 100 Villages, International Research on Poverty Reduction, https://doi.org/10.1007/978-981-95-0549-4_16

of 4.5%. The poor population in Hainan Province is concentrated, mainly in the central and western mountainous areas and the areas inhabited by ethnic minorities. Baisha Li Autonomous County is one of the poorest areas in Hainan Province.

16.1.1 Basic Information of Baisha Li Autonomous County

Baisha Li Autonomous County is a national-level poverty-stricken county, same as the Qiongzhong Li and Miao Autonomous County, which is also a national-level poverty-stricken county in Hainan Province, was once nicknamed as "both economically poor and culturally blank". Baisha County is located in the central west of Hainan Island, the northwest foot of the middle section of the Limu mountain range, the upper reaches of the Nandu River. The total population was 195,300 people in 2016, and the resident population of 171,600 people, of which mainly Li and Han people, including 121,700 Li population. There are 11 townships, 82 villages (residential) committees, and 428 natural villages in the county.

In the 1990s, Baisha County benefited from the cultivation of natural rubber and once took off the hat[1] of the national-level poverty-stricken county, but due to the decline of rubber prices, it returned to be the national-level poverty-stricken county again in 2012. 22 administrative villages in the county were rated as poor villages when targeted poverty alleviation was carried out in 2015, involving 30,834 officially registered poverty-stricken members, and the poverty incidence rate was the second highest in Hainan Province. Due to its location in the central mountainous region and its weak industrial foundation, agriculture is located in a prominent position in the economic development of Baisha County, of which natural rubber serves as the pillar industry of Baisha County.

The development of rubber industry in Baisha County has experienced a difficult process of expansion. The rubber tree is a long-cycle cash crop, which needs about 7 years of non-production period to yield the benefits and requires night work, so farmers are not highly motivated to plant rubber. Initially, only a few village cadres planted rubber in response to the call of their superiors, and only later did farmers gradually follow and develop it. The 1990s saw rubber enter the production period and the benefits started to appear. In view of this, Baisha County was not included in the national poverty alleviation and development work of poverty-stricken counties in the period of "Seven-year Program"[2] in the 1990s.

After 2001, natural rubber prices rocketed wholly from RMB 8189 yuan/ton to RMB 34,086 yuan/ton in 2011. After that, the price plummeted from RMB 20,053 yuan/ton in 2013 to RMB 14,854/ton in 2014, but still higher than the level in 2001.

[1] Hat metaphorically means poverty. When it is recognized a poverty-stricken one, the one will wear a hat; while one is lifted out of poverty, the one will be taken off the hat. – Trans.

[2] In 1994, the state council decided to launch the poverty alleviation program, i.e. the Seven-year Program for Lifting 80 Million People Out of Poverty (1994–2000).

The rapid rise in prices has boosted farmers' enthusiasm for rubber planting. For example, from 2001 to 2014, the rubber planting area in Da'an Township increased by nearly two times, and the output increased by 3.3 times; in 2013 alone, the new rubber planting area reached 17,368 mu.[3] Some farmers who planted more rubber constructed the buildings and lived in the "rubber buildings".

With the decline of rubber prices, farmers' income also began to decrease, and in March 2012, Baisha County was included in a new round of national key counties for poverty alleviation and development. The 11 townships and 53 administrative villages in Baisha County became the focus of poverty alleviation work.

In 2015, Baisha county formulated the targeted poverty alleviation plan according to the development plan of "three-year poverty alleviation battle and two-year consolidation and improvement" during the 13th Five-Year Plan: in 2016, it will realize the goal of 2684 households with 11,365 people getting out of poverty, and 8 poverty-stricken villages will be promoted as the whole. In 2017, 11,800 people will get out of poverty, and 7 poverty-stricken villages will be promoted; in 2018, 8771 people will get out of poverty, and 7 poverty-stricken villages will be promoted. Da'an Village was included in the whole village promotion plan in 2018. In order to ensure that poverty alleviation measures can be implemented, Baisha County has formulated the following poverty alleviation policies.

16.1.1.1 Education Security Policy

Baisha County plans to invest 96.75 million yuan from 2016 to 2018 to improve the conditions of schools for compulsory education with weak foundation in poor areas and to subsidize poor families from kindergarten to full-time undergraduate education.

16.1.1.2 Medical Care Policy

Comprehensively improve the level of medical care for the rural officially registered poverty-stricken households, prevent returned poverty caused by illness, and provide health care for the poor people.

16.1.1.3 Housing Security Policy

According to the standard of maximum 61,000 yuan/household, the renovation of dilapidated houses for officially registered poverty-stricken households will be implemented.

[3] 1 mu equals 1/15 hectare. – Trans.

16.1.1.4 Industrial Poverty Alleviation Policies

The Implementation Plan for Agricultural Structure Adjustment and Industrial Poverty Alleviation in Baisha Li Autonomous County (2016–2018) sets out targets for industrial structure adjustment, industrial development targets, and industrial poverty alleviation targets. The industrial adjustment proposes to reduce the area of sugarcane by 63,000 mu and basically discard it within 5 years; build 500,000 mu of core rubber plantations (including farms), promote the full-cycle intercrop model of 20,000 mu, strive to increase the yield by more than 3.0%, and stabilize the total production capacity of about 18,400 tons.

16.1.2 Basic Information of Da'an Village

Da'an Village is located at the site of Da'an Town Government, 14 km away from Baisha County, including 6 village groups and 1 village economic farm. The six village groups are Da'an, Changling, Yuanzheng, Baoer, Keyaxincun, and Keyajiucun, with a total area of 22.35 square kilometers, and a resident population of 1396, and a total of 305 households, of which 272 households with1054 people are of Li ethnicity. Among the 61 randomly selected households, only 3 were Han households and the rest were Li households.

Da'an Village has 970 mu of arable land, of which 315 mu is effectively irrigated; 3853 mu of garden land, mainly planted with fruits, cucurbits and vegetables, mulberry trees, betel nut, and other crops; 3803 mu of forest land, including 82 mu of returned fallow forest and 30 mu of aquaculture. The forest land is mainly planted with rubber trees. As Da'an Village is located in the upstream of the water source protection area of Hainan Province, it is included in the ecological protection zone, and since 2000, rubber has been expanded on a large scale, and some rubber trees are planted in the ecological protection zone, now this part of rubber trees is prohibited to be renewed.

Da'an village is situated in the flat land between mountains, except for a few kiosks and one farmhouse, there are no other non-agricultural industries in the village, and the income of local farmers is mainly from farming. Of the total 1396 people, 23.5% of villagers were in poverty. In 2016, the per capita disposable income of farmers in Hainan Province was 11,843 yuan, and the per capita disposable income of Da'an Village was 4800 yuan, which was only 40.5% of the provincial average. The annual per capita income of some poor households is seriously lower than 3305 yuan under the current standard, and they are in extreme poverty.

Since the implementation of targeted poverty alleviation in 2016, of the total 305 households living in village, 78 were officially registered poverty-stricken households (including consolidated households and officially registered households), and according to the current poverty line standard, the actual number of poor households is 65, with 274 people living in poverty. In addition, there are 12 households enjoying minimum living guarantee, involving 37 people; 2 households enjoying the five guarantees, involving 2 people; 30 people were illiterate and semi-literate; and 18 disabled people.

Under the overall deployment of the county Party committee, county government and Da'an Town Government, Da'an village has changed the poverty status of poor households through poverty alleviation measures such as industrial poverty alleviation, employment outside the village, renovation of dilapidated houses, and education subsidies. Among all the poverty alleviation measures, industrial poverty alleviation is one of the major features of Da'an Village.

16.2 The Dominance of the Natural Rubber Industry in the Villages

Compared with Qiongzhong and Wuzhishan, Baisha has industrial advantages and has formed an industrial system mainly based on rubber, and basically every household in rural areas has an industry, including 4.6 mu of rubber trees per capita, as well as economic crops such as sugar cane, cassava, and betel nut. Before 2016, poverty alleviation and development mainly focused on planting rubber, betel nut, Alpinia oxyphylla, sugar cane and cassava, and there was a lack of farming. After 2016, we started to adjust the industrial structure, mainly developing the under-forest economy, breeding bees and five-legged pigs, and planting Alpinia oxyphylla, ginger, and mushrooms.

Baisha's natural rubber scale-planting began in the 1950s, mainly by the various state-owned farms under Hainan's agricultural reclamation. After the land contracted to households, in order to develop the economy and encourage farmers to get rich, Baisha County began to call on farmers to plant rubber.

Before the family contracting of land, the economic income of Da'an Village was mainly based on cassava and sugar cane, and the products were mainly self-sufficient, even if there was a small surplus, as there was no stable market to ensure the sale of the products, many farmers' lives had difficulties and their income was only enough to maintain subsistence. In 1982, after the land contracted to households, in order to respond to the superior call, the village cadres of Da'an Village and the village collectives took the lead in planting rubber and they encouraged farmers to plant rubber. However, as rubber cutting needs to be done at night, which is inconsistent with the traditional working hours of farmers, it was difficult to promote the rubber planting in the early stage of development, and only a small number of farmers had a try. With the passage of time, the benefits of planting rubber highlighted, the first farmers who engaged in planting rubber obtained considerable income, thus forming a good demonstration effect, and some farmers began to follow.

After 1994, the state lifted the market price control of natural rubber, and the price of natural rubber began to rise sharply. Driven by the interests, farmers began to plant rubber trees in large numbers, and by the end of 1990s, almost every household in Da'an Village planted rubber trees, from as few as 400 to as many as 2000. From

2001 to 2011, the overall price of natural rubber steadily increased from 8189 yuan/ton to 34,086 yuan/ton, and this period was also a period of expansion of rubber tree area in Baisha and Hainan as a whole. Especially around 2011, when rubber prices reached a record high, if a farmer planted 1000 rubber trees, he would earn more than 1500 yuan a day from cutting rubber if all of rubber trees were put into production, and would earn nearly 30,000 yuan or more a month (based on 20 days of cutting rubber). Rubber production has led to a rapid rise in the living standards of farmers, and many of whom have built houses and bought cars.

The important advantage for farmers who engage in rubber production is that no need to worry about the marketing, as Yuanlong Rubber Co., Ltd., set up a rubber collection station in Da'an Town, responsible for the acquisition of glue and film, so that rubber products only have the difference between high and low prices, and there will be no problem with the sale. Even if farmers go out to work, rubber trees will not cause any serious losses due to the absence of management. As long as people cut rubber, the daily income from the sale of rubber can sustain their family living expenses. In the Da'an Village, each household leaves 1–2 people to take care of the rubber trees, and the rest of the laborers can go out to work. In a household, if someone goes out to work for a long time, the income from work outside will account for a large part of the income, but such farmers are very few.

The rubber trees are cut from April to the end of December every year, and the farmers, both men and women, basically cut the rubber. It takes two to three hours to cut the rubber and three hours to drip the rubber, and around 8 a.m. the rubber is collected and sent to the collection station.

Since there are many rubber collection stations around Da'an Village, farmers can sell the glue directly after they collect it from the rubber plantation, instead of storing it at home for a long time or pressing it into rubber blocks or lumps, so the storage cost is lower. 91% of the farmers in Da'an Village sell the glue once every two days, and a few of them sell it once every three days, which means that they can trade once every two to three days. The large number of transactions ensures that farmers can earn income every two or three days. Compared with most crops, which are traded once a year, the capital liquidity is high and the transaction risk is low.

On average, each household in Da'an Village owns 18.9 mu of rubber forest, with an average annual dry rubber production of 89.2 kg per mu. The average rubber price in Da'an Village in 2017 was 10.4 yuan/kg, with an average annual income of 17,533 yuan per household from natural rubber.

Natural rubber industry is an important source of household income for farmers in Da'an Village. More than 60% of the farmers in Da'an Village have rubber income accounting for more than 80% of their annual household income, and more than 80% of the farmers have rubber income accounting for more than half of their household income. Especially from 2009 to 2012, when the national rubber price was around 30 yuan/kg, 1000 rubber trees cut in Da'an Village could bring an annual income of about 80,000 yuan, and rubber farmers bought motorcycles, household appliances and furniture, and built "rubber buildings". The expansion of rubber planting has brought about the replacement of other crops, and the planting of cassava and sugar cane is decreasing year by year.

Natural rubber is also an important source of collective income for the village. Before 2000, the collective income of Da'an Village was very meager, only about 500 yuan per year. Since 2000, the village has been planting rubber trees on a large scale and relying on rubber tree rental, the village collective economic income has grown to 3000 yuan per year. Each village group also has collective income through rubber planting, for example, Changling village group relies on rubber tree rental to obtain collective income of 12,000 yuan per year.

There are also risks for villagers who rely heavily on natural rubber for their income. Natural rubber is mainly used for industrial production, and the market price is influenced by the fluctuation of supply and demand, which is also a potential risk for farmers who rely heavily on rubber planting. After 2012, rubber prices began to decline, and in 2015 the market price fell below 10,000 yuan/ton, and the purchase price of some purchasing stations was once only 6 yuan/kg. The persistently low rubber price not only dampened farmers' production enthusiasm, but also made farmers' family income face difficulties, and many farmers had problems with food and clothing, and housing, medical, and education problems also plagued farmers' families, which produces new poor households.

Due to the characteristics of the crop itself and the limitations of farmers' industrial choice, the rubber industry is temporarily difficult to be replaced in Da'an Village and even Baisha County. Baisha County has a private rubber area of 630,000 mu, per capita ownership of rubber area ranks first in the province; planting rubber is also the main source of income for farmers. According to the deployment of the county Party committee, based on ecological resource advantages, the county vigorously developed ecological agriculture, focusing on the under-forest economy and green industry, and strove to achieve "lucid water and lush mountains are invaluable assets". By developing an environmentally friendly natural rubber industry and enhancing policy support for the industry, the government is aiming to strengthen the pillar industry.

In 2017, Baisha County began to explore natural rubber "insurance + futures". The "insurance + futures" model can change the way of risk transfer of natural rubber price and state subsidies, and effectively play the role of futures market to undertake, transfer, and disperse the natural rubber price risk. The first domestic natural rubber futures insurance policy was issued in October 2017, providing risk protection for all rubber growers in Nankai Township, Baisha County, with an annual output of 1483 tons of rubber, and finally receiving a payout of 504,100 yuan.

At the beginning of the pilot, the natural rubber futures price insurance specified the first the insured included the officially registered poverty-stricken rubber farmers and those individual retail rubber farmers with weakest ability to resist risks, as a measure to help fight poverty. This protection transformed the market risk of rubber, once borne solely by rubber farmers, into one shared by multiple parties, which is conducive to improving the anti-risk ability of rubber farmers, reducing the risk of returning to poverty due to insufficient response to rubber price fluctuations, and playing a role in protecting the economic interests of the majority of rubber farmers and improving the enthusiasm of production.

Baisha County became aware of the benefits of the success of Nankai Township's natural rubber "insurance + futures" pilot and also got the affirmation of Hainan Provincial Government. In 2018, Baisha County promoted the "insurance + futures" model in the whole county, specifically set up a working team for natural rubber price insurance, and assigned a deputy governor as the team leader. In 2018 and 2019, Baisha County government invested 4.7 million yuan and 3.79 million yuan, respectively, to subsidize natural rubber price insurance, and received compensation of about 13 million yuan and 16.72 million yuan, respectively, in two years, directly increasing the average household income of farmers by 1000 yuan.

16.3 Special Industries to Alleviate Poverty

As the leading industry of natural rubber is in the market downturn, how to drive farmers to develop the economy, and help poor households get out of poverty? Da'an Village has made many attempts. For example, developing under-forest economy, courtyard economy, and free distribution of piglets, chicks, baby goose, Alpinia oxyphylla seedlings, betel nut seedlings, fertilizer, etc., to encourage farmers to develop production, but the more successful is still the special industry poverty alleviation project.

16.3.1 Project Categories

The special industrial poverty alleviation projects in Da'an Village were determined under the overall planning of the county and Da'an Township, based on various factors such as village characteristics and farmers' needs.

16.3.1.1 Mulberry Cultivation and Silkworm Breeding

Under the unified deployment of the town Party committee and government, each village in Da'an town has formed a "one village, one product" project according to its geological characteristics. The development of mulberry cultivation and silkworm breeding is the key development project in Da'an Village. This project is determined and implemented by Hainan Meiya Industrial Co., Ltd., which is the fixed-point assistance provider of Da'an Village.

In 2016, Meiya Company sent a poverty alleviation resident work team to carry out poverty alleviation work in the village, and after holding several special meetings on poverty alleviation, it determined the poverty alleviation initiative of "taking mulberry cultivation and silkworm breeding industry as the main industry poverty alleviation, supplemented by other poverty alleviation initiatives", and organized more than 30 villagers from Da'an Village to visit Qiongzhong County for study. In

March 2017, the first batch of 45 mu of mulberry leaf planting demonstration base was established in Da'an Village, and the head of each village group gave demonstration, arranging one group leader with eight women for business management. Da'an Town government and Hainan Meiya Industrial Co., Ltd., jointly invested in the construction of 150 square meters of cocoonery. In June, it officially began to raise silkworms. As of July 2018, 5 pieces of land totaling 165 mu were planted with mulberry trees, 25 cocoonery were built, and 30 poor households participated in mulberry cultivation and silkworm breeding.

The technology needed in mulberry cultivation and silkworm breeding is provided by Hainan Qiongzhong Silk Co., Ltd. The company has a workstation in Da'an Village, responsible for technical guidance and cocoon recovery. Each silkworm bed produces 90–120 catties of cocoons, with an average price of 20–22 yuan/catty. It is approximately 4 mu of land that raises a silkworm bed. Each batch has four or five silkworm beds, and it can sell two to three batches of silk each month. Mulberries and silkworms can be grown in all other months except for the two or three months in winter season. In August 2017, the mulberry cultivation and silkworm breeding project began to yield benefits, with a net income of more than 30,000 yuan. After seeing the benefits, farmers asked to join, and even villagers from nearby villages applied to join.

The land required for mulberry planting is mostly abandoned land, which is coordinated and transferred by the Anding Planting and Breeding Professional Cooperative and contracted to farmers for planting. The old and weak family laborers can participate in the relevant production, such as silkworm feeding and sanitary management. The village also carries out training on the preparation of silkworm beds for poor households through TV night school and organizes poor households to weave silkworm beds, and the products are recovered by the cooperative at a price of 5 yuan per sheet (the cost is about 1 yuan), and the average earning is about 100 yuan per person per day.

16.3.1.2 Beekeeping

The beekeeping industry is an industry driven by capable people in Da'an Village. The village is located in a mountainous area with rich nectar source, which is suitable for developing beekeeping industry. Zhang Dezhi, a big beekeeper in Da'an Village, and member of village supervisory committee, CPC[4] member. In 2014, Zhang Dezhi led the establishment of Baisha Haitong Beekeeping Cooperative, with 5 members, 4 of whom were relocated from Guangdong and 1 of whom is a household enjoying minimum living guarantee in the village. And each member has 10–80 hives.

Zhang Dezhi started beekeeping since he graduated from junior high school in 1994, and through gradual exploration and years of experience, he now has nearly 300 hives. At the end of 2016, Zhang Dezhi started helping poor households, using government funds to purchase 100 hives of bees to help nine poor households in

[4] Communist Party of China. – Trans.

Da'an Village with beekeeping, of which two households have 15 hives and seven households have 10 hives. Under normal circumstances, each hive of bees produces about 10 catties of honey, and the income from each hive is 500 yuan except for other expenses. The poor households either buy shares in the form of the hives and receive dividends at the end of the year according to the agreement, or raise bees together with Zhang Dezhi, who provides technical guidance.

As the number of beekeepers increased in recent years, there was a shortage of honey, so beekeeping production began to relocate. During the relocation, Zhang Dezhi loads a truck with his own bees and the bees of poor families in order to follow the flowers. The relocation sites are located in the province, and it often needs to relocate three times a year. Due to the significant driving effect, the number of hives from poor households increased to 200 in 2018.

The majority of beekeepers sell honey by themselves, with regular customers. They also have individual Taobao stores and WeChat shops, and the government also gives support when there are problems with market sales. For example, in 2016, when seven beekeepers in Da'an Town encountered sales difficulties, the township government subscribed for honey by holding a "Crowdfunding for Love" campaign, selling a total of 51,000 yuan of honey.

16.3.1.3 Porcupine Breeding

Porcupine farming is also an industry driven by capable people, which was developed by Yang Heshun, a villager from Yuanzheng natural village in Da'an village.

Yang Heshun started to breed porcupines in 2015, and bought 5 groups of piglets (one male and two females in one group) from a porcupine farm in Qionghai, totaling 15 piglets. At that time, the piglets were 1500 yuan/ pig (10–15 catties). Every group of piglets was raised in one pen (2 square meters per pen), and there will be 2 litters per year, 2–3 piglets per litter, and sometimes 1 piglet per litter. The porcupines have strong immunity, so no vaccination is needed, and the main feed is corn, grass, groundnut leaves, etc., and the farming management is relatively poor.

The whole body of porcupine is a treasure, with delicate meat and delicious taste, which is favored by people and known as mountain treasure. It also has high medicinal value, as the pork, brain, fat, viscera, and quill can be used for medicines, and it has the effect of reducing blood pressure, relieving pain, activating blood circulation, and dissipating blood stasis. Even the feces can be used as fertilizer for rubber trees. In 2018, the market price of live pigs is 70–80 yuan/catty, and the net pork is more than 100 yuan/catty, and the products are mainly sold to major hotels. 32 poor households in Da'an Town participated in the porcupine raising in July 2017, including 4 households in Da'an village, and the government invested 210,000 yuan in industrial poverty alleviation funds accordingly.

The porcupine farm house is located in Da'an Village, with 800 square meters and a breeding capacity of up to 1000 pigs. There were 335 pigs bred in 2017. Due to the significant benefits, 19 more poor households in Da'an Village started porcupine farming in 2018.

Yang Heshun is very confident about leading poor households to breed porcupines. As he said, "I am happy to lead poor households to get rich, and at the same time, I can expand the scale, so it is a win–win situation".

16.3.1.4 Tea Tree Mushroom Cultivation

Tea tree mushroom cultivation adopts the model of "leading enterprise + cooperative + farmers", which is a poverty alleviation project planned by the town, involving two poor villages in Da'an Town, including Da'an Village. There is one plant in each of the two village, and each plant covers an area of 2 mu, with 200,000 bags of mushroom seeds, and the products are purchased by the same company. All 65 poor households in Da'an Village participate in the tea tree mushroom cultivation project, which started in May 2017 and started to harvest mushrooms in August for 6 months. Poor households can either buy shares of cooperatives to gain dividends or engage in collecting mushrooms to earn service rewards which is paid by company. In 2017, the poor households received a dividend of 104,600 yuan.

16.3.2 Play the Role of Cooperatives in Poverty Alleviation

As cooperatives have a strong driving effect on farmers, Baisha County has developed incentives for cooperatives: 100,000 yuan of awards will be given to each cooperative with significant industry driving ability and sales revenue of more than 10 million yuan; 300,000 yuan for each cooperative with sales revenue of more than 50 million yuan; 500,000 yuan for each cooperative with sales revenue of more than 100 million yuan. Each cooperative that had completed the "three products" certification (pollution-free products, green products, organic products) will be awarded 50,000 yuan. Cooperatives that meet the certification requirements of county-level agricultural leading enterprises and pass the certification are awarded 50,000 yuan; cooperatives that meet the certification requirements of provincial-level agricultural leading enterprises and pass the certification are awarded 100,000 yuan; cooperatives that meet the certification requirements of national-level agricultural leading enterprises and pass the certification are awarded 150,000 yuan; cooperatives that meet the certification requirements of international-level agricultural leading enterprises and pass the certification are awarded 200,000 yuan. Most of the special industrial poverty alleviation projects in Da'an Village are developed by cooperatives to drive poor households to develop production.

The mulberry cultivation and silkworm breeding project relies on the Baisha Anding Planting and Breeding Professional Cooperative. *The cooperative was established in July 2016 with the purpose of developing the collective economy of the village and carrying out targeted poverty alleviation. The cooperative is promoted by the villager's committee to carry out the mulberry cultivation and silkworm breeding project to drive poor households out of poverty. The land used for planting mulberry and breeding silkworm is the marginal land or wasteland of villagers in Da'an Village, which is transferred through the cooperative and then subcontracted to farmers who are willing to plant and breed.

The beekeeping is based on the Baisha Haitong Beekeeping Cooperative, of which Zhang Dezhi is the head. When the cooperative was established in 2014, the government of Da'an Township supported dozens of hives of bee species to help expand the breeding scale. At the end of 2016, the government used poverty alleviation funds to purchase 100 hives of bees, and the cooperative helped nine poor households in Da'an Village to keep bees. After the contract of 4 years expires, the poor households can choose to quit, or keep bees on their own, or continue to keep bees with the surrogate cooperative. Under normal circumstances, each hive produces about 10 kg of honey, and the income is 500 yuan except for other expenses, and the dividend is 250 yuan per hive. Some poor households do not want to cooperate with the cooperative and want to get all the profits and keep bees by themselves, but the success rate is not high and the results are not good. As a result of helping poor households to keep bees, the government subsidized the cooperative with 3000 yuan in 2016. The cooperative has also registered its own trademark—Qun'e Brew.

Porcupine breeding relies on Baisha Yeshu Porcupine Breeding Professional Cooperative. Porcupine breeding cooperative was established in June 2017, with 7 members and 813,000 yuan of investment, mainly for breeding base construction and introduction of porcupine species. The head of the cooperative is Yang Heshun. Although the cooperative was not directly supported by government funds when it was established, the government gave great support in advertising and promotion. All porcupines are bred collectively by cooperative, and members will get distribution according to their shares. In July 2017, the cooperative started to drive poor households to breed porcupines. Poverty-stricken households join the cooperative in the form of buying shares with their industry poverty alleviation funds, and the cooperative and the poor households sign a one-year contract with a fixed profit share of 12.5%, except in case of natural disasters.

Tea tree mushroom farming relies on Baisha Zhongmin Edible Mushroom Professional Cooperative. The cooperative is a town-level cooperative, established in 2017, with poor households in the two villages in the town, i.e. Da'an Village and Nanda Village, as members. Poverty-stricken households use industry poverty alleviation funds to buy shares and enjoy dividends according to industrial income. The cooperative buys each mushroom spawn bag at 6 yuan and sells it at 6.93 yuan, with a net profit of 0.93 yuan for one bag. 10% of the cooperative's profit is kept in the cooperative for daily management, of which 5% goes to the village collective, 5% goes to the cooperative board, and the remaining 90% is distributed to the poor households in the form of dividends. In order to ensure the stable development of the cooperative, the agreement stipulates that once the shares are bought, they cannot be withdrawn within three years. In 2017, the cooperative invested 1.2 million yuan to plant 2 mu of tea tree mushrooms, driving 65 poor households and 272 people, with a dividend of 104,600 yuan that year.

16.4 Effectiveness of Poverty Alleviation and Problems in Existence

16.4.1 Effectiveness of Poverty Alleviation

Based on the stable development of the leading industry of natural rubber, the poverty alleviation work in Da'an Village has achieved good results through the development of special industries. Poverty-stricken households have obtained stable income from the rubber industry through the "insurance + futures" model. Also, they gained stable income of special industries from cooperative that they join. In 2017, 222 people from 51 poor households in Da'an Village were lifted out of poverty. Of those 14 households who still lived in poverty, some were enjoying minimum living guarantee as their families have elderly, weak, sick, or disabled members with a lack of labors, who are in need of social security as their minimum living guarantee; some were under the standard of poverty elimination due to their poor housing condition, as the local customs of Li people and traditional tattoo discouraged the poor households from not building houses in that year, and their houses were not secured. At the end of 2018, the incidence of poverty in Da'an Village was reduced to 0, and all poor households were lifted out of poverty.

16.4.2 Problems in Existence

In general, the poverty alleviation work in Da'an Village is relatively solid and the effect of poverty alleviation is remarkable, but there are also hidden worries, mainly in the following aspects.

16.4.2.1 Shortage of Arable Land May Hinder the Development of Special Industries

Baisha County is located in a water conservation area in Hainan Province, and the main source of Hainan's first river, Nandu River, is in Baisha. There are many nature reserves in the county, in addition to the protective forest belt along the rivers and waters, and other ecological sanctuaries are also scattered, so the economic development is affected. For example, Da'an Village has abundant rubber woodland resources, but since part of the woodland is ecological forest, the use cannot be changed at will. Some poverty alleviation projects, such as mulberry cultivation and silkworm breeding, require more arable land, so the scale of farmers' participation is limited, and thus their industry-driven effect will be reduced. In view of this, we can explore the expansion of farmers' ecological environment income, strive for ecological compensation, and issue direct ecological subsidies, so that poor people can benefit from ecological construction.

16.4.2.2 Poverty Alleviation May Create New "Imbalance" Problems

Targeted poverty alleviation requires changing the original "pepper-spreading" type of poverty alleviation, and carries out the targeted identification of poor households and targeted assistance. In reality, the income disparity among residents in villages is not remarkable, and it is difficult to accurately count the household income of villagers, so the identification of poor households is rather vague. The research found that poor households were much more cooperative with the research than non-poor households, and some non-poor households had negative feelings about the poverty alleviation policy. Villagers living near the poverty standard line do not have substantial differences in living, but those below the standard line can enjoy various policy support, which can lead to dissatisfaction and psychological imbalance among non-poor households, thus making up a discordant factor in the village.

16.4.2.3 Cooperative Development and Leadership Issues

In the practice of poverty alleviation in Da'an Village, industrial poverty alleviation is the main way to drive poor households out of poverty. Though the drive of capable people in planting or breeding, centered on the specific industries, the cooperative is established and encourages the poor households to engage actively in the cooperative. The government collectively invests the poverty alleviation funds and materials to the poor households allocated by the higher level into the cooperative, and all is operated and managed by the cooperative. The cooperative provides the poor households with an agreed percentage of dividends every year. In this process, the grassroots poverty alleviation departments of the government actually play the role of agents for the poor households, making agreements with the cooperatives on the yields allocated to the poor households, and supervising the operation and management of the cooperatives to make sure the consistent goals among government, cooperative director. and poor people, that is, cooperative will make profits, and help the poor get out of poverty. However, the ultimate achievement of the goal depends on the stability of the cooperative's internal management and operation on the one hand, and the sustainability of the principal-agent relationship between the government and the cooperative on the other hand. Problems in any one of these areas can affect the sustainability of poverty alleviation.

16.4.2.4 Insufficient Endogenous Development Motivation for Some Villagers

The Li people have a peaceful and happy attitude toward life and a leisurely life style. Li men like cigarettes and wine, and usually do not want to go out to work after cutting rubber, and take the money from selling glue to buy wine and drink, so the endogenous development motivation is not enough. For example, some villagers' rubber trees produce very little rubber, and an important cause is the lack of management. When rubber trees' leaves just open, it is needed to spray sulfur so as to prevent the leaves of the tree from falling off after the sunlight shines, and to apply more fertilizer can also produce more rubber, but some farmers who mind trouble do not spray sulfur, neither fertilize the trees. Beekeeping needs relocation to follow flower in order to get a good source of honey. However, some farmers do not relocate their hives after receiving government support, which will affect their beekeeping income. Some villagers have a serious mentality of "passively longing for national assistance, expecting government grants and claiming for poverty reduction funds", and voluntarily stay at home in order to get policy support, which automatically lowers their family income in order to get the "treatment" of poor households. Insufficient endogenous motivation makes it difficult to ensure the sustainability of their development even if they rely on external forces to get out of poverty for a while.

References

[India] Amartya, S. (2001). Poverty and Famine, translated by Wang Yu and Wang Wenyu, The Commercial Press.

Chen, Z., Bi, J., Wu, G., He, X., & Wang, Z. (2019). The Current Situation and Evolution of Poverty Alleviation in China and the Vision and Strategic Focus of Poverty Alleviation after 2020. *China Rural Economy*, No. 1.

Hu, H., Si, Y., & Wang, L. (2018). The impact of industrial poverty alleviation policies on the livelihood strategies and income of poor households. China Rural Economy, No. 1.

Huang, Z., Gao G., Teng F., Pan B., Song J., and Li A. (2019). Long-Term Poverty Reduction in China, Where is the Road? Poverty Reduction Strategy Foresight after the Completion of Poverty Eradication in 2020. *China Rural Economy*, No. 9.

Liu, F.-L. (2018). Local Knowledge and Targeting Bias of Precise Identification. *China Rural Observer*, No. 5.

Pan, J. (2011). *Yanzhuang Village: Economic and Social Changes in a Labor Outflow Village*. China Social Science Press.

Pan, J. (2016). *Honglin Village: Economic and Social Changes in a Beijing Suburban Mountain Village*. China Social Science Press.

Pan, J., Zhang, D., et al. (2018). *Targeted Poverty Alleviation and Targeted Poverty Removal in Hundred Villages Research - Da'an Village Volume*. Social Science Literature Press.

Tang, X. W., & Li, C. G. (2010). A Review of Economic Vulnerability of Poverty and Poverty Reduction Strategies. *China Rural Observer*, No. 5.

You, L., Liu, J., & Huo, X. (2018). Desire, Investment, and Poverty: A Theoretical Analysis Framework. *China Rural Observer*, No. 5.

Zhang, D., & Yin, Z. (2018). Financial Inclusion, Risk Response, and Rural Household Poverty Vulnerability. *China Rural Economy*, Vol. 4.

Zhang, J. (2003). Nutrition, Health and Efficiency—Evidence from Poor Rural China. *Economic Research*, No. 1.

Jin Pan is a researcher and editorial director of the Institute of Rural Development, Chinese Academy of Social Sciences. His main research interests are rural organizations and institutions and rural development.

Chapter 17
From Household to Village: Development Changes and Poverty Alleviation Practices of a Poor Herding Family in Saiding Village, Gansu

Hong Lin

Abstract Based on field surveys and personal interviews, this paper places a family's development over the past 40 years in the analytical perspective of village, local society, and national development changes, presenting the process of mutual embedding of individual, family, and village poverty eradication dynamics and national poverty alleviation practices at different development stages. On the one hand, national poverty management actions form the basic support for households' poverty alleviation actions through targeted measures on household and whole village poverty alleviation; on the other hand, households show a high degree of self-adaptation to various drivers of change in the process of national and social development. As this herdsmen family developed from a "point" pattern to a "network" pattern, the life narratives of three generations of this family concentrate on the historical process of national, social, and village development to a large extent.

Keywords Herder village · Poor families · Village community · Social change · Saiding Village

As the basic unit of social organization, the family is the constituent cell of the family-state system, and the base and carrier of social transformation. Understanding the changes in the family can not only provide insight into the behavior and philosophy of individuals, but also grasp the evolution of society as a whole. In this paper, we take the family development of a poor household in Saiding Village over the past 40 years as the starting point to trace the social change of poverty governance.

Special Note: The real names of the household cases cited in the text have been anonymized; in addition, interviews with relevant persons have been coded to facilitate the anonymization of information related to the interviewees and the citation in the text.

H. Lin (✉)
Institute of Sociology, Chinese Academy of Social Sciences, Beijing, China

Case Studies of Targeted Poverty Reduction and Alleviation in 100 Villages, International Research on Poverty Reduction, https://doi.org/10.1007/978-981-95-0549-4_17

17.1 Perspectives on Change: From Society, Village to Family

Saiding Village is the only officially registered poverty-stricken village under the jurisdiction of Kangle Town, Sunan Yugur Autonomous County, Zhangye City, Gansu Province. As a traditional livestock county relying on natural pastures for grazing, Sunan County is the only autonomous county of the Yugur ethnic group in China, and one of the 28 counties identified by the State Council as having a small population of ethnic groups and included by the Gansu Province as one of the counties to enjoy the support policy compared with those Tibetan areas.[1] The village is located in the hinterland of Qilian Mountains, with 121 households totaling 348 people, all of whom are ethnic minority households, mainly engaged in livestock production, with a per capita net income of 11,927 yuan in 2016; 20 poor households totaling 60 people were officially registered poverty-stricken households in 2014, and the poor population reduced to 7 households and 20 people in 2015, and reduced to 2 households and 4 people in 2016, all of whom are poor due to diseases; at the end of 2017, the last 2 officially registered poverty-stricken households were lifted out of poverty. The whole village of Saiding was free from poverty. The last two households lifted out of poverty were all suffering from major illnesses in their families, and it took a relatively long period of time for treatment and family economic recovery.

The family of Wang Jianrong is one of the two officially registered poverty-stricken households lifted out of poverty in the end. When the family got out of poverty in 2017, after the poverty alleviation supporting cadre worked through the family annual financial circumstances, the outcome was "there were 4 family members, with the annual per capita net income 9625 yuan in 2017; the total annual family income was 103,500 yuan, including 77,000 yuan (22,000 yuan for wool and 55,000 yuan for lambs) for breeding industry, 15,000 yuan for working outside, and 11,500 yuan for policy income (3351 yuan/person, 1.39 yuan/mu for grassland ecological incentive subsidy funds); annual family expenses totaled 65,000 yuan, including 40,000 yuan for production and 25,000 yuan for living expenses".[2]Such a family income and expenditure level is the general level of local herder families. A cadre stationed in the village said, "The highest income in the village this year (2018) is more than 150,000 yuan, the lowest is 80,000 yuan, and most families' income is around 100,000 yuan; but the pastoral expenses are also very large, and the net income is very little, which is not easy to calculate, and the herders do not know how to calculate either".[3] Wang Jianrong further explained the annual family financial situation that the poverty alleviation cadres assisted in sorting it out.

Our family is poor due to disease. My daughter-in-law was diagnosed with malignant lymphoma in 2010 in Zhangye and was treated with chemotherapy for five and a half years

[1] Website of the People's Government of Sunan Yugur Autonomous County, Sunan Overview, October 29, 2018, http://www.gssn.gov.cn/sngk/sngk/201810/t20181029_126803.html, accessed April 18, 2019.

[2] Interview code: 20171030GYQNO1.

[3] Interview code: 20181031PJPNO1.

until 2016, when there was no way to treat her with chemotherapy anymore and started to take conservative treatment, mainly using some native methods to control her condition from deteriorating. The family has small pastures, few sheep, and little income from animal husbandry, so we have been trying to find ways to increase income. Our family was the first to engage in tourism in the village, so the income from tourism was better at that time, but even in the worst year we could also have 50,000 to 60,000 yuan of income, while the net income from animal husbandry is only 20,000 to 30,000 yuan per year. We engaged in the tourism industry for seven years (2007~2014), then we encountered environmental protection rectification, and stopped tourism. In 2017, the family's sheep were contracted out, just to break even, the year's wool and lambs were contractors. In 2017, the livestock products prices are high, so in 2018 we recovered the sheep and pasture, so the income of herders were mainly from livestock production. Our family sold almost 30,000 yuan of wool this year (2018, the same below) and less than 60,000 yuan of lambs, which is the main income. In previous years, our eldest son rented pasture outside to herd sheep, and only this year he herds sheep in his own pasture; our youngest son has been working outside, but this year he came back to grazing, and now he rents pasture outside to herd sheep and paid 14,000 yuan for renting pasture, and he purchased forages with more than 20,000 yuan this year alone. I have worked for a power station since June 1, 2017, and can not rest on Saturdays and Sundays, with a monthly salary of 2,500 yuan as I just got a pay raise in August this year. Before, it was 2,200 yuan per month. Our family have to tighten our belts this year, because we need to pay back the targeted poverty alleviation subsidized loan given by government of 50,000 yuan which is due this year; and there is a 60,000 yuan of credit cooperative loan which is not urgent, as it is due in August 2019, then we will transfer the money from others, pay back and get the loan again, so it can be extended to 2020. Now, our couple, in addition to living off our son, have to work odd jobs; there are also some minimum living guarantee for us, and our status will be rated once every three years, as we passed this year so we are qualified for the minimum living guarantee.[4]

Based on Wang Jianrong's statement and the field research, we found that the factors affecting herders' household income could be basically categorized into the following three areas.

The first is the policy stability. Wang Jianrong said bluntly, "for our herders, the policy has the greatest impact, and the new policy directly affects the old herders, such as the ban on grazing relocation, as the elderly can not go out to work, so there is no other source of income, while the young people can do better, as they can go out to work. A few years ago, the government promoted tourism, and my eldest son and I together engaged in tourism. At that time, the government also criticized us, the herders, for not being open-minded, and then the herders changed their mindset, and began to pull horses, sell ghee, open restaurants during the tourist season, but the policy suddenly came and all were demolished. For the attractions my family newly built, I took out a loan of about 100,000 yuan, and now there are still 60,000 yuan left to pay back; my eldest son took out a loan of 300,000 yuan, which has not been repaid, and the annual interest costs a lot of money. The price of sheep has only gone up this year, and in previous years sheep-raising was always losing money, and herds are now raising sheep for the credit cooperative".[5]

The second is less production materials. Take Wang Jianrong's family as an example, "You can not develop production with less pasture. The large families

[4] Interview code: 20181029GYQNO2.

[5] Interview code: 20181029GYQNO2.

with a lot of pastures, do not need to spend money every year to buy forages, and rent pasture. In 1983, when household-responsibility system was initiated, we were couple, and the eldest was born in 1984 and we had no pasture, and when the next two sons also were born, we still had no pasture; at that time, the distribution of pasture to our family was for two people's living, but now we are a family of eight people living on the pasture for two people".[6]

The third is major diseases. Wang Jianrong believes: "Poverty due to illness is the real problem, and nothing else can be said to be a real poverty problem. In 2011, 2012, 2013, the individual payment for cooperative medical care was minimal, so the reimbursement ratio was very low, and there was no other way to reimburse. In 2015, the individual payment for cooperative medical care was higher, and coupled with the preferential policy for the households enjoyed targeted poverty alleviation, the reimbursement ratio for medical treatment was increased to 60%-70%. The cost of seeing a doctor is very high. There was no hospital providing chemotherapy in Zhangye, and only radiation therapy could be done. Yet my wife's disease could only be treated with chemotherapy, so she had to go to Lanzhou for treatment. At first, chemotherapy was done once a week, then once every half month, and finally once a month. In those years, we had to make more than a dozen trips to Lanzhou every year to see the doctor. From last year to this year, she had to take conservative treatment, but just taking Tibetan medicine a year would also cost more than 20,000 yuan. This year, the cost is less, and we have spent more than 10,000 yuan. To see a doctor of traditional Chinese medicine and take traditional medicine can not be reimbursed by cooperative medical care. Over the years, our family has spent more than 400,000 yuan on medical care, and the reimbursement of major medical aid, cooperative medical care, as well as some subsidies for poverty alleviation, all of which were added up to a total reimbursement for 30% to 40% of expenses, a full calculation of almost 150,000 yuan, and the rest of the expenses is borne by ourselves, all of which added up to about 250,000–260,000 yuan, mainly paid by our own previous savings, and the loan".[7]

For a herder family, if the policy is unstable and there are many uncertainties at the level of implementation, coupled with the small size of the family's pasture and the major illnesses of family members, and the result, as Wang Jianrong said, "is that there is no way to say that it is completely out of poverty". At the same time, the current situation of Wang Jianrong's family also confirms one of the characteristics of Chinese family changes in the past 20 to 30 years, that is, the continuity of the family function is greater than the changes, although it is in the process of drastic and profound transformation in all aspects of society. This continuity of family function, under the circumstances of the lower level of economic development and inadequate public welfare and public services, is only a strategic choice of the family, "intergenerational interdependence still exists in economic and non-economic

[6] Interview code: 20181029GYQNO2.

[7] Interview code: 20171030GYQNO1.

aspects, and resources remain complementary and reciprocal, allowing the continuity and maintenance of the stem family model and even the joint family model."[8]

17.2 Keeping up with the Times: The Developmental Pulse of a Family

The continuity of family function is concretely presented through family size, intergenerational transmission, livelihood patterns, living arrangements, and other developmental elements. Taking Wang Jianrong's family as an example, from a family of two when the family was formed in the early 1980s to a family of eleven in 2018, three generations of the family have experienced significant differences in education, occupation, and residence. In other words, the great changes in the development of the country, society and village over the past 40 years are concentrated in a vivid way in the struggle of three generations of the family to get out of poverty and create a better life (Table 17.1).

As the first generation of the family, Mr. and Mrs. Wang Jianrong have witnessed the development of the family over the past 40 years of hard work to get out of poverty and gradually get rich.

> *My family was very difficult when I was a child. At that time, in the pastoral area, we lived in the felt house in summer, and house built of stone in winter. Before 1983, we were a large collective, and my parents, my sister and I lived together as a family of four, with one brother who got married early and left. I got married in 1982, and in 1983, when the household-responsibility system was formed, our family was distributed with the pasture for my father, mother, sister and I. After my father died in the spring of 1983, I was separated from my family. My mother was looking for a son-in-law, and my sister was also looking for a son-in-law, so we had no choice but to divide the four pastures of us into two.*
>
> *It was only in the 1990s that people gradually began to find ways to earn money. Before that, people in the village also had little awareness of earning money, and they did not know what to work, so only kept their own family pasture. Our village had power supply in 1989, and later each family was also supplied. At that time, if people had some money in hand, they would engage in fencing, pulling barbed wire, otherwise on the pasture adjacent to each other, the livestock of neighbors' would graze on each other's grass, and it would affect the relationship between neighbors. In the past, people lived in earth houses or stone houses. In 1984, our family built two houses on the winter field, and in 1989, we rebuilt five brick houses, inside of which were paved with bricks, and now we are still living there. The area of homestead is also confirmed. We plan to renovate the houses before, but the ban on grazing came, and the environmental protection policy required to report before house renovation. In 2010, our family bought a house in the county, and then my wife was diagnosed with a disease; the loan to buy the house was repaid by tourism income, and then we relied on the loan when she did not have enough money for medical treatment. I am now dividing pasture, pasture houses, water cellars into two sons, keeping only this building for our couple.*
>
> *In 1987, our family bought an old motorcycle from people in the farming area, which cost more than 1,000 yuan and consumed a lot of fuel, so the payment was divided into twice*

[8] Yang, Juhua, and He Zhaohua, "Changes and continuity of families in the process of social transformation," Population Studies, No. 2, 2014.

Table 17.1 Family member profile

Name	Family role	Year of birth	Ethnicity	Level of education	Occupation	Residence
First generation						
Wang Jianrong	Father	1959	Yugur	3rd grade of primary school	Keeper at hydropower station	Sunan County
Pi Yuhua	Mother	1962	Tibetan	2nd grade of primary school	Herding (retired)	Sunan County
Second aeneration						
Wang Chengning	Daughter	1984	Yugur	Junior secondary school	Salesperson at boutique	Zhangye City
Chen Jun	Son-in-law	1972	Han	Senior secondary school	Director of township family planning office	Zhangye City; Huangcheng Town
Wang Chengjun	Son	1986	Yugur	1st grade of junior secondary school	Herding, livestock dealer	Kangle Pastoral Area, Ganjun Pastoral Area, Kangle Town, Zhangye City
Zhao Lan	Daughter-in-law	1989	Yugur	Junior secondary school	Herding; her father's ethnicity is Han	Kangle Pastoral area, Ganjun Pastoral Area, Kangle Town, the county
Wang Chengfu	Son	1988	Yugur	Junior college	Herding, used to work in the industry park	Kangle Pastoral Area, Ganjun Pastoral Area, Kangle Town, the county
Qi Fangling	Daughter-in-law	1991	Tibetan	Senior secondary school	Herding, used to work in the industry park	Kangle Pastoral Area, Ganjun Pastoral Area, Kangle Town, the county
Third generation						

(continued)

Table 17.1 (continued)

Name	Family role	Year of birth	Ethnicity	Level of education	Occupation	Residence
Chen Huihui	Granddaughter	2006	Yugur	3rd grade of secondary school	Student	Zhangye City
Wang Xuanlin	Granddaughter	2011	Yugur	2nd grade of primary school	Student	Sunan County
Wang Yuanchao	Grandson	2016	Yugur	Preschool	Kid	Sunan County

before it was fully paid off. Before that, everywhere we went by walk, or we ran on two legs or rode horses, and relocated by cattle, and people rode on donkeys to herd the sheep. I rode the old motorcycle for nearly 5 years, and bought another motorcycle, and then replaced it with the third motorcycle, until now this motorcycle is still good to go. In 2016, my youngest son bought a car. I do not have a driver's license, but I know how to drive a car.

I started herding at the age of 15 and stopped going to school in the third grade because I couldn't pay for my living expenses and school fees, so I started working in the village to earn work credits. My sister herded sheep, and I worked as a mobile laborer, building roads and pens, quarrying and carrying rocks in the summer, and splitting and carrying wood in the winter, and I did everything. I worked in this way until 1983 when the household-responsibility system was initiated. After that, I still herded sheep, and gradually renovated houses. After 1987, I started to build fens, water cellars, and repaired pens. I was busy working. Around 1990, power supply came, and I bought the pole and wire, connecting electric wires to every household with mutual assistance. At that time, we needed to repair the water cellar, but only the people in farming areas knew how to do it, so we followed them to learn. And we came back to repair the water cellar by ourselves. The main income of my family is from animal husbandry. I worked as a village cadre for 16 years, from 1989 to 2004. At the beginning, the salary was very low, and there was also voluntary labours, so the village cadres were exempted from voluntary work; at the beginning, the annual salary was not much, and it could almost offset the village advanced reserve fee; until 2004, the annual salary of village cadres was only more than 3,000 yuan. The village advanced reserve fee was abolished in 2000, and the former village cadres became toll cadres. The pastoral fee (collected since 1983), special production fee (collected since 1983), and slaughter fee (collected since 1992) are three kinds of fees paid to the state, while the advanced reserve fee is collected by the village as public welfare funds for village public welfare expenses such as the households enjoying the five guarantees in the village, and every household has to pay them. The pastoral fee was previously collected according to the number of people, and in 1989 it was collected according to the pasture area. Since 2000, the three fees and the advanced reserve fee has been canceled. From 2004- 2005, the state began to provide subsidies to farmers, but not herders, so there were 7 households in our team who engaged in planting enjoyed the subsidies. In 2006, there was a five-year round of grassland subsidies, and it was provided for 12 years, and the state subsidized herding households in the form of subsidies, with the aim of using grass for limiting storage and reducing the number of livestock. There are also subsidies for children's schooling, which also started in 2006 and has been implemented for more than ten years.

I have been herding livestock at home after I resigned from the village cadre since 2004. In 2006, I started to engage in tourism until 2014 when I sold the attraction, and I have been doing it for 8 years. In the past, there was a medicated bath pool that I contracted and made it a tourist attraction; as the collective pasture paid the rental, most villagers did not complain, yet there were a few who reported this thing to the villager's committee. In 2014, I sold the attraction and rebuild a new attraction on my own pasture. In January 2015, it started to build and it encountered environmental protection rectification in June when there were many formalities unfinished so we were not allowed to continue the work and it was locked all the time. In September 2017, it was demolished. When we built the attraction, my elder son's family and my family took out a total loan of more than 400,000 yuan for this attraction.

It's not an easy life. In general, the national policy has brought great benefits to us herders, but the policy is unstable, especially the environmental protection thing, which makes people frustrated. Because our place is in the functional area of the national park, now all kinds of projects in the area of the reserve have to get approved; individual construction is not allowed like before as it forbids the groundbreaking project. The high altitude places in our village are all summer pastures, which are designated as the core area, and the periphery is the experimental area and buffer area. Many people's winter pastures are in the experimental zone, autumn pastures are in the buffer zone, and summer pastures are in the core zone. If the summer pastures were banned on grazing, and there were only the pastures in the experimental area and the buffer zone, then there is no way to graze, let alone the animal husbandry. This is a place left by our ancestors, so it is good to engage in national parks, but there is no income-generating industry, so we do not see where the future is for us herders.[9]

As the second generation of their family, Wang Chengning, Wang Chengjun, and Wang Chengfu have had a very different life course and livelihood development from their parents.

(Wang Chengning) I was born in 1984 and went to school in Minle in 1991, because my parents were very busy herding sheep and there was no one to look after me, so I was sent to my uncle's house and went to school. In 1995, I went back to elementary school in Kangle. As my uncle's family moved to Xinjiang and I had no place to stay, so I returned to Kangle, and went to school with my two younger brothers. As I remembered, in 1997, when the school asked for a sheep as the advanced reserve fee, the three of us, covered in plastic, went to drive the sheep in the heavy rain, and the three children pulled and pushed a sheep. Although our clothes got wet, the sheep was driven to Kangle. I graduated from junior high school and started herding sheep at home, then I went to Hong Shiwo township and served as a clerk, and then ran to Qifeng. In 2006, I got married and gave birth to a child, and I has been home to raise the child. In 2010, I went to Zhangye to work. I sold jade ware for three years, and now I sell clothing.[10]

(Wang Chengjun) I was born in 1986, only studied in the 1st grade of a junior high school and then quit, because the family conditions are not good, as there was small pasture. When we went to school in the old district, we, the three siblings rented a house of the forestry farm, and cooked our own meals, and our parents went to visit us once every ten days or half a month. At that time, the tuition fee for one semester was more than 360 yuan, and the family income at that time was only 2,000 yuan a year, and the family had to pay a year of advanced reserve fee. At that time, the tuition fee was high and I felt that it was useless to study, so I might as well work directly to earn money. I went out to work at the age of 13 and went to Qifeng to herd sheep, earning 4,400 yuan a year. After that, I returned home and it was said

---

[9] Interview code: 20171030GYQNO1.

[10] Interview code: 20181102GHYNO1.

that I could join the army but it did not happen. Then, I went out to work again and started to herb others' sheep. After a year of herding, I paid off the debts for my family, bought a TV, and equipped my house with the large solar panel. Afterwards, I bought my own sheep. As I sold 40 of my family's cattle, bought some goats and there were more than 200 of my own sheep, later the number increased to more than 400. In 2005, I began to engage in tourism on the Macha Beach, and worked with my parents when my family did not have a penny on the account. It just happened that someone quit the attraction business, so I bought all the canvas tents, tables and chairs, and began to build attraction with the donkey cart in March 2006. The first business earned more than 4,000 yuan, and the investment in the attraction was only 20,000 yuan at that time, and the family was very happy. When we opened the attraction, the officials from county tourism bureau will come around here from time to time, and they also took us outside to visit and learn from other places, then I came back and renovated the attraction. At that time, we spent every bit of savings to make renovation, and the attraction expanded little by little. In those days, business was good, customers paid a deposit and waited in line to come. My wife met me in 2008, and we got married in 2009, but the third year after the marriage we were separated from my parents. In the first year of our separation, my mother got sick, so we took care of the family, and my father took my mother to see a doctor. The attraction continued to open. In 2014, I sold the attraction for 360,000 yuan. Although it was sold for so much money, my mother was sick, and my children were sick too. And the 360,000 yuan was distributed to my father 100,000 yuan, me 140,000 yuan, and my brother 120,000 yuan. I was thinking of buying a car or a house, but my long-term plan was to rebuild the attraction. When I just rebuilt it and encountered the new environmental policy, so had to leave it there until the spring of 2017 when it was said to be torn down. It took me a long time to build the attraction, but it was torn down in just 3 days. I spent a total of 460,000 yuan to build the attraction, and after it was torn down, I had to find a new way to survive. The main pressure I'm under is the loan, as there are still more than 300,000 yuan, and the interest for one year is a lot of pressure. This year, the children are studying in the second grade, of whom my parents take care, and we herd sheep, but also do some livestock trading. As long as the attraction compensation funds pay off the loan, our lives will be better.[11]

(Wang Chengfu) I was born in 1988 and graduated from junior high school in 2004. At that time, I heard that the school in Hunan would guarantee the employment with high salary, and I went there; I attended a one-year preparatory course and spent three year in a junior college, specialized in Digital Control of Machine Tools; and then went to Yunnan to find a job there. I did not graduate and worked in a solar energy factory with less than 2,000 yuan per month. One year later, I went to Shenzhen, and stayed there for a year, engaging in medical equipment with a monthly salary of more than 3,000 yuan. At the end of 2009, I returned home and stayed at home for more than half a year, and in September 2010, I went to work for a mining company in an industrial park and worked for four years, with a salary of more than 2,000 yuan a month at the beginning, and later the salary increased to more than 4,000 yuan. In 2014, my mother was serious ill, and she could not take care of the sheep. I came home and herded sheep in August 2014. The price of sheep was not good for the next two years, so the family rented out the pasture and contracted out the sheep, and then my wife and I went to work in Jiayuguan, and came home in autumn 2018, when the price of sheep was good enough so I recovered the pasture and sheep, and herded sheep by myself. I got married in 2013 and met my wife when I was working outside. After getting married, I wanted the stability. I didn't know much about sheep grazing at first, but I herded sheep for more than a year and then knew how to do it. If there is a ban on grazing, than I have to re-plan; I want to do some business close to home, but also do not know what to do.[12]

---

[11] Interview code: 20181102GHBNO1.

[12] Interview code: 20181102GHJNO1.

Compared to the first generation of the family, the second generation is gradually moving away from pastoral production and life, and also has more choices. From Wang Jianrong to Wang Chengning, Wang Chengjun, Wang Chengfu, and even the third generation who are still in school, the intergenerational differences among the three generations of a family largely concentrate the process of national, social and village development, and confirm the observation of a county cadre stationed in the village, "The youngest people who are still herding livestock are now the 'post-80 s'. The youngest people who are still herding are now 'post-80 s', and the younger ones don't herd anymore. There are not many 'post-80 s' people in the village, and very few people are still grazing. For young people, the ban on grazing or not actually has little impact on life, but there is a compensation for the ban on grazing. It is mainly the older herder generations that have been engaged in livestock herding for generations, and after relocation, they have no skills, they can't farm, and they can't do anything else, so survival is a big problem".[13]

The three-generation living pattern of Wang Jianrong's family largely echoes the dramatic changes that have taken place in Chinese families over the past four decades, that is, from the traditional "point" family to the "network" family. When Wang Jianrong was a child, he lived with his parents, sister, and brother-in-law in the same house, but the younger generation of his children has moved between the city and the countryside, with family members living in multiple places depending on their needs for production, education, retirement, and medical care. The location of residence has made them more mobile, as family members are connected to each other in a network, and the intergenerational living arrangement is more adaptable and open according to actual needs. "With the deepening of reform and opening up, industrialization, market-oriented development, and the migration of migrant workers to urban areas have become important mechanisms for changing social and economic life. To adapt to such changes, peasant families are changing more quickly and thoroughly toward small-sized families. In the process, many peasant families have been fragmented into urban–rural 'split families'".[14] However, the negative effects of the shift from "point" to "network" families are also evident. On the one hand, the density of relationships among family members has gradually weakened, leading to a weakening emotional ties among family members; on the other hand, this externalization and socialization of the family has led to a weakening functional support among family members, revealing that the ability of families to cope with potential social risks such as poverty has also been weakened, and suggesting that social construction needs to improve social support systems for individuals and families.

[13] Interview code: 20181031PJPNO1.

[14] Wang Tianfu, Wang Fei, Tang Youcai, et al. "Land Collectivization and Structural Transformation of the Traditional Rural Extended Family," Social Sciences in China, No. 2, 2015.

17.3 In the Same Boat: The Village as a Community

The basic logic of whole village poverty alleviation is that the village as a community is both a grassroots unit of the national administrative system and a geo-social organization composed of individual families as cells. The attributes of the village as a local community are mainly reflected in three aspects: the first is the attribute of emotion. As a kind of identity label for villagers, the village provides the basis for the emotional identity of individual villagers; the second is attribute of function. As a small social system, the village has mutual utilitarianism among each family and even individuals in the system, and the village needs to provide support for villagers and households to resist social risks; the last is attribute of institution. The village development follows different institutional logic, such as clan, elders, and administration, and villagers are both practitioners and constructors of the institutions. However, these three community attributes of villages are gradually weakening in the larger process of national and social development, and are fully reflected in the retrospective narratives of several generations of village cadres, and the narratives of the history and current status of village governance in comparison.

> *In 1971, I started to work as a finance captain, responsible for the team's financial income and expenditure and lending money to the community members. When I was a village cadre in the time of big collective, I was given 7 workpoints a day, took 36 days of workpoints a year, and I earned 1.8 yuan a day, so I could earn nearly 70 yuan a year; after the initiation of big contract*[15] *in 1983, I relied on the village advanced reserve fee as a village cadre, with a salary of 90 yuan a month, and from 1983 to 1993, it was 90 yuan a month all the time. Afterwards, it was difficult to collect village advanced reserve fee as community members did not cooperate, saying village cadres did not work a lot, just organized some meetings, and accompanied the superior leaders, so it should not distribute the money of community members to village cadres as their salaries. Before 1983, the village cadres had to develop the economy, carried out basic construction, collected the village advanced reserve fee, and considered how to distribute the money and how to make the economic construction better. At that time, village cadres thought about more things than the cadres now. They needed to manage the village annual income, decided how much livestock to raise, how much to sell, and it was needed to make plans for how much to spend money. And the whole village was like a big family. For community members, how to live a year was a problem. They could not just rely on livestock, but also engaged in side businesses. The village arranged the boys to hunt outside, dig coal, dig herbs to sell, as we set up a team dedicated to side business outside while girls were engaged with milking cows and herding sheep. After 1983, the village cadres gradually lost their power and could not get involved in the village economy but followed the policies coming from the superior. Livestock development and economic sources will not bother the village anymore, as the village cadres mainly take charge of some village public affairs, such as village infrastructure construction, building the road, fence, house renovation, repairing covered pen, etc. And the village cadres are needed to organize and coordinate. There was a household enjoying the five guarantees in our production team, and the village used to have a public welfare fund, so it could also give subsidies, and the department of civil affairs could also give subsidies, so people could live on, but after the initiation of household-responsibility system, no one cares.*[16]

[15] I.e. the household-responsibility system. –Trans.

[16] Interview code: 20181030TCYNO1.

I have been a village cadre from 1989 to 2004. Before 1983, the village was a large collective, and implemented the unified revenue and expenditure. From 1983 to 2000, the state collected three fees, and the village had to collect the advanced reserve fee, which was mainly used as public welfare fund for the public welfare of the village, such as the households enjoying the five guarantees. The village advanced reserve fee includes public provident fund and public welfare fund. The public provident fund comes from the village collective economy and is accumulated every year; the public welfare fund is collected at the end of each year and spent every next year, and a budget is made at the beginning of the year for how much money is needed for several households enjoying the five guarantees and how much money is needed for public feed, which is paid by each household, and there was money paid as money was spent at the same time. All the money coordinated by village was used to build roads, dig water cellars, etc. It was collected at the beginning of the year and borne by every household while now it is invested by the state and there wasn't the case at that time. The village established a collective ranch after 1983, with a yearly income of about 20,000 yuan, which is the main source of income for the village collective. In 2000, the three fees and the village advanced reserve fee are no longer collected. In the past, the village had autonomy, but now the village cadres do not have the power to spend money. In 2010 or so, it began to implement the system of the county's accountability for the village director, so the township set up a unified accounting, to carried out unified management of village finances. If the village needs any expenditure, the community meeting will take a vote, and then report to the township for approval, submit an expense accounts, and accept the supervision. Now the government's investment is bigger, unlike in the past when village cadres ran around asking for money to do things for the people, they could not get money and projects if they were not diligent, but now they can implement the projects as long as they apply for the projects that the township government will set up. After 1983, there were voluntary workers in the village as one labor must offer a 10-day voluntary work every year, and this was not canceled until 2000. Now the people in the village are not active, and there is no sense of self-conscientiousness, so it simply can not mobilize people to build roads. All depends on people's self-determination and conscientiousness, as you do not want to come, then do not come. In the past, this was a compulsory work, if you did not come, then the salary would be reduced. Now the village has no money, and loses the ability of mobilizing people. Now the government is strong, and many affairs have been taken care by the government, but from the village's point of view, the village loses the grip on the whole village. Although there are village rules and regulations, the constraints are not strong; before, there were voluntary work and money to restrain people, but now it is not the case. These years, the village cadres have nothing to do. The village only has a collective pasture to rent out, and the rental is used to buy forage, and then the forage is distributed to each household; if the villager does not respond to the call for work, then whose forage will be deducted.[17]

(2017) Among the village cadres, the Party secretary, the village director and the director of the supervisory committee have financial salaries, which they receive twice a year. At the beginning of my term as Party secretary, my annual salary was more than 8,000. This year, my salary increases, about 30,000 yuan. In fact, this salary in the pastoral areas is not enough to spend, and a year's salary of the village cadres is not enough to pay off the (car) gas money. Today the superior gives you a notice of a meeting, no matter how far the meeting place is, you have to come there, and no matter how you come, there are also phone bills that you have to pay a lot. No one in the village is willing to do this job, and I did not want to do it last year, as the entire team members of the three committees[18] *were changed, but I was not changed, and the town also came to me to persuade me into doing it. The candidates for village cadres are nominated by the community member assembly to vote, according to the*

---

[17] Interview code: 20171030GYQNO1.

[18] It refers to the village Party branch committee, Villager's committee and the Village supervisory committee. – Trans.

number of votes to determine the candidate. The election of the three committee members mainly depends on the ability of the individual, and whether or not the candidate really take care of the village affairs. This year, there is more work in the village, as almost every month there are inspection teams and inspectors to visit our village, especially the targeted poverty alleviation, including poverty alleviation projects acceptance, the examination of expenditure on the accounts and many other tasks.[19]

There are two factors that can be seen from the above interviews as the causes to the gradual weakening of the power of village governance subjects in terms of people, affairs, and money. One factor originates from the top-down implementation of villager autonomy and the rule of law in national governance on the one hand, and the other factor originates from the weakening of the village collective economy on the other. As the only poor village in Kangle Town, the poverty alleviation resources of Saiding Village should be targeted to the households on the one hand, and to help the village development on the other. From the identification of poor households to the implementation of poverty alleviation projects, it is undoubtedly a major village public and public welfare matter for Saiding Village. *The Organic Law of the Villagers' Committee of the People's Republic of China*[20] stipulates: "The villagers' committee is a grassroots mass self-governance organization for villagers' self-management, self-education and self-service, which implements democratic election, democratic decision-making, democratic management and democratic supervision. The villagers' committee handles the public affairs and public welfare of the village, mediates civil disputes, helps maintain social security, and reflects the villagers' opinions, requests and proposals to the people's government. The villager's committee is responsible to the villagers meeting, the villagers' representatives meeting and report on their work". And "to convene a villagers meeting, there should be a majority of the villagers over eighteen years old, or more than two-thirds of the village household representatives to participate, and the villagers meeting decisions should be made by a majority of those present". Wang Jianrong's family is a poor household from 2014 when the officially registered poverty-stricken households were initiated to 2017 when the whole village of Saiding Village achieved poverty free, "Our family was rated as a poor household mainly because my wife had a serious illness, and we were rated when the village selected poor households".[21]

All the poor households in our village were selected at the villager's assembly. 21 households were nominated at the beginning, and 7 more were selected later. Everyone has a vote so that it can prevent the conflicts effectively, and the elected ones are almost really poor people. The procedures include nomination by the villagers, review by the Party members, convening the community meeting, public announcement of the results, and reporting to the township government, and each step will go through the villager's committee. It takes several times to select poor households and convene community meetings several times to reach a consensus,

[19] Interview code: 20171106YCH-TCMNO1.

[20] Organic Law of the Villagers of the People's Republic of China, China National People's Congress, http://www.npc.gov.cn/npc/xinwen/2019-01/07/content_2070268.htm?from=timeline, accessed May 13, 2019.

[21] Interview code: 20171030GYQNO1.

and finally all the people determine a basic standard. First of all, it is family's economic income that we check. Secondly, we check whether the family has a labor force, and finally we take into account all the factors. Some families have the elderly and lack the labor, but the family pasture is large; some families have several brothers, but due to historical problems they only have small pasture, so the family economic income is small, and it should also be taken care of. Overall, the selection was fair and reasonable.[22]

From 2015 to 2017, Wang Jianrong's family received various supporting resources, including: ① 3000 yuan from temporary relief of departments of civil affairs to improve living conditions (supporting project type F); ② 12,500 yuan from subsidies for renovating dilapidated houses to improve living conditions (supporting project type E); ③ support from the Agriculture and Animal Husbandry Commission to assist 17 ewes to help develop industries (supporting project type D); ④ assistance from the Construction Bureau to build 28 square meters of color steel house to improve living conditions (type E); ⑤ 50,000 yuan of subsidized loans for targeted poverty alleviation to help develop industries (type B); ⑥ 11,500 yuan of grassland subsidies to improve living and production conditions (type F); ⑦ 6100 yuan/year of rural minimum living guarantee (type F); etc.[23]

Poverty alleviation resources not only benefit the poor households, but also the whole village. 37 out of 61 households interviewed in the *Questionnaire of the Hundred Villages Studies of Targeted Poverty Alleviation and Targeted Poverty Elimination* in 2017 responded that they had directly enjoyed poverty alleviation policies, and the villagers benefited the most from the implementation of poverty alleviation policies at the village level was the house purchase subsidy in the settlement. The result of the *Hundred Administrative Villages Studies of Targeted Poverty Alleviation and Targeted Poverty Elimination is that the poverty alleviation resources benefit the whole Sading Village and make achievements include:* more than 60 km of the internal village roads have been built, which benefits 121 households; 108 water cellars have been newly built, which benefits 80 households; the power grid has been renovated in 6 places, benefiting 74 households with power supply; the dilapidated houses of 4 households have been renovated, and the living environments of 46 households have been improved; 2 special industries have been developed with support, benefiting 10 households; 1 village cooperative has been cultivated, benefiting 10 households; 2 farm stays have been supported for rural tourism, with a total investment of 700,000 yuan from credit funds; 24 villagers have attended training sessions related to health and family planning; 121 households in the village have the access to radio and TV services; 1 village cultural activity room has been built; 100% coverage of cell phone signal has achieved. The source of funds for these development inputs is mainly the financial special poverty alleviation funds, and the pairing supporting resources such as manpower, funds, and materials from various industry departments at the county government level have been integrated. Villagers generally believe that "a series of infrastructure constructions such as water, electricity, dilapidated house renovation

[22] Interview code: 20171106YCH-TCMNO1.

[23] Interview code: 20171030GYQNO1.

and roads have brought great changes to the village".[24] Grassroots cadres believe that "the first step of real poverty alleviation should be to improve the infrastructure, and it should improve the general environment, as the general environment can be improved to stimulate poor households to find their own way out of poverty unless he himself does not feel ashamed".[25]

Saiding Village has the largest population and the largest number of households among several surrounding villages. The poor households in the village are selected through the community meeting, so there are basically no conflicts or disputes. At the beginning of targeted poverty alleviation, the village often held community meetings to select poor households and mobilize community members to work together on village construction. For example, people were mobilized to renovate the houses built in the 1970s in the settlement as many of which were dilapidated. The mobilization work is still very effective, as long as the policies and matters are explained clearly to the community members.[26]

Xi Jinping stressed in his speech at the symposium on poverty eradication in deep poverty areas that "we should organically combine the consolidation of rural grassroots Party organizations with poverty eradication, in selecting a good leader, strengthening the leadership team. Especially, it is determined to resolve the problem of weak and slack grassroots leading teams, and play a good role of village Party organizations in poverty eradication as militant bastions". From the perspective of the historical threads of village governance, the emotional attributes of villages are gradually weakening, the original institutional attributes are also weakening in the process of being incorporated into the national rule of law, and the functional attributes of villages are also gradually weakening due to the weakening power of village governance subjects; however, with poverty alleviation as an opportunity, the attributes of villages are also gradually rebuilt in the process of participation by all parties, and the functionality of villages as a local support system is somehow strengthened, which is the origin of the force that helps reduce poverty throughout the village.. In the process of household targeted poverty alleviation, the selection of officially registered poverty-stricken households at the village level has largely reproduced the emotional attributes of the village and the functional support of the village community for poor households based on emotions.

Of course, from individual to family, from family to village, from village to the country and even globally, historical processes are projected on macro or micro subjects in different ways and from different directions. In the past 40 years of reform and opening up, China's family development has shown many new features, such as "smaller family size, changing residence patterns, the emergence of non-traditional types of families, and the increasingly profound impact of aging and population migration and mobility on household registration changes". At the same time, the family change throughout the world has been accompanied by development, presenting a continuous diversification in recent decades, as emerging youth groups, technological revolution, economic uncertainty, narrowing gender gaps, longer life

[24] Interview code: 20171030GYQNO1.

[25] Interview code: 20170616HBESNO1.

[26] Interview code: 20171106YCH-TCMNO1.

spans and lower fertility rates, as well as global flows of information, goods and people, are all drivers of family change in low- and middle-income countries, and families have adapted to these changes in a variety of ways. The different dimensions of these social changes, from global to Chinese, from Gansu Province to Sunan County, from Saiding Village to Wang Jianrong's family, and different directions of anti-poverty practices, are finally concentrated in individual actions and life narratives.

References

Xi, J. (2017). *Speech at the Symposium on Combating Poverty in Deeply Impoverished Areas (June 23, 2017)*. People's Publishing House.

Yang, J., & He, Z. (2014). Changes and Continuity of Families in the Process of Social Transition. *Population Studies*, No. 2.

Wang, T., Wang, F., Tang, Y., et al. (2015). Land Collectivization and Structural Transformation of the Traditional Rural Extended Family. *Chinese Social Sciences*, No. 2.

Peng, X., & Hu, Z. (2015). Contemporary Chinese Family Changes and Family Policy Reconstruction. *Chinese Social Science*, No. 12.

Pesando, L. M., the GFC Team. (2019). Global Family Change: Persistent Diversity with Development. *Population and Development Review, 45*(1), 133–168.

Hong Lin is an assistant researcher at the Institute of Sociology, Chinese Academy of Social Sciences. Her research interests are in socio-cultural anthropology, mainly related to ethnic groups, environment, and health-related research topics.

Chapter 18
Where Does All the Money Go? An Examination of Poverty Elimination and Home-Based Entrepreneurship in Niuhong Village, Yunnan

Jing Luo and Xufeng Zhao

Abstract This paper examines the path of poverty alleviation for farmers in a Hani village under the jurisdiction of Honghe Hani and Yi Autonomous Prefecture in Yunnan Province. Through interviews and participant observation of the process of implementing Targeted Poverty alleviation in Niuhong Village from 2016 to 2019, the author found that farmers in Niuhong Village were unable to accumulate enough money to live long term in either rural or urban areas by going out to work, forming a cycle of "work-consumption-being penniless-work again". The article concludes by considering how traditional farmers can become "new farmers" under the control of the "invisible hand" of the market and custom.

Keywords Returning home · Rural revitalization · Targeted Poverty alleviation · New era · Niuhong Village

18.1 Introduction

Since the reform and opening up of China, farmers working outside have been considered in practice as the most important way to help farmers get out of poverty, and farmers' income from non-agricultural work far exceeds that from agricultural production. The author's field research in Niuhong Village, Honghe County, Honghe Hani and Yi Autonomous Prefecture, Yunnan Province, found that farmers' employment elsewhere has enabled them to earn a large amount of cash income, but this income has not been successfully transformed into capital for farmers to develop industries in rural areas, and only a very small number of farmers have successfully settled in towns and cities, while most farmers have to wander between cities and

J. Luo
Institute of Chinese Borderland Studies, Chinese Academy of Social Sciences, Beijing, China

X. Zhao (✉)
River College, Beijing, China

Case Studies of Targeted Poverty Reduction and Alleviation in 100 Villages, International Research on Poverty Reduction, https://doi.org/10.1007/978-981-95-0549-4_18

villages year after year. At present, many farmers who go out to work are already in the second or even third generation, and many of them have returned to their hometowns after working outside for more than ten years. The difference from their parents' lives is that they do not need to repeat their parents' lives, and they do not need to making a living from the land. They strive for new rural life with working experiences and accumulated capital, but the results in reality are not so much good. The life and labor of these farmers seem to fall into a cycle: go to work—exhaust consumption (investment)—go to work again. In this paper, we present a few specific cases in Niuhong Village to explore: what do the farmers spend (invest) the money they earn from working outside the village? Why did the working outside not continue to drive the villagers in Niuhong Village to prosperity after helping them to get out of poverty? How can farmers in the new era sustainably develop (get out of poverty) and become new farmers?

18.2 Village Profile of Niuhong Village and the Causes of Poverty

Niuhong Village is located in the southeastern part of Yunnan Province, Diema Township, Honghe County. It is part of the Honghe Hani Yi Autonomous Prefecture, is one of the most isolated Hani villages in the prefecture, and is also a targeted poverty alleviation village in Yunnan Province. Niuhong Village is part of the Diema Township, which is located at the junction of Honghe prefecture, Yuxi city and Pu'er city, and is one of the farthest townships under the jurisdiction of Honghe County, 123 km from Honghe County. The government of Diema Township is 28 km from the No.213 and No.323 national highways (intersect between Yuanjiang and Mojiang section), and the infrastructure such as the road is underdeveloped. The road of 28 km to the national highways was a dirt road before the year of 2018, making it very inconvenient for farmers to get in and out, and becoming a "bottleneck" for the development of Diema Township.

Niuhong Village is the most impoverished administrative village of the six administrative villages under the jurisdiction of Diema Township. The arable land (paddy) area per capita is less than 1.5 mu, and all the lands are terraces distributed in the half way up the mountain. Although farmers still have scattered dry land in the mountains to grow corn, buckwheat, and other crops, the dry land is insignificant for the livelihood of the Niuhong people. The villagers of Niuhong Village depend on the weather for their livelihood, and the food grown on the land is usually only enough to feed the whole family for half a year. Therefore, in general, there are more people with less land and the barren land is the main reason for the poverty in Niuhong Village. As of December 2016, at the beginning of the implementation of targeted poverty alleviation, there were 638 households and 3280 people in the 15 natural villages under the jurisdiction of Niuhong Village, of which 415 households and 1834 people were officially registered poverty-stricken households (members) and the proportion to the total population was as high as 65%, with a very large poverty coverage.

Food in Niuhong Village is grown in the traditional Hani terraces. The Hani terraces are mainly located in Honghe Prefecture in the south of Yunnan Province, China, which was officially listed as a globally important agricultural cultural heritage conservation pilot by the Food and Agriculture Organization of the United Nations in 2010 and became a world cultural heritage project in 2013, which is the 45th world heritage site in China. The Hani terraces in Honghe Prefecture are mainly located in Yuanyang County, where is also the main concentrated area of the tourism support of the Yunnan Provincial Government, so it is difficult for other areas in Honghe Prefecture to share the "cake" of tourism income, not to mention the remote townships like Diema Township, which is far away from Yuanyang County. The red rice produced in the Hani terraces of Niuhong Village has very low output, with a yield of up to 300 kg per mu in good years, and in bad years, the people of Niuhong Village have to pay back the money for fertilizer and seeds to grow red rice with a loss of 40 yuan per mu of rice. In such a case, the red rice produced by one and a half mu of field per capita is only enough to maintain half a year of food rations, and the people of Niuhong Village cannot solve the basic sustenance by growing food. Although the villagers rely on side businesses such as farming ducks and local small-eared pigs to support their families, but due to the closed and remote location, the return from agricultural production is only a drop in the bucket. Therefore, for a long time, having enough to eat has been a big problem for the people of Niuhong. Even so, Hani families have to set aside some grain of their meager agricultural output each year to "bake liquor" for consumption during important festivals, which makes the problem of food shortage even more serious.

The crop income of Niuhong Village cannot solve the problem of food and clothing, so the villagers need to buy food from the market with cash. In fact, it is very difficult for the people of Niuhong Village to obtain cash income in the local market because of the remote location of the market, which makes it difficult for outside traders to come in. The homogeneity of local agricultural products makes it very difficult for villagers to sell them, which limits the villagers of Niuhong Village in the local market to make money by exchanging commodities and labor.

Niuhong Village, as an entirely Hani village, has inherited the Hani tradition of having more births and rearing more children. We found in our research that it was very common for the younger generation of families to have four children, while the older generation of families generally have six to seven children. Due to the large number of children and the long-term poverty, families in Niuhong Village generally do not pay attention to the education of their children, and our sample survey results showed that the illiteracy rate in Niuhong Village was as high as 60%. The elderly in the village basically cannot read or write, not to mention speak Mandarin, and even many of the young women cannot read or write. This situation has some change only with the increased national investment in rural education in recent years.

Due to the causes above, many villagers of Niuhong Village have to "beg" for cash income. In 2011, a public welfare campaign called "fighting abduction on microblog" brought a large number of begging children from Diema Township into the public eye and drew the attention of all sectors of society. Niuhong Village became known as a "beggar village". After the children begging incident was reported in the spotlight, the poverty situation in Diema Township drew the attention of the Honghe Prefecture government, which increased its investment in infrastructure construction in Niuhong Village, which had access to electricity in 2012 and built a road in 2017. At the same time, the Diema Village government conducted special labor skills training for villagers, and the government organized labor export for villagers to enhance their connection with the outside world. Since then, the number of people in Niuhong Village going outside to work has also increased gradually. Now almost every family in Niuhong Village has laborers working outside, the labor income has been the most important source of income for villagers in Niuhong Village, Zhou Raobin, head of Diema Township said, "Our township's first major industry is working outside".

Since the 18th National Congress of the Communist Party of China, the life of the villagers in Niuhong Village and the basic appearance of Niuhong Village has undergone a radical change: food and clothing is no longer a problem that plagued the villagers of Niuhong Village, the enrollment rate of children in compulsory education has reached 100%, and now there is no dropout in Niuhong Village. Niuhong Village is no longer a beggar village. At present, the Hani terraces cultivated by the people of Niuhong Village only serve as a supplement to the family's source of income, and are no longer the main livelihood on which the villagers depend. In addition, under the leadership of the local government, the people of Niuhong Village have taken various ways to get rid of the "beggar village" hat,[1] such as developing farming and setting up new cooperatives. Nonetheless, during our research, the surplus labor force of Niuhong Village employed outside is still the most important means for the villagers to get out of poverty and get rich. In fact, the local government also guides villagers in working outside and takes it as an important measure to get out of poverty, and puts forward the slogan of "one person goes out to work, the whole family gets out of poverty and gets rich". With the trend of working outside, almost every family in Niuhong Village has its young and strong laborers working outside the village, and they jokingly say that those who stay at home are the "38, 61, and 99[2]" (i.e. women, children and the elderly). According to the staff of Diema Township, there are more than 17,000 people in the township, and nearly 4000 people work outside the village all year round, so according to the size of 3000 families in Diema Township, each family has at least one migrant worker. In our research, we learned that a villager who worked outside could send home about 10,000 yuan a year, and for families with more workforce, the remittance can reach 20,000–30,000 yuan, and the money remitted to the rural credit cooperative in Diema Township alone is 30 million yuan before the Spring Festival each year. From our field survey, the income of Niuhong Village families working outside is relatively the same, and there is no "big migrant household" in Niuhong Village, only a handful of farmers who

[1] I.e. label. – Trans.

[2] 38, 61, and 99 refer to the date of International Women's Day, International Children's Day, and the Double Ninth Festival which is celebrated on the 9th day of the ninth month on the Chinese lunar calendar, a traditional holiday for showing care and love to the elderly. – Trans.

can drive excavators have an annual income of 50,000–60,000 yuan, while the rest families have the annual income of 10,000–30,000 yuan. The cause why there is no "big households" in Niuhong Village is that the education level of Niuhong Village farmers is low, and they are engaged in unskilled work outside, so their income is not high. Technical work requires at least a high school education, but there are very few people in Niuhong Village who have received a high school education.

A large number of young and middle-aged people in Niuhong Village went out to the non-agricultural labor market, which is indeed conducive to increasing farmers' income and improving villagers' living standards. However, the further development of Niuhong Village and individual villagers after getting out of poverty is still a problem that plagues the township government and villagers. For the future development of the Niuhong Village, there is a difference in understanding between the township government and individual farmers: on the one hand, the main leaders of the Diema Township think the future development requires the creation of non-agricultural employment opportunities in the local Diema, so that Niuhong people do not have to go far from home to work, and the township government actively seeks foreign investment in the Diema Township to build a "Menguo Wine"[3] winery, hoping to industrialize agricultural products with Hani traditional characteristics by taking advantage of the government. However, the villagers are not optimistic about the winery in the township to achieve the future development and getting rich, nor are they enthusiastic about the development of rural industries, as they are still working outside, and take it as the main source of income, but also hope to return to hometown and start their own business.

In the plan for returning to hometown and starting business, the villagers of Niuhong Village mainly want to get rich by expanding their agricultural production scale. Our sample survey of Niuhong Village shows that villagers think the most urgent thing for future development is "lack of capital", with the proportion being 53.85%, followed by "lack of labor" (9.2%) and "lack of skill "(9.2%). We learned from the interviews that the reason for why villagers considered "capital" to be the most important constraint to their future personal development was they hoped to have capital to invest in their own agricultural production, especially in large-scale farming. After 2006, Niuhong villagers did not pay agricultural tax, and they were subsidized by the government for growing crops, buying machinery, etc. These measures are conducive to improving farmers' livelihoods and increasing their enthusiasm for agricultural production, but farmers still need their own financial investment to expand agricultural production. Our survey found that since the villagers in Niuhong started to work in large scale in 2012, after several years of accumulation, the medium-sized families basically have some savings, but the villagers still said they had no funds to expand the scale of agricultural production, so where

[3] Menguo wine is a traditional Hani practice of making wine, and is a daily necessity for all Hani families. The menguo wine of Diema Township is very famous in Honehe County. When we left Mengzi for Diema Township, the teachers of Yunnan Honghe College learned that we were going to Diema Township and asked us to bring back some local menguo wine, which suffices the fame of Diema's wine production.

did the remitted 30 million yuan every Spring Festival go? Why hasn't this money helped farmers to develop the local agricultural production?

18.3 The More to Raise, the More to Earn? – Agricultural Production Logic and Market Economy

People in Niuhong Village go out to work in order to improve the living conditions of their families, so those who go out to work in Niuhong Village rarely squander their income in the city, and try their best to bring all the money back home. Our survey shows that at present, the villagers' children's schooling does not constitute a family burden, mainly thanks to the state's strong support for compulsory education in rural areas, which not only exempts the students from tuition fees, but also almost all of the students' lunch fees are borne by the government. Many migrant workers in Niuhong Village bring their income home to invest in agricultural production. They are full of affection for their hometown and expect to earn higher returns from investment in their hometown, and henceforth take root in the village without going out to work. They either join with their friends outside or raise money together with their relatives to invest in expanding agricultural production. However, the difference between individual family farming and large-scale farming is not only an increase in quantity, but also a change in production logic, from which farmers do not realize the difference. Also, these weak individual farmer investors have to face extremely high risk of investment in the market with only a passion and lack of the appropriate knowledge of modern market rules, and the high probability of investment failure.

18.3.1 How to Calculate the Account of Farming: The Divide from the Individual to the Scale

Many young villagers working outside want to return to Niuhong Village for agricultural investment, whose insight and experience are richer than the average person, and they are the "capable person" of getting rich and "economic elite" of Niuhong Village, and they have a higher education than the average villagers. They are also hardworking people good at using their wisdom, and they love their hometown. Their working experience in the outside world makes them want to do something great in their hometown, but their entrepreneurial process is also quite difficult. In Niuhong Village, there are only a few local breeding households, whose farming scale is very small, with a dozen pigs at the most. During our research, I also met two more competent and experienced entrepreneurs who returned to the hometown. One is from Dujia natural village, the name is Zhu Fuguang, and the other is the rural e-commerce leader named Zhu Zhewei, from their Niuhong Village. From their entrepreneurial experiences after returning hometown and starting business, we can have a glimpse of the risks of investing in agricultural production.

Zhu Fuguang is a villager from the natural village under the jurisdiction of Niuhong Village, Dujia Village, which now has only four residents and is therefore incorporated into the Layue villager group. Zhu Fuguang is a capable person who can get rich in the village, as he went to work outside after graduating from high school, and accumulated significant savings from years of working outside. In August 2017, Zhu Fuguang and his brother-in-law (his sister's husband) were ready to make joint venture investment in a pig farm in Niuhong Village to raise local small-eared pigs. They put all their savings into the construction of the farm. In order to save money, Zhu Fuguang did not hire workers for the pig pen construction process, and he carried sand, built walls, and dug ponds at the farm site by himself. In the process of research, Zhu Fuguang's farm construction was halted halfway because the investment had greatly exceeded his budget and he had spent all his savings. He told the research group that he had no confidence about when the farm would be completed, and there was no money for the purchase of breeding pigs. Now Zhu Fuguang's house was dilapidated. He hoped the government's targeted poverty alleviation could help him renovate his house, but his family's income exceeded the national poverty line standard, so he could not be rated as an officially registered poverty-stricken household. During the survey, the Diema Township Government and the villagers' committee are still discussing how to deal with the problem of their family's dilapidated house renovation.

The research group think that Zhu Fuguang did not have a complete investment estimate for investing in a farm and underestimated the risks of farming, which was the main cause for his investment failure. Zhu Fuguang was convinced that he could make money by starting a pig farm, and his belief came from his past life practice. Taking the one head of cattle raising as an example, the price of a calf is 2000 yuan, and the price of a head of cattle sold in the market after one year is 10,000 yuan, so it can make a profit of 8000 yuan a year. The cattle are fed with grass from the mountains, and the process of raising them is just a matter of getting someone to go to the mountains every day to graze them and feed them with salt every two weeks, and there is no more investment needed. From simple bookkeeping figures, the profit of raising a head of cattle is at least 2 times, so expanding the scale of farming is the best way to make money. In fact, it is not only Zhu Fuguang who does the math, we learned in our research that almost all farmers thought of the preferred means of making wealth in the future is farming (cattle, sheep, pigs), which can also explain the majority of farmers in the sample survey thought that the limit of their wealth was "lack of funds". The general idea of farmers is to use funds to develop large-scale farming.

In fact, livestock breeding from 5 to 50 heads is not only an increase in quantity, but the production logic behind it has completely changed: large-scale livestock breeding belongs to the sequence of industrial production, which contains more than just the qualities of agricultural production, the process of large-scale feeding, and the final sale all require careful calculation. Zhu Fuguang's calculation of profitability obviously did not take these into account. And, Zhu Fuguang's ability to control the budget is also at odds with the investment ideas of modern production, as he has not even prepared the funds to operate the farm before the construction has begun. In his understanding, livestock are free to eat and do not require capital investment, so the more they are raised, the more they earn. During the research, we found that farmers with this idea are very common. There is an officially registered poverty-stricken household in Loma villagers group of Niuhong Village, who put all his savings 30,000 yuan into the construction of fish ponds. When the fish ponds were halfway through construction, he had no money to continue, and even could not pay the "new agricultural cooperation". During our research, we learned that he expected the fish pond to bring him 200,000 yuan a year after it was built, so he put all his savings into it, which is obviously a big error in the estimation of investment and output.

From the above cases, it can be seen that the knowledge, experience, and capital acquired from smallholder production and operation could not help farmers make a smooth transition into becoming large farm owners. Superficially, even the farmers themselves believe that capital is the number one constraint, limiting the scale of farming development, but looking deeper into the logic behind the scale of livestock farming, it is the transformation of family agricultural production into the industrialized agricultural production, and in fact the farmers' experience in agricultural production is not enough to cope with such a transformation, but they do not realize it, so many farmers' savings are filled into such a chasm. From the above two cases, it can be seen that the transformation of individual farmers' agricultural production from small-scale farming into large agricultural production cannot be solved simply by increasing capital investment. This transformation is a change from the logic of agricultural production to the logic of industrial production, and for individual farmers, such a transformation will not happen naturally, but requires the support of modern production knowledge and rules behind it.

18.3.2 *Who to Trust After Leaving the Village: Contracts, Trust, and Markets*

In the process of agricultural investment and operation, farmers also realize that they must use "external forces" to develop large-scale farming, including capital and sales, but when they cooperate with the outside world, they still follow the acquaintances society model in the village and do not have a sense of contract to protect themselves, which is one of the causes why it is difficult for individual farmers to obtain good returns in market cooperation and competition.

Take Zhu Zhewei, whom I met in my research, as an example. Zhu Zhewei is a villager of Zonghe villager group under the jurisdiction of Niuhong Village, and is also the head of rural e-commerce in Niuhong Village. He is considered the elite of the younger generation in Niuhong Village. He was born in 1986, graduated from technical secondary school, and later received a correspondence education and earned a bachelor's degree from Yunnan Honghe College. After graduating from technical secondary school, Zhu worked in Guangzhou, Sichuan, and Northeast China. He scrimped and saved, and saved up a considerable amount of money, about 100,000 yuan. Zhu later took out a bank loan of 100,000 yuan, raising a total of more than 200,000 yuan for the construction of a 760-square-meter pig farm in Niuhong Village, which was the largest pig farm ever built in Niuhong Village, and it could raise 500 pigs after completion.

During our research, Zhu's farm had been completed, but he owed more than 100,000 in debt and had no money to buy breeding pigs, so he was ready to go out to work again to earn money to pay off his debts. In the beginning, Zhu Zhewei's farm was built because of a friend whom he met while working in Kunming. Zhu Zhewei told the friend that the small-eared pigs in Niuhong Village had a lot of fame and many foreigners came to buy them, so the friend persuaded him to build a farm in his hometown, and as long as the pig farm was completed, the other things (including capital, operations, and sales) will be taken care of by the friend. However, after the farm was completed, when he needed to purchase piglets, Zhu Zhewei's friend said that something happened at home, so he could not invest in pig farms, and the farm came to a halt. When Zhu Zhewei talked about this matter, he felt helpless, and he also wanted to solve the problem of insufficient funds through the villagers' fund raising, and tried to start up the pig farm, but there were few followers.

When Zhu Zhewei was preparing to build pig farms, all the savings of him were only 100,000 yuan. In order to save money, construction materials were personally carried by himself, and many construction projects were also completed by his and his wife's own hands. Faced with the current stagnation of his pig farms, the villagers' committee also found no way out to help Zhu Zhewei. It happened that the rural e-commerce affairs in Niuhong Village needed a person in charge with knowledge and experience, so the villagers' committee decided to assign him to take charge of it temporarily. The head of rural e-commerce affairs had a monthly salary of 800 yuan, plus a certain percentage of sales as a bonus. This income is a drop in the bucket for Zhu's current debts.

The case of Zhu Zhewei illustrates that villagers face a stranger society after they go out to work, and the rules of interaction practiced in the stranger society are different from the traditional village's acquaintance society. The construction of trust between strangers requires some conditions, and buyers and sellers and even partners need the guarantee of contracts to keep the economic behaviors continue. Village society is an acquaintance society, where ancestors of generations living together is the biggest contract. The cost of betrayal between people is very high, as people who betray their trust cannot even continue to live in the village, so the trust between villagers in rural areas is very high. But the city as a stranger society is totally different. Cooperation in a stranger society requires a contract as a guarantee, and the contract also serves as a constraint for the parties involved. In the above case, Zhu Zhewei blindly believed in his friend's promised investment without any prior capital or other forms of input, and without signing any written cooperation agreement. He invested all his savings in the pig farm. On the one hand, this reflects the unsophistication of farmers and their confidence in their promise; on the other hand, it also shows that the farmers who go out of the village have no sense of contract and do not know how to protect themselves. The deeper cause is that after the farmers move from the acquaintances society to the stranger society, the rules of life have changed, but they have not transformed themselves.

In general, the rules of behavior in the market greatly exceed the daily knowledge and imagination of farmers, and it is extremely risky for farmers to invest in the market with the logic of rural smallholder production, while farmers' preconceptions about the market and investment come precisely from the logic of smallholder production, which is actually a structural risk for farmers to make investments.

18.4 The "Face" and "Heart" of the Village: Farmers and Customs

Even though the villagers of Niuhong Village spend most of their time away from home and do not live in the village all year around, their behavior still conforms to the customs and rules of the village, which involve all the families and are the "invisible hand" that has sustained the rural community for thousands of years. Historically, it was this "invisible hand" that enabled the villagers of Niuhong Village to unite together to overcome difficulties, and it was this "invisible hand" that served the function of social relief and social security for the villagers. Today, however, the social security system established by the state has replaced the social functions performed by customs in the past, but the customs in the village have not changed. There are some customs that make everyone feel stressed, but no one dares to be the first to break them, because breaking them means severing the historical ties with all the people in the village, and the consequences of that are too much for anyone to bear.

18.4.1 Running Accounts of History that Are Difficult to Sever: Fighting Against Customs

The Niuhong Village is a fully Hani Village, and the villagers still follow the Hani tradition of living today: to worship filial piety and to serve deaths as if they were alive. For this reason, Hani funerals are very grand, with at least a few cattle (1 head costs 10,000 yuan) or even dozens of cattle killed for a funeral. The villagers are expected to slaughter the cattle to entertain guests at the funeral, and the more cattle they slaughter, the more filial they are as their children. Therefore, in the Hani funeral, with a dozen cattle to slaughter at most, the average number of slaughtered cattle also is 2–3, plus other aspects of expenses, a funeral cost can reach 40,000–50,000 yuan, even 200,000 yuan at the most. This custom makes every villager overwhelmed, and many families even go into debt to prepare the funeral, so there is a local saying that "carrying an old man causes poverty for three generations". Funeral expenses are a heavy financial burden for the organizers, but no villager in Niuhong Village dares to be the first to break this custom, because it would not only be considered "unfilial" by other villagers, but also impossible to explain to the deceased elders.

Although a funeral may impoverish an ordinary family, the villagers are still happy to follow this custom tirelessly. In addition to funeral expenses, other nominal invitations and gifts in daily life (marriages, birthday celebrations for the elderly, baby's completion of its first month of life, housewarming, etc.) also lead to the consumption of the accumulated income from villagers' work elsewhere, and the funeral expenses are much higher than those for marriages.[4] These expenses, year after year, may make farmers who have just come out of poverty return to poverty again. The existence of such social culture not only poses a major obstacle to the Niuhong villagers to get out of poverty, but also discourages the villagers to invest their limited funds to improve their production and living conditions.

In the implementation of targeted poverty alleviation work, the Diema Township Government and the villagers' committee of Niuhong Village include changing social traditions and customs into targeted poverty alleviation work, and actively advocate rich provision for the aged and frugal burial for the deaths among the villagers. The government-led campaign to change social traditions and customs reduce the burden of the masses. The Diema Township Government took the lead and jointly formulated the *Village Rules and Regulations* with six administrative villages. In the *Village Rules and Regulations*, it regulates the arrangements for all villagers in preparing the red and white affairs,[5] advocating the arrangements of wedding and funeral affairs should be simple. In order to promote the implementation of the *Village Rules and Regulations*, the government of Diema Township allocated 30,000 yuan from its modest budget to reward the first three families for handling their funerals simple, with 10,000 yuan per household, which means that the following families who have funerals would not receive any subsidy. The Diema Township Government hopes to use these three "model" families to promote the change of customs in the township. We later learned from the Diema Township Government and the Niuhong villagers' committee that the villagers who received the 10,000 yuan of government incentive later bought a cattle to entertain relatives and friends, equivalent to re-arrangement of the funeral, so the result is that the money was spent and the cattle was eaten. With regard to this, the township government and the villagers' committee felt quite helpless. In the future, without the subsidies from the township government, it will still take time to verify whether the villagers of Niuhong Village will abide by the provisions of the *Village Rules and Regulations* on frugal burial. The cadres of the Diema Township Government and the people of Niuhong Village feel it will be very difficult, and the villagers' committee also feels that there is uncertainty.

Zhu Heifa, the first university student in the Layue village group under the jurisdiction of Niuhong Village, is not optimistic about the future change of the village's

[4] In fact, the local wedding costs in Diema Township are not high, as young people practice free love, they can get married as long as they want, and the wedding cost is only 10,000 to 20,000 yuan, even a few thousand yuan at the least. Compared to other places (including some Hani areas, the betrothal gifts in Honghe County are up to 100,000 yuan or more, and the nearby Mazahe Township reaches more than 100,000 yuan), the local wedding costs in Diema Township are very economical.

[5] Red affairs refer to the wedding ceremony; white affairs refer to the funeral. – Trans.

funeral customs. Although he has received a higher education and believes that the large scale of funerals has brought a heavy burden to the villagers, he does not think he has the courage to break the custom. Zhu Heifa is the only son in his family, and his grandparents, maternal grandparents, and his parents are all alive, which means he will have to carry six elderly people in the future. He is very worried about the future of "carrying the elderly" (funeral), because there are no siblings to share the cost of the funeral. According to the current village custom, a funeral costs 40,000–50,000 yuan, and he will have to go into debt to carry six elderly people. Even so, he did not have the courage to break the village custom. Because at the village funeral, villagers eat and drink a lot, and the villagers receive red envelopes and send red envelopes. This is not only an economic sense of mutual support, but more important significance is the maintenance of family and friendship. In the closed village, it means to shoulder each other's major relief, as the red envelopes for the villagers have the significance of "crowdfunding". With the improvement of living standards, "crowdfunding" has become a competition for food and drink, and the funeral gifts are squandered on food and drink, even with their own savings, so some well-off families go into debt due to the big event, which is really "carrying an old man causes poverty for three generations".

18.4.2 How Much is "Face" Worth: Competition in Local Rural Culture

The people of Niuhong Village are not only engaged in handling extravagant and wasteful wedding, funeral, marriage, full moon,[6] and other activities to invite guests to give gifts, but also in daily life, there is the phenomenon of squandering on meals. Zhou Raobin, head of Diema Township, thinks that over the years more and more villagers have been out to work. But why villagers still generally lack funds to develop production? The cause is that many people brought back all their earnings to the village, and squandered all the money on meals, and did not use the money to develop production. "Someone who saved a year of money outside came back and squandered away on meals in a few days". Therefore, the Diema Township Government took "changing social traditions and customs" as an important work in the implementation of targeted poverty alleviation, to help change the extravagance and blind competition in arranging the red and white celebrations in the Hani history with the power of the government so as to effectively "reduce the burden" of the masses.

Niuhong Villagers' craze for competition is prevalent. In addition to the big funeral, the luxury housing is also a phenomenon that has emerged in recent years. In recent years, the village has built a number of small two- and three-story western-style buildings, the scale of which is no inferior than the buildings in the town, and has become a "model" for villagers to follow and emulate. The traditional house

---

[6] Full moon refers to the baby's completion of its first month of life. – Trans.

in Niuhong Village is built with "bamboo and grass adobe", and people use local materials and make their own bricks with the mud from the mountains, and the labor required for this process is all self-employed. Relatives and neighbors also come to help, so the cost of building houses is not high for the locals.

Now, villagers are starting to build small western-style houses as those in the town, and it costs at least 100,000 yuan to build a house, and many even cost 200,000 yuan. The cost of building new-style buildings in Niuhong Village is very high, mainly because of the remote location of Niuhong Village, and construction materials must be transported from far away with transport costs much higher than the cost of materials. In the research, we found that there are a lot of unfinished two-story "open-air rooms" or "unfinished" house without windows in the Niuhong Village. Some houses have been in existence for a number of years, and head of household can only "live" in the "open-air room" because no money to complete the construction. Niuhong Village director took me to visit an officially registered poverty-stricken household. The family lived in a newly built two-story building, but in my view it belonged to the "unfinished" series. Although the house is built with brick-concrete structure, the door and windows are completely exposed. On the wind and rain day, a wooden board will be used to keep off a little, the walls of the house are red brick walls completely exposed, and the ground is completely mud floor. The village director said that this family became an officially registered poverty-stricken household due to the loss of the main labor force, and their original house was close to collapse and it was impossible to live, so the family took on debt to build the current new house. When I asked: since the funds are limited, can't you build a one-story building? The villager replied: there are newly built two- or three-story buildings in the village. If I build one-story bungalow, I will lose "face". The village director told me that it took at least 200,000 yuan to build such a house, and not only the raw materials needed to be transported from outside, but also the price of labor was relatively expensive, so only farmers with good conditions could afford such a house. The fact that the officially registered poverty-stricken household took on debt to build such housing beyond their capabilities shows the serious competition culture in the village.

Traditionally, Hani houses have two floors: the upstairs is used for storing food and the downstairs is for living or raising livestock. Now farmers believe that only houses like those in towns and cities are authentic buildings, so they take this as the goal of their lives, and the way of life they admire. There is nothing wrong with farmers building new-style housing, but many farmers tool on dept to build new "western-style buildings", and the permanent population is not big, so most of the rooms are unused, and even used to stack miscellaneous things, which, in fact, is very wasteful. Such housing has more significance to the villagers "face" than to the actual living.

18.5 It's not About Money: The New World and the Old System

At present, the farmers in Niuhong Village have solved the problem of food and clothing by going out to work, and have achieved "Two Assurances and Three Guarantees[7]", and the money remitted by the workers every year (30 million yuan) greatly exceeds the financial income of the township (the annual financial income of Diema Township is less than 300,000 yuan). However, this money has not become the "original accumulation" for the farmers to continue their development, but has been depleted due to various circumstances. At present, farmers think that the bottleneck of development is "capital", but the above case shows that "capital" cannot solve the current constraints of farmers' development, and the traditional smallholders are faced with two structural contradictions in their transformation into modern farmers with large-scale production: the contradiction between farmers' personal knowledge, cognitive structure, and the rules of modern market economy; and the contradiction between the current social system construction in rural areas and traditional customs. The above two pairs of contradictions are inevitable in the process of transformation in rural areas from closed communities to open communities, and are also structural obstacles in the transformation of villages from traditional societies to modern societies, which are the collision of the new world (modern market economy) and the old system (traditional customs and personal knowledge structure). The two "invisible hands" of the modern market economy and traditional village customs may change slowly over time and eventually become integrated, but this process will bring about a very high personal and social cost. The "visible hand" of government, if properly exercised, will reduce these unnecessary costs. The following two areas are worthy of experimentation.

First, the government's "visible hand" can help rural communities establish a new lifestyle and institutionalize the new style, so that farmers will refrain from making extravagant arrangements for funerals, weddings, and other traditional ceremonies. The township government can try to set up a special funeral (wedding) committee to organize funerals (weddings) with some supporting funds to stop the excessive and wasteful ceremonies. This move can solve the worries for each family. At present, a large number of rural workers in all parts of China are staying away from home for long periods of time, causing to some extent the collapse of the traditional social structure of the countryside. Traditionally, the countryside was a community of mutual aid tied by blood, and this is a choice that farmers have long made to work together against natural disasters and various unforeseen situations in order to maximize the common interests of the village and individual interests. However, in today's rural areas, traditional agricultural production is no longer the main source of livelihood for farmers, and the establishment of a sound social security mechanism by the state in rural areas has replaced many functions of the old village community. As a result,

[7] The Two Assurances and Three Guarantees refer to assurances of adequate food and clothing, and guarantees of access to compulsory education, basic medical services, and safe housing for impoverished rural residents. – Trans.

many of the customs that used to sustain villagers' relationships in villages have become anachronistic, but are difficult to dismantle in a short period of time. In this situation, the "visible hand" of the government has to invest in the construction of rural communities in addition to building a new style of life.

Second, the government provides targeted guidance and helps farmers to return to their hometowns to start their own businesses. Farmers return to their hometowns with local sentiments to start their own businesses, but are at a competitive disadvantage in market-oriented conditions due to the limitations of knowledge structure, experience, and capital. The risks behind farmers' simple pursuit of large-scale farming based on their traditional experience in smallholder production are very high. In fact, there is a set of rules of modern society behind the large-scale production and market-oriented operation of agriculture, and although farmers are involved in some of them, many structural barriers are difficult to overcome when it just relies on the power of individual farmers to make large-scale agricultural production.

The revitalization of the countryside is a major national policy and a guiding light and dream for the future development of hundreds of millions of farmers in China. The revitalization of the countryside is not only a matter for farmers, but also a matter for the overall development of the country and the future and hope of the whole society. After more than 40 years of reform and opening up, the living standard and freedom of farmers in China have been unprecedentedly improved, but farmers are still in a disadvantaged position in the market rules, so the future wealth of farmers and revitalization of the countryside need the support and guidance of the whole society. In the *Opinions on Implementing the Rural Revitalization Strategy*, the state emphasizes that "the main position of farmers should be adhered to. Fully respect the will of farmers, and effectively play the main role of farmers in rural revitalization". In fact, in the process of taking farmers as the main body of development, grassroots governments and even social welfare organizations still need to effectively guide farmers in specific investment projects, helping them to make production and investment in accordance with market laws and also to protect themselves in a market way.

China is a large agricultural country with a mature and long history of agriculture, which is why Chinese culture has a unique sense of hometown. After farmers go out to work, even though their physical ties to the village are reduced, the countryside is still the emotional homeland of farmers and the place where they will return as fallen leaves return to the roots of the trees in the future. Farmers have a strong desire to build their hometowns and to obtain a sustainable livelihood in the countryside through agriculture, which is the social foundation for the revitalization of China's countryside. To make agriculture a promising industry, to make farmers an attractive occupation and to make the countryside a beautiful home to live and work in peace and happiness is not only the government's expectation for rural revitalization, but also the farmers' personal pursuit.

References

Fei, X. (2016). *Vernacular China Vernacular Reconstruction.* Qunyan Press.

Honghe County History Office, Honghe County Yearbook 2016, Dehong Nation Press, 2017.

Honghe County, Yunnan Province: Honghe County, Yunnan People's Publishing House, 1991.

Li, P. (2018). Attaching Great Importance to Two Issues in Rural Revitalization. *China Rural Discovery*, No. 4.

Li, P. (2019). *The End of the Village—The Story of Yangcheng Village.* Life - Reading - Xinqi Sanlian Bookstore.

Lin, J., & Ma, G. The Development and Changes of Chinese Villages in the Past Forty Years of Reform and Opening Up. *Social Development Research*, No. 2.

Lu, D. (2018). The Reconstruction of Rural Life in China in the Era of Great Changes. *Culture Vertical*, No. 3.

Song, W., & Wu, J. (2016). *Hani Terraces: Historical Status, Ecological Environment, and Sustainable Development*. Science Press.

Wang, Q. (1999). *On Terraced Culture.* Yunnan University Press.

Xinglong, L. H., Hu, Y., et al. (2017). A Study of Chinese Rural Society in the Collectivization Period. *Open Times*, No. 5.

Yin, S. (1991). *A Controversial Cultural Ecosystem—A Study of Slash and Burn in Yunnan.* Yunnan People's Publishing House.

Yu, J. (2001). *Yuechun Politics: Changes in the Political Structure of Rural China during the Transition Period*. The Commercial Press.

Zhuang, K. S. (2016). *Silver Wings: Local Society and Cultural Change in China.* Life - Reading - New Knowledge.

Zuo, W. (2017). Hengqu Village: Peasant Cooperation in a Vernacular Society. *Social Development Research*, No. 1.

Jing Luo , associate researcher of Institute of Chinese Borderland Studies, Chinese Academy of Social Sciences, with research interests in social change in borderlands and borderland governance.

Xufeng Zhao , professor of River College, with research interests in modern Chinese political and social history and local history of southwest China.

Postscript

Targeted Poverty Alleviation and Elimination in 100 Villages-Case Studies is the mega program implemented by Chinese Academy of Social Sciences. Since its launch in 2016, it has closely followed the great steps of poverty alleviation in China, mobilized the scientific research forces of the whole Academy and some local research institutes and universities, and conducted in-depth research in the front line of rural areas, so as to carry out research on the motherland. This Case Studies Volume is one of the series achievements of the project "Investigation and Research of Targeted Poverty Reduction and Alleviation in 100 Villages Book Series". Based on the research reports of villages, 18 representative villages are selected, and the authors of the cases tell the typical cases on the way to poverty eradication from the perspective of village observers, with qualitative analysis and vivid examples.

Compared with the separate village research reports, the eighteen cases in this book further focus on the people and events in the villages. By telling the actual examples of poor villages and poor households that have experienced poverty eradication, as well as the typical projects, typical families, or typical roles of the villages in poverty eradication, we make the smallest cases reflect the situation of poverty eradication and socio-economic development trends of poor villages at the forefront of the battle against poverty. The villages selected in this casebook, such as Shibadong Village, Jiangjia Village, and Chixi Village, are distributed in the regions of Jixi,[1] Jiangzhe,[2] Mindong,[3] Huguang,[4] Dianqiangui,[5] and Qingganning,[6] covering various ways of poverty eradication, such as Party building leading, industrial poverty alleviation, relocation for poverty alleviation, and tourism and ecological construction. The content is substantial, real and vivid. This casebook reflects to a certain extent

[1] Geographically it refers to the Western Hebei. – Trans.

[2] Geographically it refers to Jiangsu and Zhejiang. – Trans.

[3] Geographically it refers to eastern Fujian. – Trans.

[4] Geographically it refers to Hubei and Hunan. – Trans.

[5] Geographically it refers to Yunnan, Guizhou, Guangxi. – Trans.

[6] Geographically it refers to Qinghai, Gansu, Ningxia. – Trans.

Case Studies of Targeted Poverty Reduction and Alleviation in 100 Villages, International Research on Poverty Reduction, https://doi.org/10.1007/978-981-95-0549-4

the great practice of targeted poverty alleviation and targeted poverty eradication in China and witnesses the great contribution.

This casebook is compiled by the program coordination office of "Investigation and Research of Targeted Poverty Reduction and Alleviation in 100 Villages", and written by Liu Yanhong, Jiang Wei, Sunsalahan, Xu Haijun, Zhang Zongshuai, Dong Yanmei, Lv Fang, Ning Yafang, Wang Hong, Wang Yuejin, Li Jing, Li Xin, Wang Shaoju, Geng Yu, Fang Sumei, Liao Yongsong, Wei Peng, Liu Tongshan, Zeng Junxia, Liu Xiaomin, Song Lidan, Long Cunying, Nie Jun, Chen Yi, Pan Jin, Lin Hong, Luo Jing, Zhao Xufeng, etc. The editorial team of Social Sciences Academic Press (CHINA) has worked hard for the publication of "Investigation and Research of Targeted Poverty Reduction and Alleviation in 100 Villages Book Series".

Authors.

October 2020.

GPSR Compliance

The European Union's (EU) General Product Safety Regulation (GPSR) is a set of rules that requires consumer products to be safe and our obligations to ensure this.

If you have any concerns about our products, you can contact us on ProductSafety@springernature.com

In case Publisher is established outside the EU, the EU authorized representative is:

Springer Nature Customer Service Center GmbH
Europaplatz 3
69115 Heidelberg, Germany

Batch number: 09460260

Printed by Printforce, the Netherlands